Health Visiting and Elderly People — a health promotion challenge

For Churchill Livingstone:

Publisher: Mary Law
Editorial co-ordination: Editorial Resources Unit
Production controller: Nancy Henry
Design: Design Resources Unit
Sales Promotion Executive: Hilary Brown

Health Visiting and Elderly People – a health promotion challenge

Mary E. McClymont MSc RN HV QN HVT RNT

Freelance Lecturer; formerly Principal Lecturer in Health Studies, Stevenage College, Stevenage, Herts

Silvea E. Thomas EdD MPH RN HVT RNT CertEd

Assistant Professor, City University, New York; formerly Senior Lecturer in Health Studies, Stevenage, College, Stevenage, Herts

Michael J. Denham MA FRCP MD

Consultant Physician in Geriatric Medicine, Northwick Park Hospital, Harrow, Middlesex; President-elect, British Geriatrics Society

SECOND EDITION

CHURCHILL LIVINGSTONE
EDINBURGH LONDON MELBOURNE NEW YORK AND TOKYO 1991

CHURCHILL LIVINGSTONE
Medical Division of Longman Group UK Limited

Distributed in the United States of America by Churchill Livingstone Inc., 1560 Broadway, New York, N.Y. 10036, and by associated companies, branches and representatives throughout the world.

First edition 1986
Second edition 1991

ISBN 0-443-04228-4

British Library Cataloguing in Publication Data
A catalogue record for this book is available from the British Library.

Produced by Longman Singapore Publishers (Pte) Ltd.
Printed in Singapore

Preface

In this revised version of our text, we have endeavoured to address the many changes taking place in the care of older people. These encompass changes in demographic structure, and radical reforms in social policy and legislation. The changes in professional thinking, education and development call for a renewed approach to the preparation of professionals who will be caring for older persons in the next decade and beyond.

In an effort to represent current practice and opinions, we have consulted widely, and have collated material drawn from visits to innovative practices, conferences on the care of elderly people, interviews with professional personnel at both field and policy-making levels, literature reviews and personal experience.

Many of our initial concepts and beliefs about the importance of fostering optimum ability among older people, maintaining their well-being and improving their quality of life have been retained. Consequently, the format of the book follows the previous pattern. However, considerable expansion has been possible, in some directions, because of additional research in the intervening period. Hence, we have not only updated statistics but have elaborated on theoretical perspectives in several chapters, particularly 2, 3, 7 and 8.

Most tables and illustrations have been revised and new ones added. Chapter 4 examines current controversies on the direction which health visiting might take in future, and Chapter 5, on models and frameworks of care, has been expanded in the light of new developments. In Chapter 6 we have explored the relationship of the WHO targets to the care of older adults, endeavouring to link international policies to local activities, as expressed through primary health care and neighbourhood nursing.

New thinking on the role of health visitors as health promotion specialists has led us to extensively revise Chapter 7, which highlights issues in retirement, and to incorporate a new chapter (Ch. 8) on group health promotion, theories, strategies and topics.

Recent research on informal carers and on the disabled has enabled us to delineate more clearly the role of the professional practitioner with these groups (Chs 8 and 10).

The focus of Chapter 9 is on the medical needs of older people, taking account of new findings on relevant disorders. The specific needs of ethnic minority elderly, and of frail, vulnerable old people are addressed in Chapter 10, where we have extensively revised the section on mistreatment of the elderly. Chapter 11 confronts the future.

Throughout the text we have tried to include practical suggestions on the care of older persons, within a health context, and have considered the role of health visitors in relation to targeting, teamwork, inter-sectoral activities and cost-effective practice.

This book does not pretend to be completely comprehensive in coverage; its selections and omissions reflect the thinking of its authors, who, however, believe that it will serve to fill part of the gap currently existing in the literature on the health visiting care of older persons. Although addressed primarily to health visitors, it has application for other public health nurses and for personnel working with elderly people in clinical as well as community settings. Those others engaged in health promotion may also find it useful.

M.E.McC.
S.E.T.
M.J.D.

Acknowledgements

We wish to record our particular thanks to Queen Elizabeth, The Queen Mother, for so graciously permitting us to use her photograph, and for allowing us to point out her fine example of public service, in this, her 91st year.

As with our previous edition many individuals and groups have given us time and help, and we wish to record our deep appreciation. Particular thanks are accorded to the Nursing Officers at the Department of Health; to Dr Christine Victor, Ms Sue Phillips and Dr Lisbeth Hockey.

We are indebted to Miss Nancy Roper, Miss Winifred Logan and Dr Alison Tierney for so generously sharing their knowledge with us and allowing us to use their Activities of Living Model. Also to Professor Wallston and his co-authors for granting us the opportunity to include the multidimensional scale for the Health Locus of Control.

As before, we have drawn heavily on library resources at The Royal College of Nursing, The Lister Hospital and The School of Nursing; we are greatly indebted to Sally Knight, Lois Collings and their colleagues and to the Health Information Service staff. The Office of Population, Censuses and Surveys was generous in granting us the use of much data, and we thank OPCS and the many other organisations who assisted us.

Jenny Densham, Gillian Smith, Sandra Betterton and Kate Brettell gave considerable support and help, as did the members of the HVA Special Interest Group for the Elderly and The Scottish HVA. To them, as to Sarah Colles, Elizabeth Cotton, Carol Jones, Gwen Sharp and Ann Stanton, we record our gratitude. Thanks, too, are due to the staff of the Medical Illustrations Unit, Northwick Park Hospital.

Inevitably, our families and friends have had to bear much inconvenience while we have given time to this revision, and we are grateful for their understanding and patience.

We acknowledge the help of the staff of Churchill Livingstone in Edinburgh.

Age Concern and the Derby Evening Telegraph kindly provided the photograph of Mrs Hardy Constant that appears on the back cover. In her 80s, she continues to swim to raise money for various charities.

Most of all we thank all those older persons whose example has taught us so much.

M.E.McC.
S.E.T.
M.J.D.

Contents

CHAPTER CONTENTS

1

Setting the scene

The United Kingdom population is slowly, but steadily, ageing. This trend, discernible in the first half of the century, accelerated from 1951, so that by 1987 the number of those *aged 60 years and upwards*, of both sexes, had grown from 7.9 million to 11.8 million. Moreover, the most marked increase took place in the older age groups, with those aged 75 years and upwards increasing from 1.8 million in 1951 to 3.8 million by 1987. By contrast the child population (under 15 years), decreased from 11.3 million to 10.8 million over the same period (see Fig. 1.1).

What is the significance of these changes? They certainly emphasise an improvement in the life survival chances for more older people. This gives cause for some celebration, but not complacency. They also indicate that the country is faced with increasing numbers of old persons, and possibly fewer younger persons may be available to care for them. This has caused some observers and policy makers concern, but other researchers and commentators see no real cause for alarm (Victor 1987, Jefferies 1988). It is important to get these facts into perspective and to be realistic in attempting to interpret them. In the following pages we discuss these demographic fluctuations and trends in greater detail. Suffice it to say here that those aged 65 years and upwards formed 15% of the total population in 1987 and are likely to remain so until 2001 (OPCS 1989). A 3% increase is then predicted by 2025.

Although many of these older people will continue to live active lives within the community,

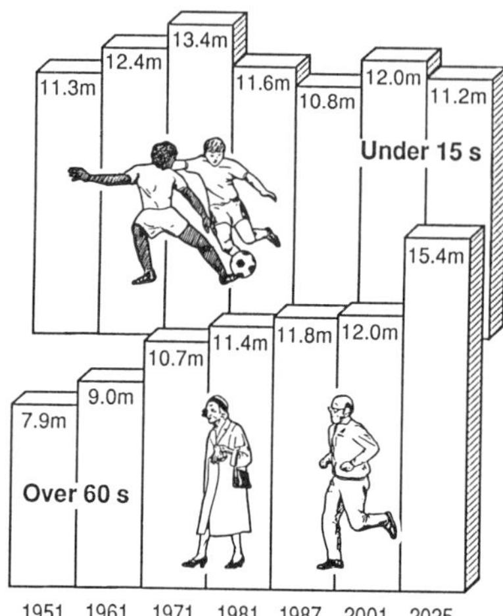

Fig. 1.1 The population is slowly but steadily ageing (Based on data from OPCS 1989; Crown Copyright.)

able to give younger generations the benefit of their experience and companionship, some will require community support to enable them to maintain their independence and quality of life. Thus there is likely to be a considerable social, economic and political impact, which will require a realistic appraisal of needs, matching allocation of resources, and creative responses. The continuing development of the health visiting service will need to take account of these issues.

WHO ARE THE ELDERLY?

In 1981 attention centred on the death of Mr Harry Shoerats, who at 111 years of age was then thought to be Britain's oldest inhabitant. However, by August 1989 his record had been broken by a 113-year-old Cleveland woman. Possibly her achievement will soon be superseded. These outstanding survivors and their centenarian peers, numbering some 2600 to date, have attracted much interest and are likely to continue to do so (Thatcher 1981, Bury 1986, Norton 1988). Their survival is attributed to several causes, including genetic make-up, hard work, an absence of undue stress, a good diet, good health, limited alcohol intake and high levels of activity. Such examples of longevity prompts the question, at what point in a person's life-cycle does he or she become 'elderly'?

There is no simple answer, as Lesnoff-Caravaglia (1987) shows. Ageing is a complex and gradual process, with psychological, social and biological characteristics varying so broadly that they do not necessarily synchronise with each other, nor with chronological age. Furthermore, when the question is placed into an historic context, other aspects emerge. A century ago when the average expectation of life was 40 for a male, and 43 for a female, those exceeding these ages would have been considered 'old'. Today such individuals would be classified very differently.

Traditionally the official retirement age has provided the demarcation line between 'the elderly' and 'the non-elderly'. In the United Kingdom this currently means 60 years for women and 65 years for men. However, since these ages were very arbitrarily determined more than a century ago, they are now being questioned as outdated and illogical. Most international documents currently use 65 years as the baseline for describing the elderly of both sexes, so it is important to note which age is being used when comparing data.

The Concise Oxford Dictionary defines the term elderly as 'getting old', thus conveying the notion of process and continuity. 'Old' is in turn regarded as 'having existed for a long period, or being advanced in years'. Whilst this emphasises relativity, it may hint at value. Old wine, old gold, old furniture are often highly prized. Old people sometimes share their status. These definitions thus outline a period of time which begins with being elderly and culminates in old age. The phrase 'later maturity', to cover this last developmental period, is the phrase preferred by Murray et al (1980). This term possibly captures the idea of continuity and experience bound up with this period and may therefore prove a more acceptable one for many people.

The elderly population, however, should not be regarded as a homogeneous entity, particularly as the period from retirement to death can cover more than 40 years, a far longer era than most other sections of the life-span. A person of 95 may differ from a person of 65 more dramatically than does a person of 35. For this reason many researchers and statisticians are increasingly differentiating between the *'young elderly'* (those aged 60/65–74 years) and the *'old elderly'* (those aged 75 years and above). A further distinction is sometimes made which categorises those aged 85 years and over as *'the very old'*.

DEMOGRAPHIC TRENDS

It should not be assumed that the ageing of the population is confined only to the United Kingdom, nor even to the Western world. Estimated statistics show that by the year 2000 the world population of elderly people will have grown to 600 million. Furthermore, by then, approximately *60%* of those aged 60 years and upwards, and *46%* of those aged 80 years and upwards, will be living in the developing countries. This is because, although the trend towards ageing is characteristic of both the developed and the developing nations, the relative rate of increase is greater in the latter. This increase in the population of older people will be particularly marked in Asia, mainly because of the increased number of aged people in China and India. By 2020 these two countries alone are expected to have a further 270 million elderly people. Large increases are also expected by that date in Brazil and Indonesia, and to a lesser extent in Mexico, Nigeria and Pakistan (WHO 1989).

In the Western world much smaller absolute increases are anticipated, primarily because the population ageing began much earlier. This expansion of the overall elderly world population, and the rapid displacement of developed countries by developing ones in the ranking order of countries with the largest 60+ groupings, will have enormous socio-economic implications. Urgent strategic planning is thus required.

It is difficult to grasp such vast figures, but perhaps even more importantly it is necessary to comprehend that population *shape* is most affected by the proportion of older people within it. Currently in parts of South-East Asia, in spite of the increase just discussed, those aged 65 years and over account for less than *6%* of the population. By contrast in parts of the developed world it is *20%*. This is partly explained by the continuing high birth rates in developing countries, coupled with the differential mortality rates, which although very disparate between less- and well-developed countries, still favour the young in each population.

These continuing high birth rates also account for the differential *ratios* which prevail between the young and the elderly populations in various countries. Thus in South-East Asia there are approximately *15 children to every elderly person*, whereas in Europe, Japan and the USA the ratio is nearer *1.5 children to 1 older person*. It is the ratio of younger to older people which indicates the nature of the problems a country is likely to encounter and hence the type of services it will require.

Issues affecting dependence

A longer life is, therefore, now an increasing possibility for many more people. Although this is to be welcomed, the change brings fresh challenges which have implications for health and well-being. It will be appreciated that the care of children and the very old, everywhere, depends on the intervening adult population. The developed countries are still endeavouring to adapt to their lower birth rates and the 'greying' phenomenon. Now in some developing countries there is concern that the adult 'caring' section of the population is being depleted, through the migration of economically active people in the younger and middle years. Although it is both valid and realistic to recognise these potential problems and to anticipate that they may impinge upon the ability of a country to sustain adequate care for its dependants, matters should be kept in proportion. Challenges also represent opportunities. The launching of the WHO global strategy, 'Health for all by the year 2000', has created potential for health improvements in all age groups. Thus in every country there is an opportunity to reduce mortality and morbidity risks, so improving the well-being and functional ability of children and elderly, people world-wide. Effecting such improvements would in turn reduce the demands on both formal and informal carers world-wide. At the same time the immense range of technological advances in agriculture, industry and other sectors has opened up the way for increased productivity, with lessened labour intensity, everywhere.

Human individuals have a great capacity for adaptation and change. Given the necessary knowledge, many are likely to be able to make the required application and develop new skills. Given the political will, it is well within the capacity of those who possess scientific and technological knowledge to share their expertise with others presently less advantaged. In this way the socio-economic opportunities may be improved in every country to a sufficient extent to enable food, goods and services to be produced to meet population requirements. There is, therefore, tremendous scope for the harnessing of technology for social benefit world-wide.

A further point, made by both Victor (1987) and Jefferies (1988), is that the concern about undue dependency is often based on a false assumption: namely, that those who are not economically active make no contribution to the national well-being. Such a viewpoint fails to take account of the extent to which older children and elderly people play their part in family and community life, often undertaking essential tasks. Many people wish to engage in meaningful roles, to the utmost of their capacity. Older people, everywhere, are no exception. Without unduly exploiting them it is possible to encourage them to do so. If this is done, while at the same time effecting the socio-economic and technological innovations just described, it may be possible to transform thoughts of potential gloom into situations of hope and development.

Turning from this glance at the world perspective, we now consider in greater detail the position within the United Kingdom.

UNITED KINGDOM POPULATION

Age structure

The age and sex structure of the UK population, for the period 1901–2001 is illustrated in Figure

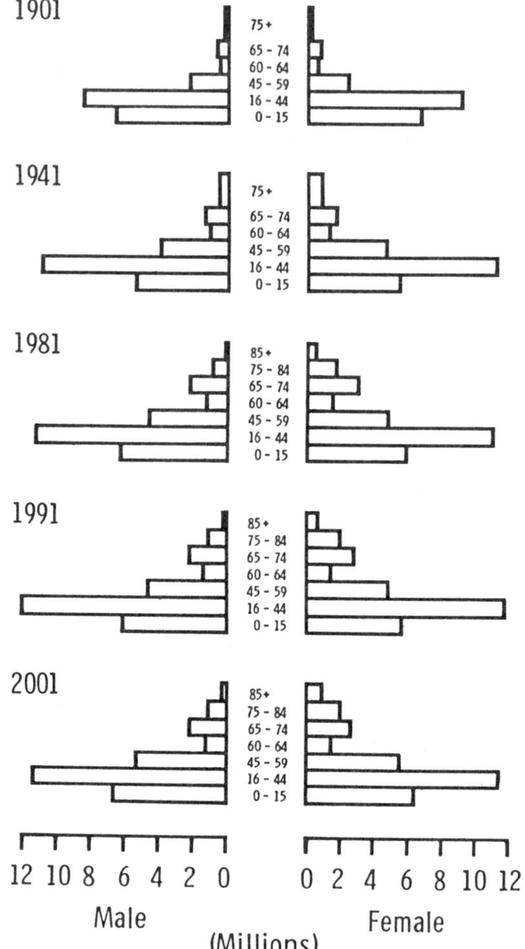

Fig. 1.2 Sex and age structure of the population of the UK for selected years 1901–2001. (Based on material from OPCS 1989; Crown Copyright.)

1.2. From the *shape* of the population profile during this time, it is clear that it has, and will, become less steeply pyramidal. This is because during the 20th century the overall population has risen by 52%, but those aged 60 years or more, of both sexes, have increased in number by 300%. Thus in the United Kingdom at present, 2 in 9 females, and 1 in 6 males are aged 60 years or more.

Absolute numbers of older people are not expected to rise appreciably in the foreseeable future, unless very striking changes occur in the mortality experience of those in earlier and middle life.

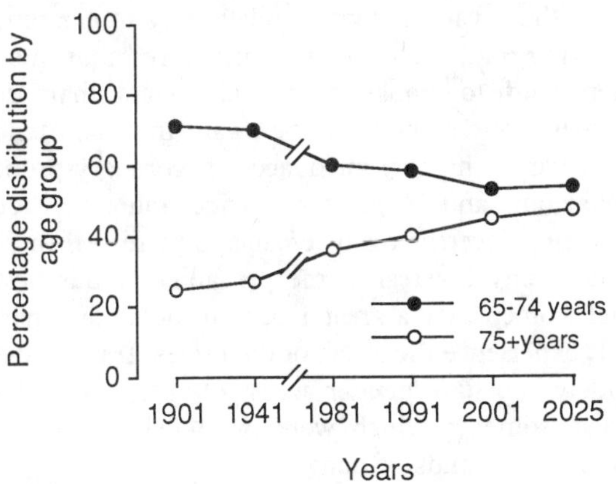

Fig. 1.3 Comparison of the proportion of the elderly population aged 60/65–74 years with the proportion aged 75 years and over. (Based on material from OPCS 1989; Crown Copyright.)

The most significant fact to grasp, however, is the relative increase in the proportion of the elderly population aged 75 years or more. In particular this shift is seen in those aged 85 years and over, as Figure 1.3 shows. This trend is likely to continue. It is projected that by the year 2025 this '*oldest old*' group will have grown from some 0.8 million in 1987 to 1.4 million, i.e. from 7% to 9% of all elderly. Even so, it should be realised that the 'oldest old' will then only represent 2% of the total population.

Nevertheless, although this confirms the assertion that there is no cause for alarm, this rapid growth in the proportion of the elderly population aged 75 years and more must be viewed in relation to the slowly falling section aged 60–74 years (see Fig. 1.3). It is this latter group of active 'younger elderly' who so often care for the very old. Furthermore this increase in the proportion of 'old elderly' must be related to the reduced numbers of non-employed women, who traditionally have been family carers and who have been the mainstay of many voluntary organisations as well.

What does this imply?

It has been pointed out that the age group 85 years and upwards is the one which suffers from the greatest physical and mental disability at present (Acheson 1981). His findings are supported by The Royal College of Physicians (1986), and by the estimates advanced from a prevalence study on disability amongst adults in Great Britain (OPCS 1988c). Thus it has been postulated that the 'oldest old' require 6 times the average resources from the health services and 26 times these from the personal social services. To date such demands have not been matched with commensurate provision, and there is concern that the gap may widen still further. Such concern prompted the Report on Community Care (Griffiths 1988), on which the Government has now announced its intentions. Improved legislation is to be welcomed, since there have been grave misgivings about community care. In arguing the case for improvements, Laurance (1988) stated that

> at a time when this policy was being heralded as a high priority, some services actually decreased. For instance the meals-on-wheels service, on which a number of older persons depend, fell in its provision over a decade and the rate of improvement in Day Centre supply has fallen since 1982.

Nevertheless, while it is prudent to note all these implications, it would be wrong to assume that all the very old are frail dependants. Figure 1.4 shows this is far from the case, giving an indication of the average pattern of activity amongst two 'reference groups', one aged 65 years and the other aged 85 years. Although there *is* declining independence with advancing years, a significant number cope well. We can all quote examples of active octogenarians and nonogenarians who continue to live full and autonomous lives until shortly before death. This is the level of independence and participation which those who offer preventive health care seek to encourage.

Sex disparity

Another significant demographic feature is the disparity between the sexes, which favours females and reflects world-wide trends. This sex difference is emphasised in each age group over 60 years. It reached a peak in 1981, when the ratio of males to females aged 85 years and upwards was 1 to 5. By 1987 this ratio had fallen slightly to 1 to 3. Overall for the population aged 60 years and upwards, it stood at 1 male for every 1.4 females, indicating the survival of more females in later old age (see Table 1.1).

Table 1.1 Distribution of the elderly population (65 years and over), shown by sex and age for 1987

	65–69 (%)	70–74 (%)	75–79 (%)	80–84 (%)	85+ (%)
Males	47	42	39	33	23
Females	53	58	61	67	77

Based upon data from OPCS (1989)

The average life expectancy rates, at birth, have shown general improvement for both sexes. Even so the average male infant can currently only expect a further 71.5 years of life, compared with 77.4 years for the average female.

It is also worthy of note that, in spite of more surviving nonogenarians and centenarians, there has been comparatively little gain in the average life expectancy for either sex after 65 years (Fries et al 1989). In fact those who did manage to survive to 65 years at the turn of the century had almost as high an average life expectancy, thereafter, as their modern counterparts. Thus in 1987 the *average* male aged 65 years could only expect a further 13 years of life, compared with 17 years for the *average* female.

Why do women live longer than men?

The answer to this question is complex. The effects of two world wars affecting this country have skewed the figures negatively for men. Both Tinker (1981) and Silman (1987), suggest part of the reason may be because women have less stressful or dangerous occupations. At present, work-related accidents are almost 50 times more common in men. Males also appear to engage in greater risk-taking behaviours. For example they are *20* times more likely to become heavy drinkers and, it is estimated, *twice* as likely to become notified drug addicts (Silman 1987). Smoking was heavily indicted as a cause of this differential in mortality a few years ago, but there are now only slight differences in smoking patterns between the sexes, with most age groups, except those aged 16–19, showing a reduction in smoking behaviour over the last 15 years. Regrettably there is still disparity between socio-economic groups, with those in lower socio-economic groups, in both sexes, having higher smoking rates (OPCS 1989). However, these various figures relate only to cigarette smoking, and it should be remembered that more men tend to smoke pipes and cigars than do women. One should also be aware that men tend to have a higher incidence of coronary-prone behaviour and a greater suicide rate than do women. Nevertheless it remains to be seen if there will be any reversal of the prevailing trends now that women play a greater part in the labour market, experience the stress of dual roles, travel more widely and have greater access to various occupations, some of which were previously barred to them on grounds of danger.

It has been postulated that women may have a biological advantage, possibly hormonal, but Silman (1987) is unconvinced. Rather he thinks there may be positive reasons for the disparity in survival. He cites the fact that women are more likely to engage in preventive health measures. Certainly they consult their doctors more frequently than do men, but this may be explained by a poorer health record on their part. This latter point is emphasised by Silman when he points out that the greater longevity experienced by women may not always be matched by a high quality of life in those added years.

There are thus several challenges for health visitors. Clearly there is a strong case for encouraging men to adopt healthier lifestyles and effect improved hazard control. There is also a crucial need to elucidate sex-related differences in ageing and to see how these affect the health status in retirement of both men and women (Cowling & Campbell 1986). Furthermore there is need for greater research and an emphasis on morbidity in women. Meantime the implications of an 'older old' population, heavily weighted to females, almost half of whom are living alone and a number of whom are chronically sick or disabled, need to be seriously addressed.

PATTERNS OF LIVING AMONG THE ELDERLY POPULATION

Marital status

Although four out of five men and two out of three

women aged 60–64 years are married and living with their spouse, there is a marked drop thereafter, especially after 70 years of age. This is due to the number of women aged 65 years and upwards who have either never married or who are widowed (Table 1.2). In fact, women of this age group account for almost half the widows in the total population, reflecting the sex disparity in later old age (Table 1.1). This is an important feature to consider, since grief, loneliness and lack of physical and psychosocial support in the home stem often from the loss of a spouse. Some older widows may also experience financial hardship, having to rely mainly on Widow's Benefit for their income. It will be seen from Table 1.2 that only 1% of men and women are separated: this is in contrast to the 2% within the general adult population. Additionally, 2% of elderly men and 3% of elderly women are currently divorced. It is likely that these figures may rise in future, in line with the steep increase in the divorce rate within the general population. Divorce and re-marriage often renders the structure of family life extremely complex. Thus an older individual may not only be affected by personal divorce and/or re-marriage, but may find his or her family and social network becoming very intricate, on account of the divorce and possible re-marriage of children and even grandchildren.

Table 1.2 Marital status of the population of the UK aged 60 years and over, shown by sex and age for 1987

Age	Single (%)	Married (%)	Wid. (%)	Div. (%)	Sep. (%)
Males					
60–64	7	83	6	4	1
65–69	7	80	11	2	NA
70+	7	68	24	1	NA
Females					
60–64	6	67	22	5	1
65–69	7	57	33	2	1
70+	11	29	58	2	NA

Based upon data from OPCS (1989)

Living alone

Whereas one in ten of the general population live in one-person households, *one in three* of the older population do so. Not surprisingly the figures differ between the sexes and with increasing age, so that *17%* of men aged 65–74 compared with *38%* of women, and *24%* of men aged 75 years and over compared with *48%* of women of the same age, live alone.

Although some people may choose to live in single households, it is worth noting that persons in later maturity may have lessened choice about doing so. Living alone does not necessarily equate with loneliness, but those who are suddenly confronted with the loss of a spouse, relative or companion, with whom they may have lived for many years, are often profoundly lonely. If they are also isolated, sick or disabled their vulnerability is likely to be increased, thus compounding their 'high risk'. Such situations frequently call for greater professional surveillance.

An added feature over the post-war period has been greater geographic mobility of families, so that some older persons, who do live alone, may find themselves without immediate, local family support. In his research Abrams (1978) found much evidence to refute the belief that families no longer care about their elderly members. He discovered 75% of older elderly who had surviving children had seen them weekly during the preceding month. However, this must be seen in the context of the 35% of older persons who have no children, and the 16% who claim 'no family at all'. In support of Abrams's finding, The General Household Survey 1986 (OPCS 1988a), shows that 72% of all older females and 64% of all older males had a visit from their family members, relatives or friends during the preceding week. In fact only 2% in this later survey said that they 'were never visited, nor could they pay anyone visits'. The majority of these respondents fell into the category of 'the very old'.

Living with others in private households

In contrast to those living alone, some 80% of all elderly men and 57% of all elderly women live with other people — either in two-person households or multi-person households. It is noticeable that the number of units of three or more persons, in which an elderly member would likely be living with a family, has fallen by one third since the 1950s. Ethnic minority elderly persons are more likely to live in three-or-more-person households, but at present they represent only a small proportion of the total elderly population. Thus, at a time when, because of earlier-age marriage, younger-age childbearing and increased longevity, we are seeing more four- and even five-generation families, the traditional picture of the three-generation family living under one roof is rapidly diminishing.

Detailed scrutiny of available figures shows that in two-person elderly households, almost 70% of older people are living with another pensioner, mostly a spouse. The remainder are living with one younger person, mostly a daughter or son (OPCS 1989). In the next subsection we take a brief glance at the patterns of living for these older people.

LIFESTYLES OF ELDERLY PEOPLE AT HOME

The pictures drawn of the lifestyles of elderly people in their own homes owe much to the work of Hunt (1978) and subsequent researchers. Helpful updating is also found in the annual General Household Survey. In her study Hunt found that there were distinct differences in lifestyle between the 'younger elderly' and the 'very old'. She therefore compared two average reference groups: one aged 65 years and one aged 85 years. Figures 1.4 and 1.5 illustrate some of the patterns and comparisons she discovered. Over a decade later the data still offer helpful insights. Figure 1.6 shows some subsequent data. Although these data are not strictly comparable, general improvement in the standards of amenities available can be discerned. Taken together the data may serve to highlight the living patterns of elderly people and so inform health visiting practice.

Examining Hunt's two reference groups (Figs 1.4 and 1.5), it can be noted, not unexpectedly, that those of 65 years appear to be more independent in daily living. They apparently have more amenities and are more likely to hold a current driving licence and to have access to a car. By contrast a sizeable proportion of those aged 85 years appear to depend on public telephones, possibly launderettes or less sophisticated forms of household washing, and probably have less adequate forms of food storage. These differences receive greater emphasis when it is realised that:

- 20% of those aged 85 years or more claimed recently (OPCS 1988c) that they cannot walk down the road without help
- 29% that they cannot cook a main meal
- 32% that they are unable to wash clothes by hand
- 10% that they are unable to open screw-tops.

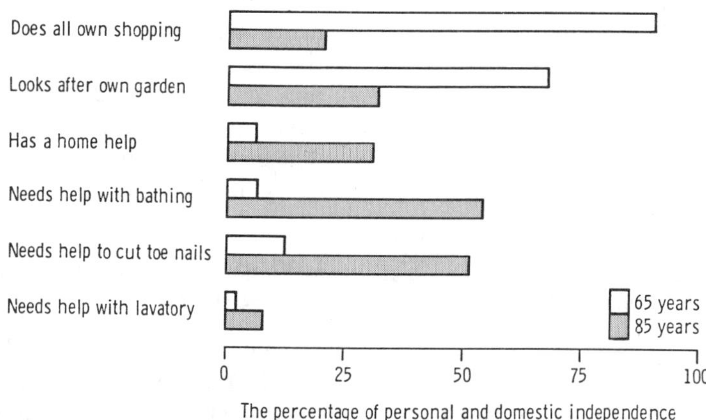

Fig. 1.4 Average pattern of activity amongst two reference groups of elderly persons: one aged 65 years and one aged 85 years. (Derived from data in Hunt 1978 and OPCS 1988a; Crown Copyright.)

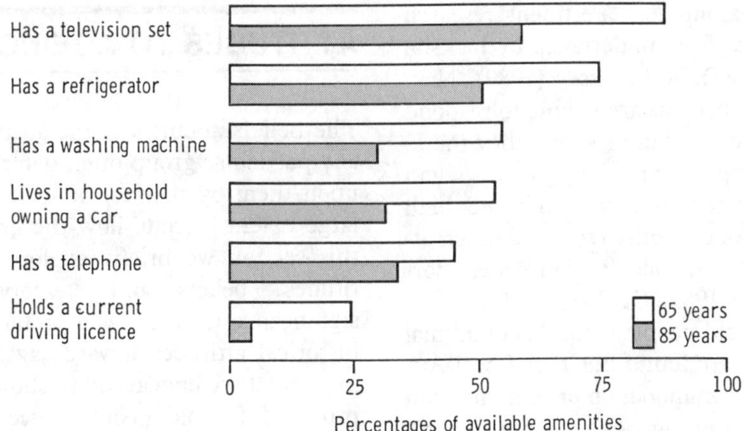

Fig. 1.5 Average pattern of activity and use of amenities among two reference groups of elderly people: one aged 65 years and one aged 85 years. (Based on data from Hunt 1978 and OPCS 1988a; Crown Copyright.)

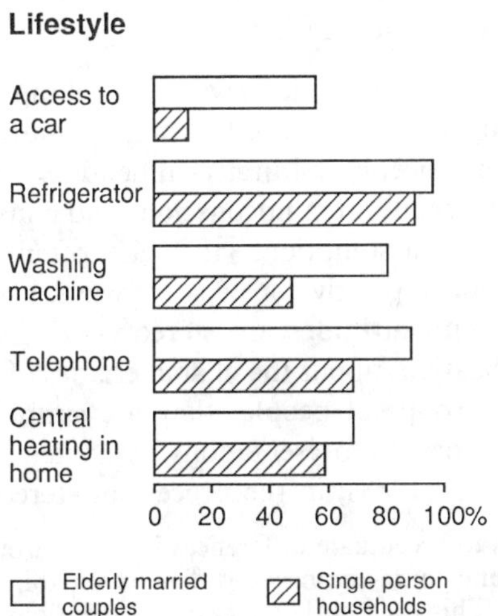

Fig. 1.6 Comparative lifestyles of elderly persons: amenities available to single-pensioner households and to married couples. (Derived from material contained in OPCS 1988a; Crown Copyright.)

Great care should be taken when examining data and endeavouring to interpret them, but while being aware that no direct comparison can be made, one cannot fail to note from these studies how many people apparently manage well. For instance, note the high proportion who *can* cook, wash, undertake personal and domestic tasks and shop for themselves, as well as get about virtually unaided.

LIVING IN COMMUNAL ESTABLISHMENTS

While a welcome trend is the increasing encouragement of older people to remain in their own homes, some inevitably cannot, or may not wish to do so. These may therefore require communal care. It is noted that only approximately *4%* of the elderly population falls within this category, although absolute numbers rise in line with population increase. Not surprisingly there is a wide age difference, with less than 1% of those under 75 years of age being found in communal establishments, compared with 18% of those aged 85 years or more. The publication of the Wagner Report (NISW 1988) and the White Paper on Community Care (DSS 1989) may affect the position of residential care in the future. Approximately two-thirds of those currently requiring communal care are found within hospitals or nursing homes. Although many of those in hospital are cared for in geriatric units, the nature of illness in old age means that a number are also found in medical, surgical, orthopaedic, ophthalmological and psychiatric wards. In fact, currently half of all the NHS beds are occupied by those aged 60 years and over. The complex challenge that an older hospital population presents to the nursing profession is discussed by Simone (1989). The emphasis of their treatment must clearly be towards restoration and rehabilitation. Pertinent research in this connection has been undertaken by Jackson (1984), Fielding (1987), and Massey (1989). Nevertheless some older persons are unable to respond to such rehabilitative programmes, and they therefore require longer-term supportive and ameliorative care. Their quality of life and high dependency needs are currently receiving much attention (see Miller 1985, Jones & Van Amelsvoort Jones 1986, Fielding 1989, Denham 1990).

Of the remaining old people living in communal establishments most are found in either Local Authority residential accommodation or in homes run by voluntary or private agencies. A few elderly persons are looked after under Boarding-out schemes. Recent trends have been to encourage further development in the private sector, on the premise that this increases client choice and reduces the risk of institutionalisation. Whilst this form of provision may result in more personalised care, there are considerably increased risks of exploitation (Challis & Bartlett 1986). Furthermore some less affluent elderly people and/or their relatives have experienced difficulty in meeting their share of the fees.

One feature, common to all residential establishments over the past decade, is the rise in the average age of residents. In some instances this has resulted in correspondingly high dependency rates, with consequent implications for staffing levels and resource requirements, as well as for staff education, training, supervision and support. In this connection one trend which may receive some impetus in the future is the work undertaken by a few health visitors in participation with staff in communal establishments. They organise seminars, workshops and short courses, working mainly as resource persons. Thus they have assisted staff in encouraging residents to form and attend exercise and fitness groups, relaxation sessions and music and movement activities. They have stimulated the introduction of creative pastimes, reminiscence programmes and the participation of residents in their own care. By assisting residential staff in reducing boredom and apathy among older residents they have contributed towards greater interaction and have thus helped to improve well-being.

ATTITUDES TO AGEING

The beliefs about, and the attitudes held towards any particular group often determine the value set upon them by the rest of society and hence, to a large extent, dictate how the group is treated. In this section we briefly explore the nature of attitudes, beliefs and stereotypes, with their significance for care, as a prelude to outlining the historical attitudes towards ageing. Placing these in context we endeavour to show how the services provided for old people reflect changing beliefs and values.

ATTITUDES, STEREOTYPES, MYTHS AND LABELS

Defined as persistent ways of thinking and responding, attitudes, whether they be individual or social, are deeply culturally-embedded. Springing from powerful, often unconscious and constraining beliefs and assumptions, they are often strongly displayed, in positive or negative ways. Closely involved with attitudes are stereotypes. As sets of generalizations about the characteristics of individuals or groups of people, they are simplistic and often distorted representations. As stated by Slater & Gearing (1988), in the process of stereotyping

> we tend to accentuate differences between groups of people and to de-emphasise differences within groups. This can subtly affect our perceptions, so that we create 'us and them' notions and hence situations.

This tendency to over-generalise, and thus categorise as homogeneous, individuals and groups who are in fact highly heterogeneous, stems frequently from ignorance and limited experience. It also arises from deep-seated fears and irrationalities, and from the often fictional images which we form about ourselves and others. However, these notions then often become taken-for-granted reality, and as such go unchallenged. Prejudice may also underlie some attitudes and stereotypes, as may myths, which are fictional narratives frequently passed on to subsequent generations.

Closely allied to stereotyping is the concept of labelling. Labels are shorthand descriptions of persons or groups, based upon perceived images and characteristics. As such they convey a social identity, which invites responses and further, often distorted, perceptions. Sometimes labelling leads to the adoption of a self-identity. An individual or group may be so conditioned into accepting the ascribed label, that they assume behaviours which fit in with the perceived image. They thus render true the label and associated stereotype. This is often described as self-fulfilling prophecy.

Duplicity towards older people

Even compassionate behaviour can create overprotection and under-estimation. Over two decades ago, Simone de Beauvoir (1970) argued that in spite of better education and the dissemination of research findings, for a considerable time, *duplicity* remains a hallmark of the adult's attitude to the aged:

> While bowing to the ethic of respect, subtle under-mining of their authority can occur, leading to their abdication of autonomy and their adoption of passive roles.

Images of ageing

Thus there are individual and societal images of ageing, and commonly held stereotypes arising from beliefs and misconceptions about social status and social roles in later life. Such stereotypes are frequently reinforced by the mass media, by those pursuing particular ideologies and/or by the attitudes of prestigious individuals or groups. Such myths and stereotypes often heighten our expectations of the behaviour of older people, causing us to react sharply when they differ from our preconceived notions (Hendricks & Hendricks 1985). These writers point out the common 'ideal type' of the elderly which we often create. One such is as follows.

> The ideal old person is white-haired, inactive, unemployed and enjoys passivity. . . . Makes no demands; is docile, accepting loneliness, boredom, and other constraints without murmur. Can live cheerfully on a pittance, having few needs. Is often slightly deficient in intelligence; tiresome in talk; usually asexual and if not is unseemly! . . . Main occupations are religion, reminiscing and attending the funerals of friends. . . .
>
> (Hendricks & Hendricks 1985)

Although this description may be regarded as a blatant caricature, there are other stereotypes which are equally demeaning. These are discussed by Comfort (1977), when he points out that assumptions are often made that the elderly can no longer exercise rational choices, should not be allowed to take personal risks, will always wish to conform and are unlikely to hold relevant views.

PROFESSIONAL ATTITUDES TOWARDS OLDER PEOPLE

Thus the personal and social attitudes shown towards older people stem from similar sources to those of all other attitudes. Nor should it be supposed that negative attitudes, or stereotypes, are confined to lay persons. Professional workers as well may have distorted notions about old people, mainly because they tend to see only those older people who have problems. Hence professionals may be the ones most *unlikely* to have their negative preconceptions disconfirmed (Slater & Gearing 1988). These writers cite several research studies and reports which demonstrate some professional attitudes — for example:

- 14% of rehabilitative staff felt that talking to old people about exercise was unimportant or a waste of time (McHeath 1983)
- Passive acceptance of old people's problems by social workers meant little attempt was made to try and achieve personal or environmental change (Goldberg & Warburton 1979)
- General practitioners may not give work with old people a high priority, because of pessimistic attitudes to ageing (Age Concern, England 1985)
- Health visitors gave a lower visiting allocation to old people (Dunnell & Dobbs 1982)
- Student nurse attitudes were reviewed by Fielding (1986) and found frequently to be negative.

Confirmation of some other prevailing unfavourable professional. attitudes towards older people are described by Norman (1987) and Victor (1987).

Personal perceptions, values and attitudes

At this juncture it may be salutary for us to review our own personal perceptions of, and values about, old age. It is suggested by Murray et al (1980) that such an exercise is an essential prelude if one wishes to undertake effective work with older people. Moreover, those of us who work constantly with those in later maturity need to regularly re-appraise our attitudes, beliefs and values, in order to discover if '*hidden ageism*' pervades our work. Ageism is one of the most covert of attitudes, all the more pernicious because its manifestations are so subtle that it may not be noticed for what it is — *a pejorative image of older people*. It is only by appreciating the uniqueness of every individual, the distinctiveness of their life-patterns and their coping mechanisms, and hence their needs, that we can go some way towards offering improved personal care.

ATTITUDES TOWARDS ELDERLY PEOPLE THROUGH THE AGES

In spite of a keen interest in longevity, shared by almost all societies, cultural attitudes towards ageing have been somewhat ambivalent. Both de Beauvoir (1970) and Victor (1987) have commented on the literary treatment of ageing. They show how even in cultures where old age was venerated, respect was sometimes interwoven with resentment, conflict and satire. Few works actually tackled the problems of ageing, while older characters rarely constituted the central theme.

At a personal level not all individuals seem to have looked forward unreservedly to old age, though many appear to have espoused the desire for long life. This ambivalence may in part be due to the heightening of awareness of personal mortality. Self-image may at times be threatened when a person's belief system does not include an appreciation of the phase of later maturity as the rounding-off of the cycle of life.

Whether old age was regarded as a blessing, a birth right, or a burden, seems to have depended largely on the age of the individual expressing the viewpoint. Personal values, life experiences, health levels and self-concept appear to have mattered as much as did the nature and frequency of a person's contact with old people. Such factors still appear operative today.

Historical equivocalness

Historically this equivocalness is well demonstrated. In pre-literate societies, where survival was the over-riding issue, the knowledge and experience of older people became highly valued. However, when they became physically or economically dependent, they were often abandoned, neglected, ritualistically killed, or encouraged to commit 'altruistic suicide'. It is as much a false assumption to believe that all old people held high prestige, or were cherished by their kin in the past, as it is to claim that they are more often abandoned in our present-day more mobile society.

Positive attitudes towards ageing were displayed by the Taoists and by the early Chinese, who regarded long life as a 'crown of development', doubtless greatly enhanced by its rarity. The Hebrews, too, revered longevity. They considered it a reward for godly living, which led them to call for great respect towards older people, and exhortations to aspirants to keep the Mosaic Law. Paradoxically, however, the most graphic lament on old age is found in Ecclesiastes, Chapter 12.

In 55 BC Cicero wrote in *De Senectute* one of the most spirited and lengthy defences of old age ever recorded. Translated by Falconer (1923), it well repays reading. One excerpt may serve to indicate the tenor of his work:

> Those, therefore, who allege that old age is devoid of useful activity, are like those who would say that the pilot does nothing in the sailing of the ship, because while others are climbing masts, running about

gangways, or working at the pumps, he sits quietly in the stern and simply holds the tiller. He may not be doing what younger members of the crew are doing, but what he does is better and much more important. It is not by muscle, speed or physical dexterity that great things are achieved, but by reflection, force of character and judgement: in these qualities old age is usually not poorer, but often even richer.

Conversely, negative attitudes were shown by the early Egyptians, who feared the physical decline of old age. They sought to defer its ravages by eating the glands of young animals — a rejuvenation theory which has had more modern resurgence within monkey-gland therapy!

The Greeks, too, held contradictory notions. Their mythology is shot through with accounts of their quest for eternal youth. Such searching often led to inter-generational conflict. Nevertheless Plato (who died over 80 years old, with pen in hand) and his fellow-philosopher, Aristotle, asserted the value of a gerontocracy. Both of them emphasised the experience and wisdom brought by many senior citizens to political and civic life.

While many of these examples were valid, it is necessary to realise that the accounts of several old worthies are the stories of the privileged few. For many people of their time, life was brutish and short. The average expectation of life was below 30 years of age, and even those who achieved the sixth decade were sometimes sick, often disabled, and especially if they were of the poorer classes, had experienced great deprivation.

Capturing prevailing ambivalence

Shakespeare immortalised much of this ambivalence when he created his classic character, King Lear. Elsewhere, in his satirical poem on the seven ages of man, he wrote his well-known, melancholic, somewhat cruel comments on the sixth age:

> The sixth age shifts into the lean and slippered pantaloon, with spectacles on nose and pouch on side. His youthful hose well sav'd, a world too wide for his shrunk shank: and his big manly voice turning again to childish treble, pipes and whistles in his sound.
>
> *As You Like It*

Unfortunately, what often is intended to be humorous, or possibly provocative, is accepted; it may then be used to fuel ageism, that subtle denigration of the elderly which is so difficult to pinpoint.

Modern viewpoints

More recently, Norton (1982), the pioneer British gerontological nurse–researcher, declared:

> Old age is the fulfilment of every individual's birth-right, which many more people will achieve over the next decade.

Amongst others her optimism is echoed by Ebersole & Hess (1985). They also quote Jones (1978), who says:

> Images of ageing are changing, as the potential of the old has been brought to public attention. Older people are becoming liberated from the negative images which bound them, and are emerging to claim their unique place in society. Continued growth, personal transformations, and creative expressions mark the lives of older people everywhere.

It may be that, in the harsh light of reality regarding the plight of some older aged, one may view these comments as idealistic and therefore misplaced. Nevertheless they represent a goal to be achieved.

SOCIAL ATTITUDES PERCEIVED IN LEGISLATION

The attitudes of society towards elderly persons are often encapsulated in legislation, and the Poor Laws (1601–1948) demonstrate the slow, often chequered move towards more humane and dignified treatment of older people, especially the elderly poor. Even as recently as the 19th century many feared the harsh routines of the workhouse. The anguish and fear of many old people was captured by Dickens and epitomised in his character, Betsy Higden:

> Oh master! . . . master!' returned Betsy, '. . . I've fought against the Parish and fled from it (the workhouse), all my life, . . . and I want to die free of it'.
>
> *Our Mutual Friend*

Current social and political attitudes towards older people

Nevertheless the principle of collective responsibility for vulnerable members of society has gradually emerged. Philanthropy, patronage and reactive concern are all shown in the different voluntary organisations formed to care for elderly people in the past, as well as in the statutory and voluntary services being established in the present. However, while it is clear that many older people have benefited from the more humane social and personal attitudes which prevail, there is no room for complacency. Revelations over the past three decades, affecting many different aspects of the [illegible] of elderly people, show *not only a lack of em-[illegible]ccountability and respect for old people, but [illegible]ss under-resourcing of essential services for* [illegible] [illegible]hereas Reports in the 1960s and 1970s focu[illegible] [illegible]utional neglect, Wicks & Henwood [illegible] that more recent criticisms have been [illegible] [illegible]he paucity of statutory [illegible]ervice develop[illegible] [illegible]lly within the community. Their comm[illegible], [illegible]hose of the Audit Commission's Report (198[illegible]) [illegible]ight some current social and political attitu[illegible] [illegible]rds elderly people.

Children are seen to have needs, whe[illegible] elderly people are often regarded only as having p[illegible]blems. Until comparatively recently, older people were a relatively invisible social group, and the most needy sections from within them were often unable to redress policies which apparently receive mass support.

There is now, however, firm evidence of a greater collective raising of consciousness. Groups and Federations of older people have been formed, better able to use the political process and to campaign for improved conditions for older adults. Amongst those now retiring there is an articulate and more affluent minority, who are well able to wield considerable socio-political influence if they wish to act on behalf of the less advantaged majority. Moreover, pressures on national governments from international organisations, or collectives such as the European Economic Community, urging conformity with European Parliamentary legislation, may create conditions for change in some countries, which might not otherwise be brought about. However, in spite of some assertive actions, both for, and by, old people, ageism continues to adopt many guises.

THE MANY GUISES OF AGEISM

Some forms of subtle denigration can be as hurtful, or more so, than overt physical neglect. For example, compare the great prestige which is currently attached to youth, physical beauty, sexual attractiveness, speed, competitiveness, aggressiveness, productivity and rapid adaptation, with that afforded contemplation, wisdom and experience. Expressed policies on age, related to job opportunities, especially in times of recession and high unemployment, often discriminate against the older worker. Stress on the use of sophisticated technological machinery, concern with materialism, and an emphasis on planned obsolence can all enhance the pain some older people feel at social relegation following retirement.

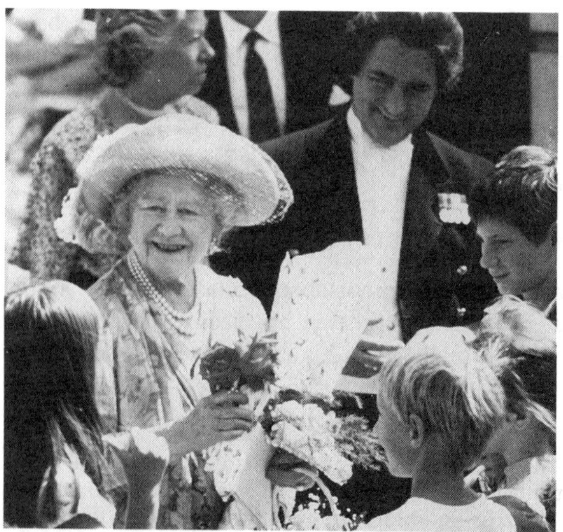

Fig. 1.7 Her Majesty Queen Elizabeth, The Queen Mother, on her 90th birthday — Patron of Research Into Ageing. Photograph by courtesy of Camera Press (Copyright); reproduced by permission.

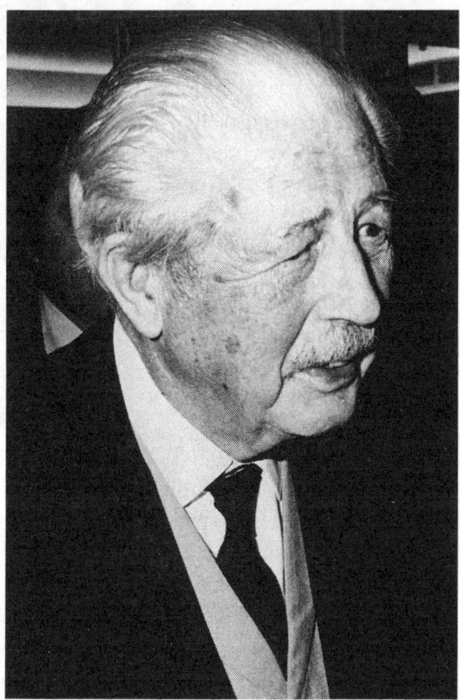

Fig. 1.8 Older people represent a great human resource. The late The Right Honourable The Earl of Stockton, OM, PC, an active member of The House of Lords in his 90s. Photograph taken at a Distinguished Company Luncheon and reproduced by permission of Research into Ageing.

Such approaches ignore the many older people who do remain fully independent; run their own households; maintain recognised and socially useful roles with their children, grandchildren and sometimes their great grandchildren, and still play a prominent and useful part in their local community and sometimes in even wider social and political life (Figs 1.7 and 1.8).

Similarly, there is often a tendency to overlook the many unifying values, which enable younger and older people to find affinity in common concerns. It may be that the changing demographic structure (which for a few years means a lower proportion of young workers), and the growing emphasis on consumer participation, self-help and community development, will accelerate the process of attitude change.

THE DEVELOPMENT OF HEALTH VISITING SERVICES FOR ELDERLY PEOPLE

Although some forms of medical care have always been available to older people, the speciality of Geriatric Medicine (which concerns the treatment of disease in elderly people) is of comparatively recent origin. Similarly the geriatric nursing services have undergone marked changes in the past half century, as reviewed by Evers (1981). However, gerontology (which is the scientific study of ageing, and the application of derived knowledge to the promotion and maintenance of well-being in later life) is a distinct field, involving multidisciplinary perspectives. It is in the gerontological field that health visiting older people finds its affinity.

Florence Nightingale (1893) appreciated the contrast between sick nursing and the education, surveillance and supportive care of the apparently well. As a result she urged the nascent health visiting profession to 'develop this new work of home health-bringing'. In recognising the need to work with the community, for its development, she was appreciating the essence of the early service and encouraging health visitors in their educative thrust towards health.

The birth of the profession

Health visiting was born in the middle of the last century, in the period of rapid industrialisation, with its accompanying socio-economic changes, marked inequalities, poverty, deprivation and degradation, rampant infectious disease, malnutrition and premature death. Influenced by the Sanitary Reform Movement and closely associated with emerging feminist groups, the early practitioners sought to visit all age-groups. Their purpose was

> to elevate the people, physically, mentally, morally and spiritually.

They co-operated closely with lay workers, often spearheading teams of volunteers, and much of their work was conducted in self-help groups and through mutual aid societies. However, they were deflected somewhat from their comprehensive ideals and universal approach by the prevailing socio-political influences.

POLITICIAL PRESSURES — PROFESSIONAL STRUGGLES

The latter part of the 19th century saw the struggle between the dominant medical profession and the emerging professions of midwifery, nursing and social work. Caught up in the politically popular and rapidly expanding maternity and child welfare movement, the limited numbers of trained health visitors found themselves under the administrative sway of the powerful, but benign, Medical Officers of Health. Thus they were channelled into a concentration of effort on child health and sanitation (MacQueen 1962, Owen 1983). Nevertheless the claims of the elderly population were pressed very firmly by Beatrice and Sidney Webb (Royal Commission on the Poor Law 1909). With two other members they wrote a Minority Report, *setting out proposals for a national health visiting service for the aged.* They were particularly impressed by three main features of health visiting, and these they wished to see applied to the care of older people. They were:

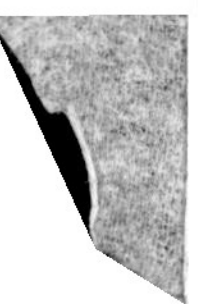

1. the humanising and educational character of the service
2. the stimulus it gave to personal responsibility
3. the active strengthening of recipient self-respect, personal willpower, participation and self-help.

The Webbs advocated:

> Just as the Public Health Authority exercises general supervision over the health of infants, so it must exercise similar guardianship over its older citizens. Through these health visitors going their daily rounds, the Authority will become aware of the aged before they are sick, neglected or lack care.

While some may feel that this approach smacks of paternalism and interference in personal liberty, others may place it in its historical context and perceive it as a genuine concern to improve the lot of a, then, very deprived group.

Health visitors will be interested to note that their role as a case-finder was clearly seen at this early stage. However, although the goals of such a proposed service were well within the remit and original aims of the profession, in the event the recommendations of the Minority Report were not accepted. Rather the care of the older person was left to the individual policies of Local Authorities, which meant some provided the minimum required. One may speculate how far the health care of older people suffered in consequence.

The inter-war years

In spite of some role extension for health visitors as a result of the Local Government Act 1929, there was little national encouragement to enlarge the scope of the work. Economic recession, and high unemployment following the 1914–18 War, meant few efforts were made to enlarge the workforce between the two wars. Nevertheless, because of the statutorily prescribed duties in the maternity and child health, school health, and child life protection fields, as well as responsibility for care and after-care services, demands for health visitors outstripped their supply. Care and after-care services at that time mainly involved work with those suffering from infectious diseases (many of which were rife and serious), and with the mentally subnormal. Because of these strained manpower resources, few authorities or practitioners could exercise a preventive health function for other age-groups, including the elderly. Medical services remained both curative and custodial. A few health visitor pioneers, however, managed to keep a corner of their caseload for work with older people in their community.

THE ADVENT OF THE WELFARE STATE

The introduction of the National Health Service in 1946 was considered by Lamont (1954) to be the gateway of opportunity for the health visitor. It provided the legislative base for widening and enriching the role, through work with all age groups. It not only gave greater scope for home visiting and liaison activities, but enabled work to be undertaken in other settings as well. Statutory duties now included the promotion of health, the prevention of disease, and care and after-care functions. These were largely for those suffering from chronic infectious diseases such as tuberculosis (which then presented a major public health problem), the aged and the mentally disordered. The subsequent National Assistance Act, 1948, brought the end of the Poor Law, and gave additional chance for innovatory care to be given. This included visiting elderly persons in residential accommodation, as well as participating in their health promotion through the new provisions for recreational, diversional and social welfare facilities.

Unfortunately, the depressed levels of health visitor recruitment during the 1939–45 war meant that the remaining practitioners were often unable to seize the opportunites which the new legislation offered. Furthermore the local authorities, which then administered the service, often had policies which were not conducive to development. There were many financial claims on different services in post-war Britain and those such as housing took priority. In some areas a few practitioners developed initiatives such as forging links with the then-new Old People's Welfare Committees, and offering health education programmes in the newly developing Elderly Persons Clubs. A few became involved in health advisory clinics for the middle-aged and elderly, where progressive medical officers facilitated them. Others ran community programmes with Health Education Officers, which included courses to prepare persons for retirement, prevent accidents in later life, or assist carers to meet the needs of their ageing friends or relatives.

THE INTRODUCTION OF ATTACHMENT SCHEMES

During the 1950s and early 1960s, further diversification took place. Ministry of Health circulars re-emphasised the all-purpose, family health care role of the health visitors. Certain Medical Officers of Health and County Nursing Officers encouraged policies of attachment to general medical practice, hospitals and university departments. Such changes were hotly debated. Hitherto, health visitors had been perceived as relating to defined geographic communities, with the major thrust of their work towards primary prevention. (This is defined as all those efforts undertaken to promote health and increase human resistance to disease. Thus it includes maintaining good nutrition and healthy lifestyles, encouraging social well-being, fostering optimum development, teaching about specific protection and the measures necessary to make the environment safe and less favourable to human-disease-agent interaction.)

There were those who feared that attachment schemes would divert practitioners from primary to secondary prevention, or even tertiary prevention. Although health visitors had always played a part at these latter two levels, they had not constituted major components of health visiting work. Secondary prevention is defined as all action taken to identify deviation from the normal. Thus it includes early diagnosis and prompt referral for treatment, so that the period of disorder may be shortened. Activities comprise individual and mass case-finding measures, screening surveys and selective examinations of aggregates within the population.

Tertiary prevention, on the other hand, occurs at a later stage in the disease process, when disorder is well established. At this level the goal is to reduce the effects of the disorder, prevent complications, aid restoration, and prepare the community to support and use the rehabilitated person whenever possible. Exponents of attachment schemes argued that they were but extensions of earlier health visiting activities, and that they would facilitate access to other vulnerable groups, especially elderly or handicapped people. Hence the three levels of prevention were seen by them as inter-related and complementary.

THE FIRST ENQUIRY INTO HEALTH VISITING

The first enquiry into health visiting was undertaken by the Jameson Committee. In their Report (Ministry of Health 1956) they offered some clarification of the scope and range of the role, by stressing that the main functions of the health visitor were 'health education and social advice'. They itemised the duties they felt were included. Those functions relating to the care of the elderly are:

- health education to individuals, groups and communities
- supportive visiting to older people, to facilitate independence and mobilise services
- ascertainment and supervision of specific health problems
- assessment of psychosocial and economic need
- liaison with, and assistance to voluntary bodies working with the aged
- supportive help to the staff of Welfare Departments
- special attention to the elderly sick, infirm, or needy, in collaboration with the general practitioner and/or district nurse. This, however, excludes specific curative duties.

In arguing that the major role for health visitors should be health education and social advice, the Committee stressed that the care of elderly persons must begin in earlier years, and be intensified in middle-age to avoid a disease-oriented approach to ageing. Although modifications of some of the welfare-directed services occurred with the expansion of Social Services Departments after 1970, these duties have remained substantially the same. They were elaborated in The Mayston Report (DHSS 1971).

THE FORMATION OF THE CETHV

With the formation of the Council for the Education and Training of Health Visitors (CETHV) in 1962, great changes occurred in the education of health visitors (Wilkie 1978, Batley 1983). A broadened curriculum led to more theory being included on gerontological principles, the physical and psychosocial aspects of ageing, current health problems, and policies affecting older people. Written examination questions on older people were included in all sections of the syllabus (see Appendix 6 for a sample set of questions). At least one of the health visiting studies required for Part II of the examination had to cover the care of an elderly client. Thus the ensuing decade saw some advances in health visitor contact with older people. Fieldwork Teachers, and Assessors of supervised practice, helped students to obtain more comprehensive field work experience, as a corollary to their theoretical studies, and qualified practitioners put their new skills into practice.

1974 AND BEYOND — AN ERA OF REORGANISATION

The past 15 years have seen a number of reorganisations within the NHS, each affecting both health visiting and old people. The first reorganisation took place in 1974, when health visiting services along with other community health services were removed from the jurisdiction of Local Authorities, and placed under the aegis of Area Health Authorities. The intention was to integrate curative and preventive health services, under a system of consensus management, in which nursing would play an equal part.

Impetus was thus given to the further development of liaison schemes, which allowed more health visitors to become involved in the pre- and post-hospital care of older people. Nevertheless, some observers argued that this over-medicalised the health visiting approach to health care of elderly people, and detracted from the raison d'être of the service: namely, primary prevention. It has also been argued that any increased contact with hospital personnel was made at the expense of retaining close contact with local authority staff, particularly social workers, environmental health officers, housing officers and community development workers.

The diversification of practice

There are some examples of innovatory practice during this period. For instance, Halladay (1981) described a Manchester-based scheme, headed by a health visitor, and Day & Mogridge (1981) described an experimental scheme where a health visitor was based within a social services setting, with responsibility for health education and liaison duties for older and handicapped people.

In spite of an apparent reluctance on the part of health visitors to publish their work, a few accounts are available about different and often creative schemes. They show that practitioners engaged in a variety of activities with older people, running exercise and keep-fit classes; bereavement counselling groups; health advisory clinics for older adults; screening programmes; support groups for carers, and for elderly people living in high-rise flats, or in large impersonal housing estates. Some practitioners participated in community self-help projects, workshops on retirement, or developed schemes for visiting those attending accident and emergency departments. Examples of these various activities can be found in Drennan (1984), Drummond (1984), Coupland (1986), Machell et al (1988) and Enderby (1989).

Reorganisation in 1982

Managerial changes following further NHS reorganisation in 1982 resulted in health visiting experiencing the effects of high retirement levels, when a number of senior managers left the service. At the same time financial stringencies caused lessened recruitment and secondment for education and training.

In spite of its avowed objective, 'Patients first', this reorganisation did not result in any marked extension of health visiting services for older people. Apart from staffing resources, this may have resulted from health authority policies, which continued to emphasise the role with mothers and children.

The introduction of general management in 1984

Further administrative changes followed reorganisation in 1984. Area Health Authorities were abolished and District Health Authorities reconstituted. General management was introduced and the new style meant that, in some instances, health visitors were being managed by other than their own professional heads. The effects of these and other changes affecting community nursing services are discussed by Littlewood (1987), who considers that

> they have reduced nursing power within nursing and raised the health service in Britain to a frenetic level of efficiency and production.

She related her comments particularly to the effects upon hospitalised elderly, emphasising an important role for health visitors in the prevention of re-admission following early discharge.

New patterns of data collection and information dissemination

One feature of the 1984 reorganisation was the development of new patterns of data collection and information-dissemination, in line with Körner recommendations (1984). The great potential which this change holds for health visitors was welcomed by Fawcett-Henessy (1987). However, she emphasised the need for appropriate data input. All workers in the field of preventive medicine face great difficulties in developing valid forms of prevention measurement. Health visitors have an added difficulty in endeavouring to quantify qualitative information. As yet, appropriate software packages, which seek to capture the subtle quality and ramifications of health visiting, do not seem to be available. This challenge is currently receiving some attention. Meanwhile, more precise classification of quantitative data should facilitate 'targeting', and so help to improve overall community nursing services (Hull 1989, King 1989).

THE PROPOSED REFORM OF THE NHS, 1989

Amid a welter of controversy and public concern, the Government launched its proposals for further and radical reform of the NHS (DHSS 1989). Under the title 'Working for Patients', its stated objectives were two-fold:

1. to give patients, wherever they live in the UK, better health care and greater choice of services available

2. to provide greater satisfaction and rewards for those working in the NHS, who successfully respond to local needs and preferences.

Several key measures were proposed in order to achieve these objectives:

1. reformed management bodies
2. new funding arrangements
3. self-governing hospitals
4. general practitioner practice budgets
5. more delegation of responsibility to local level
6. better audit arrangements.

Although the objectives were generally welcomed, criticism of the proposed key measures has centred on the undesirability of a market economy approach to health care; on an over-emphasis on acute and curative aspects to the detriment of preventive health care; an undue emphasis on efficiency, productivity, and cost effectiveness; and insufficient detail about effective consumer representation.

Health visitors, in company with other community health staff, welcome the proposals for greater delegation and better utilisation of professional skills. They also are glad to see some review of the cost of drugs and medications. Nevertheless, they share the concerns expressed about reformed management and reduced elected representation, as well as the unease that the proposals may militate against those with long-standing chronic illness, or disability. Older clients are more likely to fall into this latter category, and they may well suffer from larger list sizes within general medical practice, as well as budgetary limitations. On the other hand, there is general professional approval for the greater involvement of clients and patients in their own care, and for a greater choice of services to be available. Positive benefits of this kind could mean an extension of provision for the apparently well. If this were so, then health promotion and health maintenance might be afforded as much, if not more, recognition than is envisaged for those suffering from illness. Health visitors will doubtless wish to make their views known to their Parliamentary representatives and their professional organisations, so that subsequent legislation may be modified to take account of present anxieties.

THE COMMUNITY NURSING REVIEW

The last 15 years has seen a plethora of Reports — many endorsing the health visiting role with older adults They include DHSS Reports (1976a, 1976b, 1977, 1981), The Royal Commission on The National Health Service (1979), The Black Report on Inequalities in Health (DHSS 1980), and The Nation's Health (Smith & Jacobson 1988). There has been limited action on most of these, hence one of the most eagerly awaited and significant documents for health visitors was the Report of the Community Nursing Review Committee (DHSS 1986), known as The Cumberledge Report. Applied only to England, it stressed the need to:

- ensure systematic identification of the health needs of individuals and communities
- enable more effective responses to such needs through improved teamwork
- bring the management of community nursing services closer to consumers
- provide opportunity for community nursing staff to work in new and wider roles
- improve consumer participation in the planning and provision of health care.

The Committee therefore advocated the setting-up of Neighbourhood Nursing Services, in which health visitors, district nurses and school nurses could form integrated teams and function as professionals in their own right, being freely available to clients. This was seen as satisfying consumer wishes for more accessible, acceptable and available services. The Committee also urged the setting-up of local health care associations, in which consumers and professionals together could plan 'good health programmes'. One such programme would involve older people.

Although there was no central government direction on the implementation of the Report, it is noteworthy that by the beginning of 1989 over 100 of the 192 District Health Authorities concerned had schemes for modified neighbourhood nursing services, or locality management, either planned or in operation (Dalley 1989). Although these are somewhat truncated versions of the services envisaged by the Review Committee, they may go some way to improving provisions for older people.

Likewise a review of community nursing services in Wales advocated a somewhat similar development, but operating through strengthened primary health care teams (Welsh Office 1987). Some of the implications of these schemes for health visitors, especially as they concern care of older people, are discussed in Chapter 6.

REALITIES AND CHALLENGES

In spite of the evident increase in the number of people aged 60 years and over, and the emphasis upon their health needs, as seen in the various reports just discussed, the reality of health visiting involvement with this age group is limited, as evidenced by official statistics and research reports.

For instance, Dunnell & Dobbs (1982) found, in their national study of nurses working in the community, that health visitors spent only 9% of their time with those aged 65 years or more. In another study Taylor et al (1983) estimated that on average *17%* of all health visits within the United Kingdom were paid to elderly people. In more recent research Luker & Perkins (1987) found that in a stratified random sample of 1460 elderly people in Trafford, less than 1% had been visited by a health visitor in the month preceding the study.

The position is further clarified by reference to Tables 1.3 and 1.4, although the time scale in publishing data often render them currently outdated. It will be noted that whereas the number of children aged 0–16 visited by health visitors (in England only) remained fairly constant over the 10-year period, the number of older persons receiving health visits gradually fell. Furthermore the ratio of visits paid per child visited in 1986 is seen to be 3.4 to 1, whereas for the fewer number

Table 1.3 Number of health visitors (whole time equivalents), health visitor managers and student health visitors, for the period 1976–86, for England only

1976 (w.t.e.)	1981 (w.t.e.)	1982 (w.t.e.)	1983 (w.t.e.)	1984 (w.t.e)	1985 (w.t.e.)	1986 (w.t.e.)
Health visitors						
7090	9117	9350	9550	9214	10 147	10 353
Health visitor managers						
....	....	1466	1298	1491	1416	1345
Health visitor students						
947	...	1069	1023	971	866	832

Based upon data from Central Statistical Office in the report Health and personal social services statistics, 1988. HMSO, London

Table 1.4 Numbers of persons receiving health visits at home from health visitors, together with number of visits paid, shown by age, for 1976–1986, England only

Number visited and number of visits (thousands) Year:	1976	1981	1982	1983	1984	1985	1986
Children aged 0–16	2512.8	2514.0	2512.7	2516.3	2530.6	2537.8	2555.4
No. of visits paid to children aged 0–16		8727.3	8902.2	8917.3	9002.9	8982.9	8936.7
Persons aged 17–64	532.2	798.5	840.6	890.6	1005.2	1076.9	1135.4
No. of visits paid to persons aged 17–64	2340.1	2535.9	2719.6	3067.0	3300.7	3479.0	3496.4
Persons aged 65 & over	531.0	465.0	458.2	446.3	451.6	465.5	433.6
No. of visits paid to persons aged 65 & over	1407.2	1367.9	1321.0	1291.2	1265.5	1233.1	1132.7

Based on data supplied by Central Statistical Office in the report Health and Personal Social Services statistics, 1988. HMSO, London

of elderly persons visited (who presumably were the most vulnerable), the ratio for the comparative period equalled 2.6 to 1. The number of visits paid to the intervening population showed a consistent rise over the decade.

Health visitors may well wish to question this apparent inequitable distribution of health care, at a time when demographic trends show lower birth rates and a rising number of elderly people. Of course it must be appreciated that health visitors have contact with older people in many places other than the home setting. These include adult health clinics, well-persons sessions within general medical practice, clubs and groups for older persons, and contacts within communal establishments. To date these contacts may not all have been recorded. With the advent of the new computerised information systems this is likely to change, and thus a more accurate picture of work with the elderly population may be shown.

POSSIBLE REASONS FOR DISPARITY IN HEALTH VISITS

Various reasons have been advanced for the disparity in the number of health visits paid to different sections of the population. They include the following:

- historical developments within health visiting
- high case-loads with low health visitor–population ratios
- competing demands related to the time-resources available
- traditional low-priority rating for the elderly population, throughout all the health and social services
- personal inclination or disinclination
- greater job satisfaction from work with younger persons
- policy decisions and constraints from employing authorities, which militate against older people even in localities where the proportion of older persons aged 65 years and upwards is higher than that of children aged 0–5.
- inadequate information systems which make it difficult to obtain accurate, relevant data.

The length of time needed for a visit to an older person, compared with that required on average for a younger person, was considered by Dingwall (1977) to constitute a disincentive. However, Luker (1982) refuted that the time factor was a major disincentive. Instead she postulated from her research that health visitors adopt an avoidance strategy with older people, because they lack an appropriate frame of reference for dealing with this age-group. Another researcher argued, from her study, that health visitors *do* have a distinct agenda when visiting older adults and that they *do* have clear goals (Fitton 1980).

A further viewpoint was advanced by Taylor et al (1983). They considered that health visitors find the thought of visiting all the elderly within a practice population to be so daunting and impracticable in relation to their other responsibilities, that this acts as a major disincentive. They suggested a more selective approach might provide a solution (see Ch. 6, p. 138).

Certainly the sudden confrontation of 'crisis visiting' can be very off-putting for health visitor practitioners. This should act as a major argument for intervention at earlier ages and stages, to reduce the possibilities of crises developing. It seems little attention has yet been directed towards studying how far the low levels of involvement with elderly people stem from health visitor frustration at the seemingly intractable nature of some of their problems. A number of these difficulties are of a socio-environmental nature, remediable only through economic and political measures and hence rarely directly within the remit of health visiting. A few relate to medical causes, in which case perhaps closer involvement of specialists in geriatric medicine in health visitor education might have a beneficial effect.

Whatever the reasons for an unequal distribution of health visits across the population, there can be no doubt that the profession is now facing one of the most searching times in its history. Change is the order of the day — change in the structure and administration of the service, and change in established patterns of work. Some health visitors welcome this as an opportunity to be creative. Others, more fearful, would prefer perhaps to cling to tradition (Goodwin 1988). All practitioners, however, face a number of dilemmas, which have to be resolved. These dilemmas include the following.

- How to deploy their specialised skills and limited resources (particularly time and manpower) effectively, in the face of legitimate, competing and increasing demands, while simultaneously maintaining and improving standards
- Whether to retain the generic role of the health visitor, across all age groups, (which has long been regarded as a major professional strength), or whether to develop specialist skills for specific age groups. The latter might increase in-depth knowledge and expertise
- How to adequately emphasise the professional role in primary prevention, while maintaining the balance between primary, secondary and tertiary levels of care.

These dilemmas take on a new dimension in the light of changing demographic trends, alterations in the pattern of disease, the advent of nurse-practitioners in community nursing, and the proposals for reform of the NHS and Community Care. *A service geared for prevention fits uneasily into an illness-dominated framework* (Gooch 1989). Only informed and corporate debate can determine the direction which health visiting should now take.

Any increase in work with older people will likely demand a greater degree of flexibility, as well as the development and utilisation of a broader range of professional skills. This was recognised by Goodwin (1988) when she claimed that health visitors are well able to face the demands of change, by reason of their unique flexibility and versatility. She outlined proposals for the modification of practice, linked to the WHO targets for Health for all by 2000 (WHO 1985) (see also Ch. 6, pp. 116–117).

The Oxfordshire Project, described by Dauncey (1989) is a further example of such modified practice. However, this is highly child-related. Other possibilities have been highlighted by Gooch (1989) and by Lowe (1989). Furthermore the Health Visitor Association (HVA) Special Interest Group for the Elderly has initiated several innovative schemes. The Royal College of Nursing (RCN), through its Health Visitors' Forum has also carried out an exercise with its members entitled 'Change for the Better'. These various modifications are also being reflected in the individual initiatives often quietly undertaken by practitioners.

In these continuing and crucial discussions one point remains clear. Our health visitor predecessors fought hard to reduce premature death in earlier life, so that many more citizens might achieve greater longevity and improved health. In so doing they presented their successors with both an opportunity and a socio-moral responsibility: namely, how best to continue comprehensive levels of care so that those who have reached later maturity may experience high-quality life in those added years.

SUMMARY

In this chapter we have sketched in the background to the rest of the book. In reviewing the past, we have endeavoured to draw some lessons for the future. The claims of elderly people for attention and preventive health care have been outlined, in the context of world-wide increases in their numbers, and the changing proportions and ratios encountered in different populations.

The implications of changing demographic trends have been mentioned, with particular reference to the health and social services. One major emphasis has been on the resource which older persons represent, and the contribution they can, and do, make to society. While recognising that there are many who offer care to elderly people, particularly informal carers, and while stressing the need for collaborative multi-disciplinary approaches, the main focus has been on health visitors and *their* contribution to older people. Factors affecting professional attitudes, and issues regarding priorities in care, have been examined in the light of the many proposals for change. Thus the chapter serves as a prelude to subsequent and more detailed discussion about specific aspects affecting health visiting care with older people.

REFERENCES

Abrams M 1978 Beyond three score years and ten: a first report on a survey of the elderly. Age Concern, Mitcham

Acheson E D 1981 Introduction. In: Shegog R F A (ed) The impending crisis of old age. Oxford University Press, for Nuffield Provincial Hospital Trust, Oxford

Age Concern, England 1985 General Practitioners and the needs of older people: a policy paper. Age Concern, Mitcham

Audit Commission 1986 Making a reality of community care. HMSO, London

Batley N 1983 A history of the CETHV: the middle years. The Council for the Education and Training of Health Visitors, London

Bury M 1986 Living to be a centenarian. New Society 16th May: 14–15

Challis L, Bartlett H 1986 The paying patient: customer or commodity? Surveying private residential homes for the elderly. In: Phillipson C, Bernard M, Strang P (eds) Dependency and interdependency in old age. Croom Helm, London

Comfort A 1977 A good age. Mitchell Beazley, London

Coupland R 1986 Effective health visiting for elderly people: a specialist health visitor's perspective. Health Visitor 59 (October): 299–300

Cowling III W R, Campbell V G 1986 The health concerns of ageing men. Nursing Clinics of North America 2 (1) March: 75–83

Dalley G 1989 The impact of new community management structures: an over-view. Lecture given in a Conference, February 1989 'Enhancing the quality of community nursing', held at The King's Fund Centre, London

Dauncey J 1988 A change for the better. Health Visitor 61 (December): 385

Day L, Mogridge J 1981 Health visitor who stayed. Health and Social Services Journal 91: 1114–1115

de Beauvoir S 1970 Old age. Penguin, Harmondsworth

Denham M J (ed) 1990 The care of the long stay patient, 2nd edn: Chapman & Hall, London

DHSS, Scottish Home and Health Department, Welsh Office 1971 Report of a working party on management structures in the local authority nursing services (Mayston Report). HMSO, London

DHSS 1976a Prevention and health: everybody's business. HMSO, London

DHSS 1976b Priorities for health and personal social services in England: a consultative document. HMSO, London

DHSS 1977 Priorities in the health and social services: the way forward. HMSO, London

DHSS 1980 Inequalities in health. Report of a research working group, Chairman Sir Douglas Black. HMSO, London

DHSS 1981 Growing older. HMSO, London

DHSS 1983 Griffiths NHS management inquiry report. HMSO, London

DHSS 1986 Neighbourhood nursing: a focus for care. Report of The Community Nursing Review Committee, Chairperson: J Cumberlege. HMSO, London

DHSS 1989 Working for patients. HMSO, London

Dingwall R 1977 The social organisation of health visitor training. Croom Helm, London

Drennan V 1984 A new approach. Nursing Mirror 159 (14) (17th October), Supplement x

Drummond G 1984 Laughter is better than medicine: a support group for caring relatives. Health Visitor 57 (July): 201–202

DSS 1989 Caring for people: community care in the next decade and beyond. White Paper (November 1989). HMSO, London

Dunnell K, Dobbs J 1982 Nurses working in the community. Office of Population Censuses and Surveys, Social Survey Division, HMSO, London

Ebersole P, Hess P 1985 Towards healthy ageing, 2nd edn. Mosby, St Louis

Enderby V 1989 Ageing well in Thetford. Health Visitor 62 (2): 61

Evers H K 1981 Tender loving care. In: Copp L A (ed) Care of the aging. Recent Advances in Nursing series. Churchill Livingstone, Edinburgh

Falconer W A 1923 Translation of Cicero, De Senecute, De Amcita, De Divinatione. Heinemann, London

Fawcett-Henessy A 1987 The future. In: Littlewood J (ed) Recent advances in nursing series, No 15, Community Nursing. Churchill Livingstone, Edinburgh

Fielding P 1986 Attitudes revisited. Royal College of Nursing, London

Fielding P 1987 Research in the nursing care of elderly people. Wiley, Chichester

Fielding P 1989 The care of elderly people. In: MacLeod Clark J, Hockey L (eds) Further research for nursing: education for care. Scutari Press, London

Fitton J 1980 Health visiting the aged. Health Visitor 53 (12): 521–525

Fries J W, Green L W, Levine S 1989 Health promotion and the compression of morbidity. Lancet i: 481–483

Goldberg E M, Warburton R M 1979 Ends and means in social work. Allen and Unwin, London

Gooch S 1989 Moving forward. Primary Health Care April: 6

Goodwin S 1988 Whither health visiting? (Keynote speech at HVA Annual Conference, October 1988). Health Visitor 61 (December): 379–383

Griffiths R 1988 Community care: an agenda for action. Report to the Secretary of State for Health and Social Security from Sir Roy Griffiths. HMSO, London

Halladay H 1981 A geriatric team within the health visiting service. Nursing Times 77: 1039–1040

Hendricks J, Hendricks C D 1985 Ageing in mass society. Winthrop, Cambridge, Massachusetts

Hull W 1989 Measuring effectiveness in health visiting. Health Visitor 62 (April): 113–115

Hunt A 1978 The elderly at home. Office of Population Censuses and Surveys, HMSO, London

Jackson M F 1984 Geriatric rehabilitation on an acute care medical unit. Journal of Advanced Nursing 9: 441–488

Jefferies M 1988 An ageing Britain — what is its future? In: Gearing B, Johnson M, Heller T (eds) Mental health problems in old age. Wiley, Chichester

Jones D C, Van Amelsvoort Jones G H M 1986 Communication patterns between nursing staff and the ethnic elderly in a long-term facility. Journal of Advanced Nursing 11: 265–275

Jones T 1978 Going strong in your eighties. Quest 2: 113

King W 1989 Resource management. Health Visitor 62 (April): 115–116
Körner E 1984 Fifth Report of the Steering Group on Health Services Information, Chairperson: Mrs E Körner. HMSO, London
Lamont D J 1954 The role of the health visitor in the care of the elderly. The Medical Officer 92: 162–163
Laurance J 1988 The myths of old age. New Society 18th March: 19–22
Lesnoff-Caravaglia G (ed) 1987 Realistic expectations for a long life (Frontiers in ageing series, vol 5). Human Sciences Press, New York
Littlewood J 1987 Community nursing: an overview. In: Recent advances in nursing series, No 15: Community nursing. Churchill Livingstone, Edinburgh
Lowe R 1989 Whither health visiting? In the ideal position. Health Visitor 62 (June): 175
Luker 1982 Evaluating health visiting practice: an experimental study to evaluate the effects of focused health visitor intervention on elderly women living at home. Royal College of Nursing, London
Luker L A, Perkins E S 1987 The elderly at home: service needs and provisions. Journal of The Royal College of General Practioners 37: 248–250
McHeath J A 1983 Activity, health and fitness in old age. Croom Helm, London
Machell S, Mackenzie K, Phillips W 1988 Ageing well in Riverside. Health Visitor 61 (1) (January): 21–22
MacQueen I A G 1962 From carbolic powder to social counsel. Health Visiting Centenary Lecture, Nursing Times 58: 866
Massey E A 1989 Articulation of a nursing theoretical framework within institutional environments for our aging adults. In: Recent advances in nursing series, No 23. Churchill Livingstone, Edinburgh, p 82–88
Miller J 1985 A study of the dependency of elderly patients in wards, using different methods of nursing care. Age and Ageing 14: 132–138
Ministry of Health, Department of Health for Scotland, Ministry of Education (1956) Working party on the field of work, training and recruitment of health visitors, Chairman: Sir W James. HMSO, London
Murray R B, Huelskoetter M M, O'Driscoll D 1980 The nursing process in later maturity. Prentice Hall, Englewood Cliffs, New Jersey
Nightingale F 1893 Sick nursing and health nursing. In: Nightingale F 1954 Selected writings. Compiled by Seymer L R. MacMillan, New York, p 356–376
NISW (National Institute of Social Work) 1988 Residential care: a positive choice. (The Wagner Report). HMSO, London
Norman A 1987 Aspects of ageing: a discussion paper. Centre for policy on ageing, London
Norton D 1982 Foreword. In Anderson Sir W F, Caird F L, Kennedy R W, Schwartz D (eds) Gerontology and geriatric nursing. (Modern nursing series): Hodder and Stoughton, Sevenoaks, Kent
Norton D 1988 The age of old age. Geriatric Nursing and Home Care (June): 24–25
OPCS (Office of Population, Censuses and Surveys) 1988a General Household Survey No 16: 1986. HMSO, London
OPCS (Office of Population, Censuses and Surveys) 1988b General Household Survey No 15: Informal carers. HMSO, London
OPCS (Office of Population, Censuses and Surveys) 1988c The prevalence of disability among adults. HMSO, London
OPCS (Office of Population, Censuses and Surveys) 1989 Social Trends No 19: HMSO, London
Owen G 1983 (ed) Health visiting, 2nd edn. Bailliere Tindall, London.
Royal College of Physicians 1986 Physical disability in 1986 and beyond. Journal of The Royal College of Physicians, London 20(3) (July): 160–193
Royal Commission on the Health Service 1979, Chairman: Sir A Merrison; Cmnd 7615. HMSO, London
Royal Commission on the Poor Law 1909 (Minority Report: Webb B S, Webb S). HMSO, London, p 793–795, 919–943
Silman A J 1987 Why do women live longer than men and is it worth it? British Medical Journal 294 (23rd May): 1311–1312
Simone E M 1989 The hospitalised elderly: a nursing perspective. In: Recent advances in nursing series, No 23. Churchill Livingstone, Edinburgh, p 36–44
Slater R, Gearing B 1988 Attitudes, stereotypes and prejudice about ageing. In: Gearing B, Johnson M, Heller T (eds) Mental health problems in old age. Wiley, Chichester.
Smith A, Jacobson B (eds) 1988 The nation's health: a strategy for the 1990s. King's Fund, London
Taylor R, Ford G, Barber H 1983 Research perspectives on ageing: the elderly at risk. Age Concern, Mitcham
Thatcher A 1981 Centenarians. Population Trends (Autumn): 11–13. HMSO, London
Tinker A 1981 The elderly in modern society. Longman, London
Victor C 1987 Old age in modern society: a textbook of social gerontology. Croom Helm, London
Welsh Office 1987 Nursing the community: a team approach for Wales. Report of the Community Nursing Review Committee, Chairperson: N Edwards. Welsh Office, Cardiff
WHO (World Health Organization) 1985 Targets for health for all by the year 2000. WHO, Geneva
WHO (World Health Organization) 1989 The health of the elderly: Report of a working group. WHO, Geneva
Wicks M, Henwood M 1988 The demography and social circumstances of elderly people. In: Gearing B, Johnson M, Heller T (eds) Mental health problems in old age. Wiley, Chichester.
Wilkie E 1978 The history of the Council for the Education and Training of Health Visitors. Allen and Unwin, London

CHAPTER CONTENTS

2 Biophysical aspects of ageing

Ageing is a complex and multifaceted process, involving biological, social, psychological, environmental and spiritual components. However, when these are examined separately an artificial division is inevitably created, hence the need for maintaining an holistic perspective. This is especially so when dealing with biophysical aspects, because in focusing on cellular activity and body systems, one may lose sight of the fact that, while structures age, it is people who grow old.

One may ask the question: what is ageing? There is no simple answer. Attempts to define and explain ageing centre on the biological changes which are universal, intrinsic, progressive and decremental, and which eventually affect survival capacity (Kirkwood 1988). With increasing age there is a change from growth and evolution, towards atrophy and involution, although the rate varies according to the interplay of heredity and environment. This heterogeneity explains why some elderly people look young and full of mental vigour, while others appear 'old' before their years. What seems to be important is *how* people look and feel in old age, and their ability to carry out the activities of daily life, rather than their chronological age. A summary of the common age changes, together with some age differences is given in Table 2.1 at the end of the chapter. This table is intended to provoke thought and discussion, as a basis for determining goal-related professional activity at either primary, secondary, or tertiary level. It must be clearly appreciated that the table is limited and does not represent a comprehensive range of health visiting duties with elderly people.

BIOLOGICAL THEORIES OF AGEING

Although many biologists accept that ageing has a molecular basis, research in the field is complex, and theories abound (Hipkiss & Bittles 1989). Because the process begins at birth and continues throughout life, all age-groups have to be studied. However, since the longitudinal studies, so essential to scientific understanding, have to be conducted over such a long time-span, few researchers can offer continuity. Animal studies are useful, but cannot supply all the answers appropriate to humans, and many experiments involving them, and people, are unsuitable on ethical grounds. Furthermore, some earlier studies were conducted on older persons within institutional settings, so a somewhat distorted picture emerged. Nevertheless, much research is being undertaken at the present time (Rothstein 1987, Evered & Whelan 1988).

The normal model of ageing is time-related, involutional, irreversible and eventually damaging. Although the sequence remains the same, the rate of ageing varies (Fig. 2.1). The unique components of heredity and environment act on cellular activity, immune mechanisms and body chemistry to produce this differential yet inevitable process (see Fig. 2.2). By contrast the pathological model of ageing assumes that age differences, although equally damaging, are potentially preventable, or at least reversible or controllable, given prompt effective action (see Fig. 2.3). Thus improvements in socio-economic circumstances, personal health measures and specific protection (such as via prophylaxis) can help to stop the normal, but in-

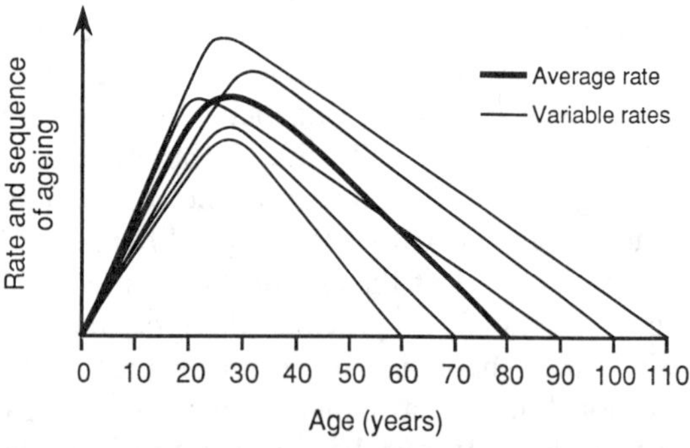

Fig. 2.1 The ageing process — the sequence and rate of ageing, with some variations in rate, though not in sequence.

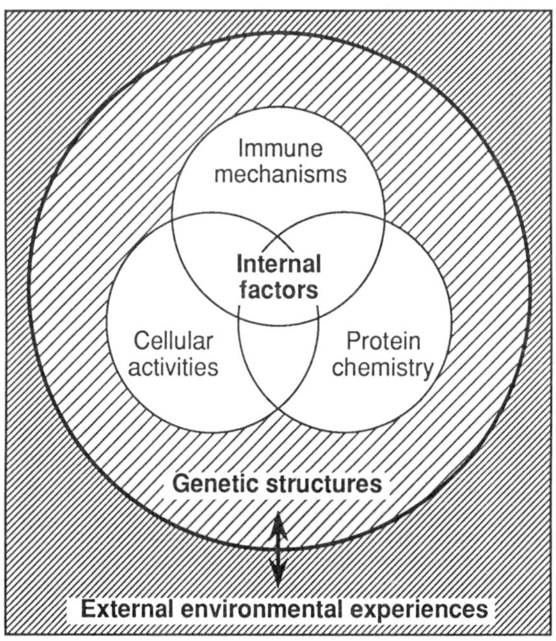

Fig. 2.2 Elements in the natural model of ageing.

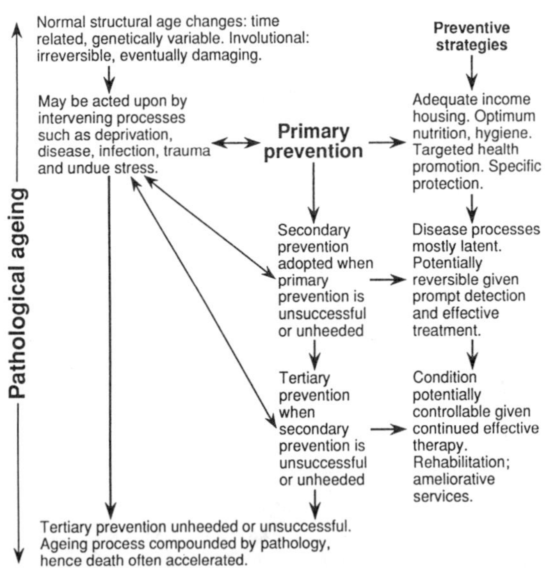

Fig. 2.3 Elements in the pathological model of ageing, showing potential for prevention.

evitable, structural age changes from being affected by disease.

Gerontological research, therefore, is aimed at reducing the rate and ravages of ageing, so that health and vigour can be preserved for as long as possible. This is an entirely different approach from that of geriatric research, which seeks to identify more effective diagnostic and therapeutic measures related to disease in later life. While both approaches are necessary, neither is concerned with the prolongation of life in a grossly diseased state — what has been called 'medicated survival'. As stated in Chapter 1, health visitors are more likely to be concerned with gerontological activities.

CURRENT THEORIES OF AGEING

Current theories of ageing are based mostly on research in the fields of immunology, molecular biology and protein chemistry. They have been classified as mainly genetic programme theories, or environmental insult theories. According to Kirkwood (1988) a more plausible idea is the disposable soma theory. This is a non-adaptive theory, which postulates that a more or less fixed level of 'investment' in somatic maintenance and repair is determined, in order to maximise reproductive capacity. Hence fitness is kept merely at the level of maintenance and repair needed to support the organism in its expected lifetime in a wild environment (Kirkwood 1981, Kirkwood & Holliday 1986, Kirkwood 1988). This notion has its analogy in the 'planned obsolescence' approach to the manufacture of disposable goods, where little is invested in their long-term durability.

To date there is insufficient evidence to support any one of these various ideas over another as a 'core theory', so that a multifactorial stance is probably to be preferred. Each idea provides some clue to the ageing process, and it is best to keep abreast of current research, so that thought can be revised in line with objective proof. Meantime the apparent relationship between the various theories should be noted.

AUTO-IMMUNE THEORY

Under this view, ageing is thought to relate to qualitative changes in the cells which mediate the immune response, as well as to alterations in the production of antibodies, including an increase in the levels of auto-antibodies (Walford 1983, Hipkiss & Bittles 1989). These latter changes in self-recognition allow increased self-destruction to occur — hence the increase in auto-immune disorders, as seen in later maturity. These changes, and the lowered levels of host resistance which stem from decline in the immune system response in old age, are attributed to alterations in the secretion of thymosin from the thymus gland, and to the action of that important organ on the production of sufficient, effective T-cells (thymus-mediated lymphocytes). Thus immunocompetence is reduced. At the same time the B-lymphocytes, which produce antibodies, appear to be less efficient in old age. They are fewer in number, and also appear less competent to deliver antibodies to the site of needed action. Hence, while circulating levels in the blood remain relatively high, respiratory secretion levels, for instance, could be low. Furthermore, the alterations which result in the production of auto-antibodies also appear to affect the cyto-toxic properties of cells, so that an increase is observed in the risk of neoplastic disease and certain circulatory disorders, such as arteritis. Maturity-onset diabetes and senile amyloidosis are other examples of conditions possibly arising from changes in the auto-immune mechanism. If this theory holds, then it is postulated that manipulation of the immune system could both slow the rate of ageing and possibly reduce the levels of mortality and morbidity which currently result from infection or auto-immune disease. (For further information see Bittles & Collins (1986), Phair et al (1988) and Hipkiss & Bittles (1989).)

'BIOLOGICAL CLOCK' THEORY

Protagonists of this theory contend that each of us has an 'internal clock' which governs the rate of cell activity, especially mitosis replication. It is believed by Hayflick (1987) that this mechanism resides in the cell nucleus, and that eventually it may be possible to control environmental 'triggering' influences, so modifying the mechanism and slowing down senescence. Variants of the theory exist. One is that embryogenesis and cell differentiation are genetically controlled. At a certain point in the life-span, it is thought, the usual 'regulator genes' are replaced by 'ageing genes', which may produce a repressor, thus effectively stopping the essential transcription of messenger RNA. As a result, subsequent protein synthesis is affected. This process has been likened to the running out of a tape on a tape-recorder, except that replay is not possible! This programmed ageing notion is discussed by Ebersole & Hess (1985). In support of the notion of an 'ageing gene' Hipkiss & Bittles (1989) describe a line of investigation which could reveal useful information. It lies in the study of transformed or tumour-forming cells.

> Transformation confers indefinite proliferative capacity and an escape from the prior cellular senescent and mortality properties. Research is therefore attempting to identify and characterise the basis of their indefinite survival. Studies of fusion between transformed and untransformed cells shows that in some cases the resultant hybrids regain their mortality: in other words, the senescence factor, (whatever it is), dominates immortality. With the aid of recombinant technology, the next few years may identify which genes are responsible.

CROSS-LINKAGE THEORY

This theory supports the view that chemically active, unwanted, migrant molecules link covalently together, creating strong bonds between molecular structures that are normally separate. Lipid, protein, nucleic acid and carbohydrate are major body chemicals which are capable of cross-linkage. Damage is caused, particularly within the bonds of the double helix, so that eventually cell mutation or cell death occurs. Cross-linkage in collagen leads to insoluble, rigid, less resilient connective tissue, while affected elastin becomes brittle and frayed. Since all materials that pass between cells and vessels must go through connective tissue, the cross-link impact on body ageing is profound. Research suggests that certain chemicals known as lathyrogens, calorific restriction and the action of penicillamine each inhibit cross-linkage formation (Sacher 1977). Protein aggregation, which is a required function during collagen and keratin synthesis, can lead to cross-linking between amino-acid residues and adjacent polypeptide chains. These cross-links are then often less amenable to removal by the enzymes usually responsible for their elimination. This is thought to be one factor in the formation of senile cataracts (Hipkiss & Bittles 1989). Evidence which supports the idea that the elimination of altered proteins decreases with age is accumulating. Whether this is a cause or effect of ageing is not fully clear. If the process of cross-linking could be prevented it might be possible to add years to life. Whether it is biologically feasible remains uncertain at present.

ERROR-ACCUMULATION THEORY

Closely allied to cross-linkage theory is error-accumulation theory, as readers will readily appreciate. The basic proposition is that genetic mutations are caused by external factors like viruses, toxins, or radiation. Successive generations of faulty cells thus develop. When mitrochondria are attacked, cellular energy is affected. If ribosomes are damaged, protein synthesis becomes disorganised. If lysosymes are harmed, enzymes become defective, with consequent mis-selection of amino acids and disruption of cell life. Cumulative errors can eventually interfere with the ability of the organism to maintain biologic function. This situation is known as error-catastrophe (Hipkiss 1989). This error process is described by Comfort (1977) as either: faults in the original blueprint, or in the copying process, or in the tools used. In each case imperfect reproduction adversely affects ageing. Both this theory, cross-linkage theory and free-radical theory would be supported by the idea of 'disposable soma' theory, as discussed earlier.

FREE-RADICAL THEORY

It is postulated that unpaired molecular fragments attach themselves to other molecules, thus damaging, or altering, their original structure or function, through oxidation. Such fragments can be generated from chemicals such as petrol, by-products of plastics and certain paints, atmospheric ozone, tobacco smoke and rapidly oxidising foods. They can cause chromosomal aberrations and intracellular havoc. Some researchers have suggested that free-radical scavengers, named mercaptans, provide protection from rapid oxidation (Sacher 1977, Walford 1983, Holliday 1986, Hipkiss 1989). These are assisted by vitamins A, C and Niacin, and by trace elements such as selenium, manganese, copper and zinc (Davies & Stewart 1987). The anti-oxidising action of vitamin E is also thought to inhibit free-radical behaviour and hence retard ageing. However, the question of the efficiency of free-radical scavengers in later life has also been raised. If this theory is as important as its proponents suggest, then the environmental control of pollution, the provision of clean air, and the monitoring of healthy nutrition should lead to healthier ageing.

HORMONAL AND ENZYME THEORIES

These theories link ageing to centralised endocrine control in the hypothalamus and pituitary glands. Some researchers also consider the thyroid gland has a crucial role. Another important hormone is somatostatin, which is also produced by the hypothalamus, as well as other tissues. Its action appears to inhibit the release of growth hormone, although the regulatory processes which govern its production and release are as yet little understood (Hipkiss & Bittles 1989). Cerebral metabolism, and the action of monoamine neurotransmitters, are other important features, since it is possible that they could bring about retardation of ageing.

WEAR AND TEAR THEORY

This view argues that repeated injuries to, and misuse of, body structures causes them to wear out and hence to cease to function. It is linked to ideas that ageing arises from the exhaustion of irreplaceable substances, and to the stress adaptation theory of ageing.

STRESS ADAPTATION THEORY

The constant bombardment of the individual by internal and external stressors is thought to lead to the accumulation of toxic metabolites and hence residual damage. The body is eventually unable to resist this process and therefore dies.

THE IMPLICATIONS OF THESE VARIOUS THEORIES OF AGEING

While some theorists, such as Comfort (1977); feel that the prospects for age retardation are bright, and quite imminent, others are concerned about the implications of such research (Hipkiss 1989). In particular, the social, moral and political repercussions are open to debate. Although a knowledge of the different biological theories of ageing is helpful in understanding the physiological manifestations which can affect the aged client, health visitors need to think very carefully about the benefits and problems which might be involved in age retardation. Furthermore it is important to consider the ethical issues of such intervention, in order to safeguard the rights, dignity and integrity of persons in later maturity (Davis 1981).

PHYSICAL ASPECTS OF AGEING

> It is important to distinguish between ageing as a long-term biological process and 'old age' as a natural and inevitable stage of human development.
>
> (Skeet 1983)

It is these natural changes, resulting from molecular and cell inefficiency, which can lead to impaired functioning in later maturity. Some of these normal physiological features have a significant effect upon the diagnosis and treatment of co-existing pathological states. For instance, the impairment of homeostatic mechanisms, which can occur with age, can affect postural control of blood pressure. Many drugs can potentiate this effect and thus can result in falls caused by hypotension. Changes in hepatic and renal function can alter the speed with which drugs are excreted, so affecting drug reactions. For this reason it is important to monitor medications and to ensure appropriate drug compliance, which may sometimes be difficult with older people.

External signs of physical ageing

Skin changes

Because of atrophy of the epidermis, sweat glands and hair follicles, and the loss of subcutaneous fat, which results in reduced body insulation, skin becomes thinned, wrinkled, dry, fragile and discoloured. The hair becomes sparser, grey or white, while some recession of the hairline occurs at the temples. Facial skin folds develop, which can cause considerable distress to some people. These may be helped by appropriate advice on cosmetic management. Pruritus may prove troublesome with some older people, particularly in those living in dry, over-heated atmospheres (Ebersole & Hess 1985). Advising against the use of strong soaps and alkalis, and recommending the use of moisturising agents and room humidifiers, can be helpful. Of course it is necessary to determine that there are no underlying pathological reasons for such skin irritation.

Height

Normally the height of the young person equals the span between the tips of the fingers when outstretched. In older people, loss of height results in the span eventually exceeding the height. This is partly due to narrowing of the intervertebral discs, with collapse of vertebrae caused often by osteoporosis, and partly to the tendency to walk with a stoop. Consequently, older people should be encouraged to adopt a healthy posture. To reduce the risk of accidents their environment should be checked to determine whether they have difficulty in reaching curtains, hooks, or cupboards, which formerly were accessible. These difficulties increase accident risks. Older people may also experience problems in adjusting to standard chair and table heights, which hitherto they found manageable. They may find this frustrating and sometimes embarrassing, and may therefore welcome some advice.

Weight

Weight tends to remain constant until the late 70s, but the proportion of fat to muscle changes — muscle being lost while fat is gained. However, fat is often lost from the face, while remaining more marked over hips and abdomen. Establishing wise eating patterns in earlier life is the most effective measure for weight control in later years. Nevertheless, some obese older people benefit from supervised dieting and extra exercise.

Sensory changes

Vision

This vital function deteriorates with age. The crystalline lens becomes less elastic and degenerative changes occur in the muscles of accommodation, making it more difficult to focus for close work. This condition is known as presbyopia. Visual acuity, i.e. the ability to distinguish objects sharply, diminishes, while depth perception also becomes impaired and visual fields may contract. The light–dark adaptation mechanism is reduced also in elderly people, which can be a factor in accidents. Consequently, some older persons may require advice about night driving or the use of photo-chromic lenses. Increased intra-ocular pressure can cause simple glaucoma, with gradual loss of peripheral vision. This is of course a pathological condition. A white line (arcus senilis) develops in the outer aspect of the iris, due to lipid deposits in the cornea. Loss of orbital fat sometimes causes the eyes to appear sunken and there may be ptosis of the lids. Again it is difficult sometimes to disentangle physiological age changes and pathological states. Sensitivity to glare and flicker may increase and colour discrimination may deteriorate. Advice may be required regarding the positioning of lights and watching television.

Hearing

It is well known that hearing is impaired with age. Tests show that hearing loss occurs over all sound frequencies, especially high tones. This is usually due to degeneration of the organ of Corti, and/or loss of neurones in the cochlea. Rigidity of the ossicles and impaired elasticity of the basilar membrane, affecting vibration, can also increase difficulties in sound discrimination. Degeneration of hair cells in the semi-circular canals contributes to the uncertainty of balance, especially during darkness, or on other occasions when visual input is reduced. Hardness of hearing can lead to difficulties in communication, sometimes generating distress, suspicion and causing social isolation. Such situations call for empathetic and supportive interventions. Facing the client and enunciating words clearly and slowly can be helpful. Much can be accomplished without shouting. Older persons need to receive regular auditory screening and to be taught how to use any supplied aids correctly. The annoying sounds which are experienced with many hearing aids result from amplification of background noise, the sounds from which are reflected back into the receiver. Unfortunately it is difficult to control this problem, but future research may result in improved hearing aids.

Nose, throat and tongue

Atrophy of the mucosa, and reduction in the number of taste buds, results in an impaired sense of taste. Similarly there is a reduction in the sense of smell. These changes can affect appetite, enjoyment and sometimes safety. Loss of elasticity in laryngeal muscles and cartilage reduces the responsiveness of the cough and swallowing reflexes, as well as altering the pitch, power and range of the vocal cords. Some older people experience unpleasant gagging sensations, for which they may require dietary advice.

Touch and sensation

Temperature and pressure responses are reduced as a result of skin, vascular and neuro-endocrine changes. Diminished touch perception may increase accident risks. Thus older people may burn themselves during cooking and fail to notice the lesions, which can then become sore and infected. They and their carers need to be informed of this risk so that they can guard against such happenings. Pain thresholds rise in some old people; therefore pain, such as from a fractured neck of femur, may be reduced. Sensitive awareness to subjective pain reaction is an important health visiting skill. The kinaesthetic sense, i.e. awareness of body position and movement, may also degenerate. Thus some elderly people may adopt very inappropriate positions. Such mal-posture can increase their discomfort through alteration of body alignment. Advice on this matter may be particularly needed when older people have experienced problems such as cerebrovascular accident. Teaching them to exercise in front of mirrors can help.

Other changes

Musculoskeletal changes

Ageing is associated with progressive bone density loss from the skeleton, and continuous remodelling. Bone becomes more porous and demineralised. Bone mass tends to diminish about the fourth decade onwards, especially in postmenopausal women — hence the disparity in fractures between the sexes. Genetic factors may help to explain why osteoporosis occurs more frequently in certain ethnic groups such as Asians and Northern Europeans.

The evidence that osteoporosis can be delayed by calcium supplementation is mixed (Gray 1986). Hormone replacement therapy has been shown to be effective in preventing the onset of osteoporosis (Ettinger et al 1987, Smith & Jacobson 1988), although the increased risk of heart disease associated with this treatment renders it controversial (Vessey & Hunt 1987). Exercise has also been shown to prevent involutional bone loss (Aloia 1981, Riggs & Melton 1988), but older persons should be cautioned about the risks of accidents. (This topic is discussed further in Ch. 8, pp. 198–202.) Some progress is being made on developing regimens that stimulate bone formation and thus have the theoretical potential of increasing bone mass, but only sodium fluoride has been widely evaluated (Riggs 1984, Riggs & Melton 1988). Another possible approach is by stimulation of bone formation through physiological growth factors (Centrella & Canalis 1985).

There are also other changes: cartilage tends to calcify, especially in the ribs; synovial membranes of joints thicken; articular cartilage becomes damaged, hence pain may occur and mobility be affected; degenerate ligaments decrease in elasticity. Nevertheless, regulated exercise and careful positioning, together with weight control, help joint protection.

Muscle power peaks between 20 and 30 years and thereafter declines. Thus older people may be unable to manage dexterous tasks as easily as when young. Progressive atrophy occurs, and the strength of the non-dominant hand is usually less than that of the dominant hand in both sexes, although power is greater in men. While decreasing power can be regarded as inevitable in ageing, keeping fit through balanced exercise undoubtedly helps to maintain strength and the sense of well-being. Incorrect use of muscles can generate tension and soreness; hence, correct posture, movement and relaxation are important.

Since the centre of gravity is changed in age, problems of balance can arise. Adaptive mechanisms for stability include wearing well-fitting, low-heeled shoes, adopting a wider-based gait, taking shorter steps with toes pointed out, and using a stick or other walking aid. It should be remembered that postural changes in turn compress body cavities, often altering cardiac, respiratory and digestive function; so prolonged sitting and shallow breathing can be hazardous in the old. Walking ability is retained in most active elderly people, although in the comprehensive longitudinal study of three cohorts of 70-year-olds in Gothenburg, Sweden, it was found that only a few 79-year-old people are able to walk at the speed needed for pedestrians to cross street intersections with traffic signals (Lundren-Lindquist et al 1983, Svanborg 1988).

Cardiovascular system

This system shows ageing changes quite separate from pathological processes like atheroma. Morphological changes in the heart appear to be a structural adaptation, in the direction of increased volume (Svanborg 1988). Echocardiographic measurements indicate that the ratio between the volume and the thickness of the heart wall remain amazingly constant (Svanborg 1988). There is an increase in fibrous tissue, which can affect the conducting system. The ability to elevate the pulse rate falls with increasing age, and therefore there is some reduction in exercise capacity. Thus, whereas most older persons can walk up a hill, not all older elderly may be able to run for a bus. However, consistent graded exercise has been shown to improve stamina in most healthy older people. Heart rhythm is essentially unchanged and the capacity for hypertrophy is retained, in sensitive response to extra loading.

Blood pressure

The dynamics of ageing are well represented in the age-related changes in blood pressure. This rises in many older people, especially those living in Western societies. It is probably a pathological process. New evidence from the Gothenburg longitudinal study shows that there are marked differences in blood pressure readings between men and women aged 70 years and over, especially in diastolic pressure. Such readings appear significantly higher in females, though how far such data can be generalised to other elderly populations is uncertain. Furthermore, inter-individual differences commonly increase with age, up to at least age 79 years. Sex differences appear to vary markedly over short periods of time, while age-cohort differences arise within 5-year intervals (Svanborg 1988). Thus clinical reference values for determining hypertension have become even more complex (Landahl et al 1986). This means that it is highly debatable whether hypertension should be treated in the elderly. Inappropriate treatment can lead to the prescribing of large doses of anti-hypertensive drugs and the consequent risks of fatigue, dizziness and postural hypotension. Blood pressure readings are notoriously sensitive to physical and emotional changes, hence at any age great care needs to be exercised when monitoring these. In view of the noted age-cohort differences within relatively short periods of time, it is important to bear in mind that current clinical reference values might not be appropriate for coming generations of older people (Svanborg 1988).

Venous system

Inefficiency in venous valves, coupled with poorer muscle tone can lead to pooling, stasis, dependent oedema, organ hypoxia and thrombus formation. However, exercise and appropriate positioning can do much to reduce such hazards. Changes in capillary permeability can cause poorer tissue oxygenation and nourishment, so care is needed to reduce the risk of tissue injury.

Blood constituents

Generally, ageing has little effect on blood constituents. The haemoglobin in older people is the same as in younger persons. Red cell life-span is unaltered. The erythrocyte sedimentation rate may rise slightly and platelets may show some diminished clotting power. There might be a slight fall in the total number of white cells. However, anaemia in the elderly is usually the result of disease.

Respiratory system

The total lung volume remains unchanged, but calcification of the costal cartilage, kyphosis and demineralisation of the rib cage impede respiratory efficiency. The lung itself becomes less elastic, and the chest muscles less strong. Total lung capacity is not significantly altered, but residual capacity increases and vital capacity decreases because of the diminished strength of the muscles of respiration. Peak expiratory volume is also reduced. Alteration in the size and number of alveoli, sclerosing of bronchi and supporting tissue, as well as degeneration of bronchial epithelium, can lead to diminished oxygen diffusion, less effective cough reflexes, faulty clearance of secretions and lowered resistance to infection. It is therefore important to assess these by objective means, such as the use of a peak flow meter. However, encouraging appropriate maximum activity, correct breathing, as well as suitable posture, can considerably improve respiratory performance in many older persons.

Digestive system

The ageing changes in the alimentary tract are well documented, but they often cause little symptomatic change. In addition to the blunting of the sense of taste, changes occur in the gingival tissue and cement. Dentine formation and pulp can also be affected, caries and tooth loss being common. However, it is debatable whether this represents normal ageing. Changes in the shape of the mouth, due to reabsorption of maxilla and jaw, can affect chewing. In edentulous states, properly fitting dentures are needed for adequate mastication and for cosmetic reasons. Loss and thickening of saliva, coupled with atrophic tongue changes, can lead to mouth dryness and burning sensations. These may cause considerable discomfort and distress to some older people and may lead to anorexia. Adequate hydration is essential, particularly if the older person is taking antidepressants, antispasmodics, antihistamines, or other drugs causing dry mouth. Regular assessment of mouth state is a guide to general well-being.

Changes in oesophageal motility and mucosal atrophy may contribute to swallowing difficulties in ageing. Reduced absorption of nutrients may occur due to atrophy of gastric and intestinal mucosa, achlorhydria, decreased digestive enzymes and altered blood flow. This can particularly affect the absorption of vitamins and iron, which can lead to energy loss, malnutrition and/or anaemia, especially where there is a reduction in intrinsic factors. Much can be done to help promote appetite through the improvement of visual presentation of the diet, flavouring foods safely, without the addition of salt, as well as attending to the appropriate consistency of items, where swallowing difficulties are present.

Elimination may also be affected as poor colonic muscle tone and decreased peristalsis can lead to delayed transit time, constipation, sometimes faecal impaction, considerable discomfort and possibly faecal incontinence. Dietary advice regarding adequate intakes of high-fibre foods and sufficient fluids, together with unobtrusive supervision, are therefore fundamental for older people.

The liver decreases in size, so that hepatic blood flow diminishes. This has some impact on drug detoxification. Decreased weight, glycogen storage and protein synthesis can also affect hepatic function.

Genitourinary system

Renal function deteriorates significantly with age. This may be exacerbated by dehydration, infection and impaired cardiac output. Thickening of the membrane of Bowman's capsule, together with impaired permeability and degenerative changes in the tubules, results in a reduction of the life-span of nephrons. Glomerular filtration rates show considerable variation among the elderly in different populations. There is slow decline from age 20, with a further decrease after 50 years, although this appears to level off after 70 (Svanborg 1988). Tests of glomerular filtration show a 50% reduction in a fit 80-year-old man compared with his 20-year-old counterpart. A two-thirds reduction occurs in the sick elderly, which has important implications for drug excretion. In appreciating the filtration, secretion, excretion and reabsorption functions of the kidney, it is important to note that reserve kidney function also declines with age.

Although incontinence is pathological, it is estimated that 1–10 women of all ages within the general population are so affected. Frequency, nocturia and stress incontinence are therefore not uncommon in ageing. Some older clients are too embarrassed to seek help, yet they welcome factual objective advice. Health visitors can help to promote continence, by modification of the environment where necessary, encouraging regular voiding habits in relation to body rhythms, as well as by teaching exercises to improve the tone of pelvic muscles. Providing information on the use of appropriate aids and protective garments, when required, can help to reduce social embarrassment.

Changes affecting sexual function

This aspect is dealt with sensitively by Shaw (1984), who shows how ageing can modify activity, but stresses the importance of continuing creative, health-giving relationships. Sexual activity is more common among the elderly than is popularly supposed, varying as much as any other characteristic. Sexuality assumes different importance at different times. As age advances, intimacy and touching may be as important as, or more important than, the physical pleasure of intercourse (Greengross & Greengross 1989). However, sadly, some older people are rarely touched. This aspect is dealt with, in a nursing context, by LeMay & Redfern (1987) and Redfern (1989).

In women the production of oestrogen, progesterone and follicle-stimulating hormones changes with menopause, resulting in gradual atrophy of the ovaries and uterus, with involution of the vagina, labia and clitoris. The vagina decreases in expansive ability, the epithelium thinning and drying, so that dyspareunia and vaginal burning may result from coitus. Regular lubrication and/or oestrogen replacement therapy may help. While breast engorgement and orgasm is of shorter duration in later maturity, it should be remembered that sexual pleasure is more than a physiological response.

In men, lessened androgen production causes the testes to diminish in size and firmness. The seminiferous tubules thicken, seminal fluid is reduced and also thins. Both erection and ejaculation are slower, and scrotal vasocongestion and muscle tone decrease. Sperm production and viability are inhibited, with some reduction in male fertility. Sexual functioning can therefore be maintained throughout life, although some modification in positioning and techniques may be required (Lewis 1985). Health visitors may be called upon to advise on psychosexual relationships in later life and should therefore be aware both of the inhibitions and prejudices which exist, and the techniques which may be helpful to older people (see Lewis 1985, Greengross & Greengross 1989).

Central nervous system

Neurones are lost, though much less than previously thought. Recent studies show these are mostly confined to specific brain regions. There is loss of function of the cholinergic system, with a decline in the neurotransmitter substance acetylcholine. By contrast the cholinoreceptor cells, which are stimulated by acetylcholine, do not appear to decline. Although serotonin does not appear to decline with age, the number of serotonin receptors does (Hipkiss & Bittles 1989).

There is considerable evidence that, even in 'normal' ageing, neuronal proteins may form aggregates called tangles, paired helical filaments and amyloid plaque. The difference in Alzheimer's disease is that these structures are formed in large quantities, from neural cells. Brain atrophy occurs, as does the synthesis of acetylcholine and serotonin. Furthermore, alterations in the oxidation of glucose lead to a 50% reduction in energy in this condition (Hipkiss & Bittles 1989).

With ageing, changes in the basal ganglia, and deposits of lipofuscin occur, with some peripheral thinning of the myelin sheaths and atrophy of fibres. The significant change is in reaction time. Performance is slower with age, so time must be allowed for response. Reflex action is also diminished, which, together with reduced vibration responses and proprioceptive ability, causes balancing problems and thus increases accident risks. However, it must be remembered that wisdom and experience have led older people to adapt, and that they are still able to develop new neural patterns, though less likely to do so. The effects of nervous system changes on cognitive and emotional states are mentioned in the next chapter.

Endocrine system

There seems little change in endocrine function with age, apart from the loss of secondary sex characteristics, and alterations in thyroid, cortisol and other hormonal levels already mentioned. However, there is considerable difficulty in differentiating between normal age changes and pathological conditions. Pancreatic changes, with modifications in insulin production and utilisation, may lead to impaired glucose tolerance. Renal threshold for glucose rises, which entails that persons with hyperglycaemia may not show glycosuria. Hence it is necessary to test blood rather than urine when screening for diabetes in elderly persons.

Temperature control

This becomes less effective with age, causing body temperature to fall, thus increasing the risk of hypothermia. This is potentiated by diminished shivering response and impaired appreciation of changes in environmental temperature. Some elderly persons with a body 'core' temperature of less than 35°C do not appear ill, but are clearly at risk.

SUMMARY

At the beginning of this chapter we stressed the need to adopt an holistic perspective, particularly when concentrating on biological *age changes*, which are complex, plural, cumulative and often eventually damaging. *Age differences* on the other hand have been seen to be vested in individuals, who are unique; hence there is variation from person to person in the rate of ageing, though not in its sequence.

The parameters of normal ageing are not yet firmly established, because the process is often compounded by pathology. Gerontological research aims to define the causes and course of normal ageing, in order to delay its progress, thus increasing vigour and activity for more older people for a longer time. However, this raises profound moral, ethical and social issues, affecting clients, professional workers and policy makers.

Health visitors share with their clients a responsibility to observe, assess and monitor biological age changes and age differences, helping to alleviate their effects and preventing complications as far as possible. Health promotion aims to give people, early in life, the information and means to control their own health and thus, in time, favourably affect their ageing. Health education seeks to change behaviour in positive ways, towards this end. In such activities, offered over the life-span, health visitors have a continuing role.

DETAILS OF AGE CHANGES

Lists of symptoms, and tables such as that presented in Table 2.1, though important, are abstract and therefore tend to be perceived as lifeless and lacking reality. The case study of Mrs A is intended to provide the balance. It demonstrates the marks of biological ageing, with which health visitors are commonly confronted. While the physical aspects of ageing are deliberately emphasised in this example, it is essential to recognise the inter-dependence of the physical, psychological, social and spiritual facets of a person's personality. This close and inseparable relationship between all parts of a 'whole' person, and the environment, are illustrated in the case study that concludes Chapter 3.

CASE STUDY

Mrs A, who is 89, lives with her 62-year-old son. Measuring 1.4 m in height and weighing 31 kg, she epitomises the title of 'little old lady'. However, her seeming frailty belies her vitality. Her marked loss of height often causes her distress, especially as she can now no longer easily see out of her kitchen window to watch the birds in her garden. She cannot reach her upper larder shelves without difficulty, so has to resort to ingenious ways of retrieving needed items, via a butterfly net and similar means. A cushion on her chair allows her to reach the dining-room table. This makes her feel childish, increasing her frustration, but she jokes this away by amplifying the ridiculous.

Her formerly glossy black hair is now silver-white and thinning, but is still well styled and groomed. Her skin is dry, wrinkling and pigmented in places, with laughter lines apparent at the corner of her eyes and over her rosy cheeks. At times she says she is bothered by her skin dryness; however, she is aware of the wise use of moisturising lotion and applies her make-up with discretion and to good effect.

She bemoans the loss of the speed and dexterity which she formerly enjoyed. The sequel to a fractured wrist is poorer fine movement and arthritis. Nevertheless Mrs A still manages much of her own housework, cooking and laundry. She indulges in short naps whenever she relaxes, because her night-time sleep is sometimes fitful. Her mastication problems, due to waning power in her masseter muscles, tend to restrict her menu choices, so she goes for softer textured foods. Retaining a strong liking for steak and kidney pie, she finds this sometimes aggravates her hiatus hernia, which causes her discomfort.

Since cataract surgery 5 years ago, Mrs A has encountered occasional difficulty with stereoscopic vision. This affects her ability to judge the depth of steps, rendering her more accident prone. Furthermore she does not always see surface dust clearly, wash plates cleanly or cope with objects under her feet. These points sometimes cause her social embarrassment and distress.

Although her appetite is now small, she eats regularly, preparing meals for her son who is not yet retired. Since she can no longer manage the walk into town, and feels too unsteady to cope with buses, Mrs A tends to shop at the small neighbourhood shops, where prices are higher and choice is sometimes limited. Mrs A is, however, very content. She prefers routine, still rising at 7 a.m. and retiring by 10.30 p.m. Frequently she sleeps in the sitting position, to afford her greater comfort. She often thinks of the past and wonders about the future. She appreciates the use of a commode at night, and experiences occasional stress incontinence by day. This did cause her some social embarrassment, but now she wears protective clothing and copes well.

Mrs A is clothes conscious, but has some difficulty finding smart suitable garments which cater for her small size and mild kyphosis. Her osteoarthritis and mild hypertension are controlled by medication and she benefits greatly from regular chiropody. In spite of a recent episode of thrombo-phlebitis and occasional bronchitis, Mrs A considers she enjoys good health.

Mrs A manages to bath herself with minimal assistance to reduce accidents. She also follows body exercises on breakfast television programmes. Although fine motor movement is less sensitive, she still crochets, knits, sews and cooks for her family, her church and many friends. Sadly her network of contemporaries is narrowing through death — she often reminds visitors that she is the sole survivor of her nine siblings. Her days are full, nights 'tolerable'. She has learned to know her body over the years and considers it has served her well.

Table 2.1 The ageing process, showing, by system, normal age changes, the pathological associations and the implications for health visitors caring for clients

System	Normal ageing changes	Pathological associations/risks	Caring for clients: implications for health visitors
Skin	Decreases in strength Wrinkling and thinning occurs Atrophy of epidermis and sweat glands Fragility and dryness Greater irritation	Skin abrasions Intertrigo Infections Pressure sores	Careful skin handling Use less soap but more moisturising creams Reduce exposure to extremes of heat or cold Teach skin care, avoidance and/or relief of pressure Encourage use of humidifiers if central heating used
	Reduction in subcutaneous fat Laxity of skin		Maintain level of personal appearance to cope with altered contours
	Less body warmth due to lowered insulation from lessened subcutaneous fat	Greater risk of hypothermia	Monitor body and environmental temperature
	Pigmentary changes: Greying hair Less body and more facial hair	Lentigo Keratosis	Explain skin changes and teach appropriate cosmetic care
Nails	Reduced peripheral circulation Thickening, ridging and brittleness	Onychogryphosis Paronychia Fungal infection	Teach suitable nail hygiene including need for regular chiropody Check for infections and refer for treatment as necessary
Eyes	Loss of orbital fat Sunken ocular appearance, ptosis of eyelids	Entropion Ectropion	Encourage regular ophthalmic examination and treatment of minor eye ailments
	Increased visual sensitivity especially to glare and flicker		Ensure correct lighting and caution against glare, flicker, or the use of sharp objects near eyes
	Changes in shape of cornea, lipid deposits increase opacity		
	Astigmatism Arcus senilis	Myopia Corneal ulcer	Encourage regular visual screening and the use of corrective lens as prescribed
	Reduced tears	Dry eyes syndrome, Stenosing of lacrimal duct Lacrimal abscess	Encourage appropriate eye hygiene If drops used, ascertain that they are correctly instilled Advise against effect of sudden cold or use of volatile substances near eyes
	Presbyopia Decreased colour awareness	Faulty discrimination of colours, leading to accident risks	Encourage regular ophthalmic examination

Continued overleaf

Table 2.1 Continued

System	Normal ageing changes	Pathological associations/risks	Caring for clients: implications for health visitors
Eyes (contd)	Reduced elasticity and some sclerosing of lens	Cataract	Regular ophthalmic examination Monitor degree of blurred vision and poor colour perception. Explain need for preoperative waiting period and support before and after surgery (lens extraction) whilst adjustments made. Maximise colour contrasts and teach safety measures. Supervise personal hygiene
	Shallowing of anterior chamber and reduced absorption of ocular fluid		
	Increase in intra-ocular pressure	Glaucoma	Monitor installation of eye-drops and supervise prescribed drug regimes which aim to reduce intra-ocular pressure and so prevent blindness Encourage annual tenometry for all high-risk clients Check that close relatives know associated risks
	Decreased blood supply	Reduced visual efficiency	Ensure adequate general nutrition and monitor general health
	Degeneration of choroid, ciliary body, iris	Refractive errors	Teach use and care of any prescribed aids
	Contracted pupils and slowed reflexes	Pupillary change may indicate systemic disease	Monitor reactions and co-ordination and teach safety measures
	Degeneration of retina Reduced visual neurones	Retinopathy and/or retinal detachment Occlusive or cortical blindness	Caution against sudden changes from light to dark, advise on wise use of sunglasses, and care during night driving Encourage – orientation – safety – use of resources for the visually impaired
	Poorer light–dark adaptation, visuospatial and depth perception	Increased accident risk	
	Macular degeneration Blurring and fading of vision	Loss of central vision	Reassure that total blindness will not usually result Teach to use aids and to view objects eccentrically

Table 2.1 Continued

System	Normal ageing changes	Pathological associations/risks	Caring for clients: implications for health visitors
Ears	Degeneration of organ of Corti Impaired sensitivity to high tone frequencies	Degrees of deafness with risk of – isolation – suspicion – depression – tinnitus	Teach auditory protection for clients of all ages Advise on regular auditory testing for elderly Teach correct use of aids, both personal and environmental Encourage lip-reading and communication Support research
	Impaired endolymph production with possible alterations in balance	Meniere's syndrome	Teach compensating posture and balancing techniques Teach management during episodic attacks and preventive measures in effort to reduce frequency – low sodium diet – diuretic therapy Monitor correct use of vasodilators if prescribed to reduce formation of endolymph
	Excess secretion of wax Impacted cerumen due to narrowing of canal and dryness of skin	Pressure	Monitor aural hygiene Refer for removal of wax by irrigation
	Diminished vibratory power Decreased hearing acuity	Conductive deafness	Teach compensating communication techniques for hard of hearing and promote understanding of the needs of elderly deaf clients
Nose, throat and tongue	General mucosal atrophy Impaired sense of – smell – taste	Anorexia	Advise on oral hygiene Review diet and improve visual presentation of food whenever possible
		Increased risk of – fire – gas poisoning – food poisoning	Explain risks and work out safety measures with client
	Neural degeneration Diminished cough and swallowing reflexes	Increased risk of aspiration or choking	Teach emergency measures in event of choking Help client eliminate foodstuffs which create undue gagging or swallowing difficulties
	Muscular inelasticity Alteration in the power, range and pitch of voice	Aphonia	Refer for general medical check Encourage general muscular relaxation

Continued overleaf

Table 2.1 Continued

System	Normal ageing changes	Pathological associations/risks	Caring for clients: implications for health visitors
Sensation and temperature control	Degenerative changes: Impaired awareness of – heat – pain – cold – touch – position and balance	Defective localisation of pain Risk of burns, hypothermia and other accidents	Monitor sensory reactions via unobtrusive measures Carry out regular checks of skin state to reduce risk of infection from unrecognised lesions, especially in existing neuropathies Alert to risks of accident and hypothermia, and check regularly on environmental temperature Teach compensating balancing techniques
Skeletal	Bone – porosity – demineralisation – reduced mass Loss of strength	Increased bone pain and fragility	Check diet and advise on adequate intakes of calcium and vitamin D, and exercise to improve bone strength
	Height decreases inversely to span Thinning of intervertebral discs leading to trunk shortening, postural changes and stoop	Backache, kyphosis, locomotor and balance disturbance	Assess and then modify environment to meet bodily changes Teach correct posture and encourage exercise Reduce hazards in home and outer environment Teach general safety measures and gait adaptation
	Calcification of cartilage Reduction in size of rib cage and in shoulder width Compression of body cavities	Impaired respiratory, cardiac and digestive functions	Teach suitable breathing exercises and measures to reduce risk of respiratory infections Advise on modifying diet to facilitate digestion Encourage appropriate exercise to strengthen cardiac reserves
		Osteoporosis Osteo-malacia Osteitis deformans	
	Brittleness of bones	Fractures	Advise on posture and movement, especially lifting techniques
Muscles	Loss of bulk Decreased power for muscular activities	Increased accident risks and greater fatigue	Safety measures Teach food-related exercise to improve stamina and strength. Avoid over-fatigue, through balanced activity and sleep and rest
	Atrophy of fibres Less flexibility, poorer co-ordination, limitation in range and speed Tremor	Personal and environmental accidents Myopathies	Teach muscle relaxation techniques Encourage full range of movement daily Re-arrange environment to improve safety and encourage use of modified equipment

Table 2.1 Continued

System	Normal ageing changes	Pathological associations/risks	Caring for clients: implications for health visitors
Joints	Thickening of synovial membrane and cartilage degeneration Loss of elasticity and resistance Aching and stiffness	Greater risk of trauma. Osteo-arthrosis, rheumatoid arthritis and gout	Encourage healthy posture and exercise Monitor weight control and prescribed drugs/medications Advise re-dangers of self-medication Recognise potential threat to independence and take positive steps to increase diversional interests whilst maintaining optimum self-help If surgery is indicated, support through waiting period and postoperatively Teach correct use of aids and appliances if prescribed
Cardiovascular	Reduced elasticity in blood vessels Increased systolic pressure	Hypertension Aortic dilatation and incompetence	Encourage weight control, non-smoking and general relaxation, balanced by optimum physical exercise related to capacity
	Increased deposits of lipofuscin – fibrous tissue – sclerosing Decline in cardiac 'stroke volume' Reduced capacity for physical work	Atheroma Ischaemic heart disease and cerebrovascular accidents	Encourage regular health checks and monitor blood pressure readings, cholesterol levels Monitor compliance in, and reaction to, all prescribed treatment, reporting and educating as necessary Supervise management and correct elimination Inculcate a positive psychological outlook, especially towards any rehabilitative measures
Other vascular changes	Reduced blood flow and vascular efficiency Reduced tissue oxygenation Altered capillary permeability	Tissue hypoxia Gravitational ulcers	Encourage aerobic type exercises unless contraindicated Teach correct use of shoes and supportive hosiery Encourage regular calf-muscle exercises and compliance with prescribed therapy
	Peripheral stasis with venous 'pooling'	Venous obstruction leading to varicose veins	Caution against excessive sitting and prolonged standing, or sudden changes of position
	Poor peripheral circulation	Dependency oedema Risk of chilblains, thrombo-peripheral disease and orthostatic hypotension	Raise resistance to infection via good diet and sound hygiene measures with regulated exercise Advise on suitable footwear and hosiery and how to keep warm in cold weather

Continued overleaf

Table 2.1 Continued

System	Normal ageing changes	Pathological associations/risks	Caring for clients: implications for health visitors
Respiratory	Alteration in size and number of alveoli Decreased vital capacity	Lowered efficiency Increased risk of infection	Maintain optimum but regulated activity Encourage adequate ventilation of environment Encourage to stop or reduce smoking and control weight. Maintain optimum nutrition
	Sclerosing of bronchi and degeneration of mucosa Reduced muscle power	Impaired tissue oxygenation and self-cleansing mechanisms Decreased reserves	Maintain general health through sound personal hygiene, adequate sleep and diet designed to increase resistance to infection
		Chronic obstructive disease	Strengthen muscles of respiration through appropriate exercises. Teach appropriate posture and measures to facilitate expectoration
	Cell alteration Increased risk of 'wild' cells	Neoplastic disease	Promote general well-being Pre- and postoperative support if surgery or other therapy, is indicated Ameliorative measures and psycho-spiritual support
Digestive and excretory	Jaw atrophy and tooth changes Altered bite, made worse if wearing ill-fitting dentures	Jaw pain Dental caries and periodontal disease	Teach sound oral hygiene and check for ill-fitting dentures if applicable
	Waning muscle power leading to altered mouth shape Mastication problems	Restricted diet leading to malnutrition Oral ulcers and stomatitis	Advise on modifications to diet which preserve nutritional elements but facilitate mastication Maintain oral hygiene Monitor adherence to prescribed regimes if therapy given
	Reduced swallowing reflex and thickened saliva Sensitivity in swallowing Dry mouth	Parotitis Dysphagia Reflux	Check diet and oral hygiene Ensure adequate fluid intake Advise on sucking ice or using sugarless chewing gum Monitor drug therapy which may contribute to mouth dryness
	Reduced oesophageal motility Choking tendencies	Hiatus hernia Oesophageal carcinoma	Teach correct positioning and movement and other symptomatic care as indicated Offer supportive intervention Monitor energy levels Reduce fat and increase fibre intake Encourage social eating Supervise remedial therapy Maintain exercise and general relaxation techniques

Table 2.1 Continued

System	Normal ageing changes	Pathological associations/risks	Caring for clients: implications for health visitors
	Atrophy of mucosa and reduced enzyme action	Decreased digestion of fat, vitamins and iron Malabsorption syndrome Iron deficiency anaemia peptic ulcer	
Liver	Decreased weight and impaired efficiency Decreased detoxification ability	Nausea and lethargy Drug accumulation and toxicity	Advise ameliorative measures Modify activity Ensure adequate nutrition, modifying fat intake Monitor drug actions and reactions
Elimination	Prolonged intestinal transit time Slowed peristalsis Constipation Formation of diverticula	Faecal impaction Diverticulitis Increased risk of colonic cancer	Ensure adequate bulk in diet Encourage regularity of meals and adequate fluid intake Supervise remedial regimes
	Poorer colonic and sphincter tone Reduced bowel control	Greater risk of faecal incontinence	Teach correct pelvic exercises and the avoidance of injurious laxatives. Advise on personnal hygiene
Genitourinary	Membranous thickening Impaired filtration Lowered renal blood flow Limited renal efficiency Lower specific gravity Stasis	Lessened homeostasis Electrolyte imbalance Greater risk of – infection – calculi – prostatic disease in males	Encourage high fluid intake — at least 2000 ml daily Modify salt intake and check diet Promote perianal hygiene to prevent infection Monitor compliance with any prescribed regime for urinary infection, or diuretic therapy Check to avoid potassium depletion
	Reduced muscle tone in bladder wall Frequency, nocturia and stress incontinence	Frank incontinence	Provide bladder training related to circadian rhythms and encourage pelvic floor exercises to improve tone Modify environment to promote continence Advise on suitable aids if required Teach appropriate skin protective care and deodorant measures where necessary
Sexual functioning	Alterations in hormonal levels		
	Females: labia and clitoris shrink and ovaries atrophy Fertility ceases	Irritation after coitus, with dyspareunia Increased risk of cystitis	Advise on modifying sexual techniques Use of lubricating cream Vulval toileting, use of non-occlusive hosiery, avoidance of potentially irritating substances such as bath foam, and care when taking hot baths Encourage adequate nutrition and high fluid intake

Table 2.1 Continued

System	Normal ageing changes	Pathological associations/risks	Caring for clients: implications for health visitors
Sexual functioning (contd)	Males: genital organs decrease in size and elasticity Seminal fluid and sperm production diminish, but fertility is retained	Scrotal irritation Prostatic enlargement with risk of urinary retention.	Advise on suitable scrotal support and use of protective cream Refer for medical aid: support client during pre- and postoperative phase where applicable Offer symptomatic advice and reassurance during period of readjustment
Endocrine functioning	Reduction in levels of activity Increased catabolism Modified fat distribution	Increased auto-immune responses	Monitor metabolic responsiveness Encourage weight and dietary controls Raise general resistance
Nervous system	Reduction in levels of nerve activity Slowed reaction time	Poorer co-ordination	Adjust pace of interaction Allow time for sensorimotor responses
	Reduced brain weight and blood flow Poorer cerebral oxygenation	Vertigo and transient ischaemia. Stroke	Teach suitable posture and movement, avoiding rapid changes of position, especially from horizontal to vertical state Monitor blood pressure
	Some neurones lost Fibres and impulses degenerate, leading to weaker reflexes Reduced proprioceptive ability	Confusion Increased liability to falls	Teach gait adaptation and improve environment to facilitate safe locomotion. Reinforce safety education. Monitor rehabilitation if accidents occur
	Neurochemical changes Impaired thermal control with diminished shivering	Liability to burns, cold and other injury Misleading presentation of symptoms	Protect against extremes of temperature Observe closely for any disregarded symptoms

REFERENCES

Aloia J F 1981 Exercise and skeletal health. Journal of the American Geriatrics Society 29: 104–107

Bittles A H, Collins C J (eds) 1986 The biology of human ageing. Cambridge University Press, Cambridge

Centrella M, Canalis E 1985 Local regulators of skeletal growth: a perspective. Endocrinol. Review 6: 544–551

Comfort A 1977 To be continued. In: Barry J R, Wingrove G (eds) Let's learn about ageing. Wiley, Chichester

Davies S, Stewart A 1987 Nutritional medicine. Pan Books, London

Davis A J 1981 Ethical issues in gerontological nursing. In: Copp L A (ed) Care of the aging. Churchill Livingstone, Edinburgh

Ebersole P, Hess P 1985 Towards healthy aging, 2nd edn. Mosby, St Louis

Ettinger B, Genant H K, Cann C E 1987 Post menopausal bone loss is prevented by low dosage oestrogen and calcium. Annals of Internal Medicine 106: 40–45

Evered D, Whelan J (ed) 1988 Research and the ageing population. Ciba Foundation Symposium No 134. Wiley, Chichester

Gray Muir J A (ed) 1986 Prevention of disease in the elderly. Churchill Livingstone, Edinburgh

Greengross W, Greengross S 1989 Living, loving and ageing. Age Concern, Mitcham

Hayflick L 1987 Origins of longevity. In: Warner H R, Butler R N, Sprott R L, Schneider E L (eds) Modern biological theories of aging. Aging series, vol 31. Raven press, New York

Hipkiss A 1989 The production and removal of abnormal proteins: a key question in the biology of ageing. In: Warnes A M (ed) Human ageing and later life:

multi-disciplinary perspectives. Research studies in Gerontology. Edward Arnold, London

Hipkiss A, Bittles A 1989 Basic biological aspects of ageing. In: Warnes A M (ed) Human ageing and later life: multi-disciplinary perspectives. Arnold, London

Holliday R 1986 Genes, proteins and cellular ageing. Van Nostrand Reinhold, New York

Kirkwood T B L 1981 Repair and its evolution: survival versus reproduction. In: Townsend C R, Calow P (eds) Physiological ecology: an evolutionary approach to resource use. Blackwell Publications, Oxford

Kirkwood T 1988 The nature and causes of ageing. In: Evered D, Whelan J (eds) Research and the ageing population. Ciba Foundation Symposium No 134. Wiley, Chichester

Kirkwood T B L and Holliday R 1986 Ageing as a consequence of natural selection. In: Bittles A H, Collins K J (eds) The biology of human ageing. Cambridge University Press, Cambridge

Landhal S, Bengtsson C, Sigurdsson J, Svanborg A, Svärdsodd K 1986 Age-related changes in blood pressure. Hypertension 8: 1044–1049

Le May A C, Redfern S J 1987 The nature and frequency of nurse–patient touch and its relationship to the well-being of elderly patients. In: Sorvettula M (ed) Collaborative research and its implementation in nursing. Proceedings of the Workgroup of European Nurse Researchers' Conference, Helsinki 1986. Finnish Federation and Nurses and Nursing Research Institute, Helsinki

Lewis C B 1985 Ageing: the health care challenge. An inter-disciplinary approach to assessment and rehabilitation. Davis, Philadelphia

Lundren-Lindquist B, Aniansson A, Lundgren A 1983 Functional Studies in 79 year olds: walking reserve and climbing capacity. Scandinavian Journal Rehabil. Med. 15: 125–131

Phair J P, Hsu C S, Hsu Y L 1988 Ageing and infection. In: Evered D, Whelan J (eds) Research and the ageing population. Ciba Foundation Symposium No 134. Wiley, Chichester

Redfern S 1989 Key issues in nursing elderly people. In: Warnes A M (ed) Human ageing and later life: multi-disciplinary perspectives. Research studies in gerontology. Edward Arnold, London

Riggs B L 1984 Treatment of osteoporosis with sodium fluoride: an appraisal. In: Peck W A (ed) Bone and mineral research. Annual 2 a yearly survey of developments in the field of bone and mineral. Elsevier, New York

Riggs L and Melton L J 1988 Osteoporosis and age related fracture syndromes. In: Evered D, Whelan J (eds) Research and the ageing population. Ciba Foundation Symposium No 134. Wiley, Chichester

Rothstein M (ed) 1987 Review of biological research on ageing. Liss, New York

Sacher G A 1977 Life table modifications and life prolongation. In: Finch C E, Hayflick L (eds) Handbook of the biology of ageing. Van Nostrand Reinhold, New York

Shaw M W 1984 (ed) The challenge of ageing. Churchill Livingstone, Melbourne

Skeet M 1983 Protecting the health of the elderly. Public Health in Europe (8). World Health Organization, Copenhagen

Smith A, Jacobson B 1988 The nation's health: a strategy for the 1990s. Health Education Authority, London School of Hygiene and Tropical Medicine and King Edward's Hospital Fund for London, London

Svanborg A 1988 The health of the elderly population: results from longitudinal studies with age cohort comparisons. In: Evered D, Whelan J (eds) Research and the ageing population. Ciba Foundation Symposium No 134. Wiley, Chichester

Vessey M, Hunt K 1987 The menopause, hormone replacement and cardio-vascular disease: epidemiological assets. In: Studd J (ed) Hormone replacement therapy. MTP Press, London

Walford R L 1981 Immuno-regulatory systems in ageing. In: Danon D, Shock N W (eds) Ageing: a challenge to science and society, vol 1: Biology. Oxford University Press, Oxford

Walford R L 1983 Maximum life-span. W W Norton, New York

CHAPTER CONTENTS

3

Psychosocial and spiritual aspects of ageing

An exploration of the psychological, social and spiritual aspects of ageing provides some contrasts to the biological facets examined in the previous chapter. Current studies show that although some faculties may wane in later life, others are retained into extreme old age, and some may improve and sharpen. Thus, later maturity has the potential to be a time of personal development and enrichment. Figure 3.1 is intended to convey this point — that while there is evidence of eventual biological decline in old age, psychosocial and spiritual growth can and does occur.

One recurring theme throughout recent literature on elderly people is the continuity of growth and the capacity for adaptation. Of course the risk of maladaptation is also present, as it is for any age group. Over the years humans have shown themselves to be both resilient and resourceful. The lives of many of those who have survived into later maturity, often bear testimony to these qualities. Integrating life experiences and reflecting on them can move one onward to greater understanding. However, it is also important to appreciate that for older, as well as younger people, a present as well as a past orientation is necessary for full living. This is emphasised by Ebersole & Hess (1985), who stress the importance of 'an awareness of both *being* and *becoming*' in relation to being old, or becoming old.

As in the biological realm, there is a great variation in the rate and manifestation of ageing in psychosocial and spiritual planes. This is partly because every old person is constitutionally unique, with potential still present to be

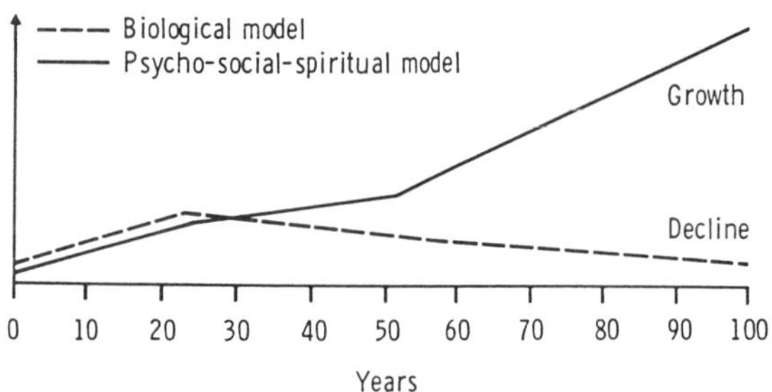

Fig. 3.1 Comparison of biological and psychosocial–spiritual models of ageing, indicating potential for growth.

maximised, and partly because the force of different life events, and the availability of solutions, produce highly individual responses. For these reasons health visitors need to be flexible in their approaches, applying their interventions creatively, in order to meet the many different needs and reactions of their older clients.

Furthermore, it is necessary to appreciate that the distinction between normal and abnormal ageing in the psychosocial realm changes as data emerges from new research. Features previously considered to be the norm may well be identified as pathological, as has been seen to be the case in the biological realm.

THEORIES OF PSYCHOSOCIAL AGEING

Theories attempt to explain and predict events and behaviour encountered in practice. However, the various psychosocial theories of ageing are at present as debatable as the biological ones. They have been criticised as being either too abstract, or as being underdeveloped, or, in the case of some developmental theories, as being rather deterministic. Nevertheless each perspective offers some helpful insights, or stimulating notions about ageing, which reward study. In the absence of a preferred theory, therefore, it is probably best to adopt an eclectic approach.

PSYCHOLOGICAL THEORIES

For the purposes of our discussion these are classified as:

- psychoanalytic and developmental theories
- humanistic theories
- continuity theory
- social learning theory and efficacy.

Psychoanalytic theories

Freud was one of the first psychologists to consider the components of personality development. He postulated that development in later life depended on psychological processes in early childhood — hence his emphasis on appropriate psychological management in the early years.

His contemporary, Jung, who stressed the differential developmental patterns shown by introverts and extroverts, asserted the importance of the last half of life in its own right. He defined the purpose of later maturity as 'inner discovery through reflective activity', contending that those who seek for personal meaning and the spiritual self are less likely to experience restlessness or disorientation in old age. Jung also taught that denying the validity of unconscious experience and the existence of the psyche could lead to intrapersonal conflict and a sense of meaninglessness in later life. While this may happen, it should be pointed out that not all individuals appear to value such psychological exploration, while some older people seem far less reflective than others.

These Jungian views were adopted by Butler (1963), when he stressed the growth potential for older people of '*life-reviewing*'. He saw such a review as a catalyst for developing identity in later maturity. It is these ideas which underlie modern reminiscent groups, which some health visitors and their colleagues have so successfully instituted. However, when using this approach, care must be taken to ensure that the techniques adopted do not trivialise experience, as this can then be detrimental (Joyce 1989).

As a development of Freudian dynamics, Erikson (1963) introduced *epigenetic theory*. He perceived the life-span as consisting of eight specific developmental stages, each with its own developmental tasks to be achieved. The last stage he considered was a vantage point from which one could view one's entire life, either with integrity or despair. He stressed that good health, sound economic circumstances, regular and satisfying social contacts and the presence of at least one reference figure, could assist older persons in achieving integrity. While acknowledging the usefulness of his ideas, critics have argued that the theory does not make clear exactly *how* an individual proceeds from one developmental stage to another, or what happens if an individual fails to achieve an earlier developmental task. Furthermore, his ideas are thought to be somewhat class and culture bound. Nevertheless, others have derived help from his ideas and have incorporated them into their own work. In his more recent writings Erikson elaborated on the concept of integrity in later life (Erikson et al 1986).

Building on Erikson's epigenetic theory, Peck (1968) elaborated the concept of ego-integrity in later life. He identified discrete tasks which he thought were necessary to its achievement, describing these as:

- ego-differentiation versus work-role preoccupation
- body transcendence versus body preoccupation
- ego-transcendence versus body preoccupation.

He asserted that to achieve ego-integrity, older people must relinquish their occupational identity, rise above any bodily discomfort, and perceive meaning in their experiences. His ideas have been criticised on the grounds that they place too great a burden on frail old people, who may not always be able to laugh at their discomforts or rise above their circumstances.

The concept of ego-integrity was also investigated by Clayton (1975). He related it to wisdom, seeing this as

> an adaptive perception of reality, whereby one draws new meanings from prior experiences.

While appreciating that wisdom often develops in later life, he questioned if individuals ever fully achieved Erikson's developmental tasks, from young adulthood onwards.

Spirituality was considered a most important part of development in later maturity by Hall (1983), who thought this is the way older people more fully realise ego-integrity. Similarly Abrahams (1983) identified 'forgiveness seeking' as a strong theme in the attempts of some older people to achieve ego-integrity. He postulated that when older persons are reviewing their life-experiences, they may feel a sense of guilt that they have not always fulfilled their earlier aspirations. He stressed that professional workers encountering such reactions should demonstrate empathy, so that older clients could be 'permitted to feel forgiven'.

Humanistic theories

Considerable research in this field was carried out by Buhler (1964). She identified three types of developmental progress which eventually affect persons in later life:

1. development dominated by bio-physical performance
2. development concerned with achievement and production
3. development characterised by contemplative activity.

Although each of these stages is important to the full rounding of the personality, stage 3 may be considered to have particular relevance for old people.

The theory of motivation developed by Maslow (1962, 1987) was also located within a humanistic framework. He conceptualised individuals as striving for full holistic growth, through a hierarchy of values/needs, which he presented in a pyramidal form (see Fig. 5.1, p. 86). The base of the pyramid he considered represented physiological and safety and security needs. These two 'survival' levels he thought demand such urgent attention that they consume an individual's energy until satisfied. Only when these needs are met can attention be directed towards affiliation and self-esteem needs and eventually to self-actualisation. These levels Maslow located at the peak of his pyramid.

From his research Maslow found younger people did not fit his model of self-actualised persons. He therefore concluded that maturity and self-knowledge, born out of life experience, is necessary for one to achieve this full growth. Such findings led Ebersole & Hess (1985) to adopt his model as having particular relevance for older people.

Continuity theory

This theory emphasises the complex inter-relationship between the biological, psychological and social influences which make for change, or stability, in older individuals. It focuses on the efforts which older persons make in order to preserve the habits, preferences and lifestyles that they have acquired over many years. Hence Ruff (1982) sees successful ageing as depending on how far these components are retained and integrated into a person's present circumstances.

Health visitors make use of continuity theory when they take account of their client's past as well as present circumstances. Enabling older clients to build on their existing skills and knowledge, and to select coping mechanisms from their life repertoire, can aid problem solving. However, one should be mindful of critical reviews of this theory. It is suggested by Victor (1987) that events such as retirement, widowhood, or children leaving home, constitute problematic role changes when viewed from a continuity perspective, since there can be no anticipatory socialisation to prepare persons for such eventualities. The theory is also criticised by Burbank (1986) on the grounds that it is unsupported by empirical evidence. She considers a phenomenological approach might prove a more productive way for health staff to study the psychosocial aspects of ageing.

Social learning theory — efficacy and self-efficacy

A social-psychological theory, thought to be highly relevant to ageing, was developed by Bandura (1977, 1986). He introduced the concepts of efficacy and self-efficacy, in the context of social learning and the part played by 'modelling' upon behaviour. He postulated that individuals acquire new behaviour patterns by observing the behaviour of others and then cognitively coding these patterns into 'memory banks', to be recalled later as guides to action. As these patterns are imitated and tried out, individuals correct their performance through feedback. Health visitors will note that such social learning clearly depends on the quality of the role models, as well as the ability of individuals to decide when a particular behaviour pattern is appropriate. In the context of this theory one might pose the question: are the present nonagenarians and centenarians the first generation to provide role models in 'older ageing'?

Another postulation by Bandura is that, through repetition of imitative behaviour, individuals learn what to do to bring about favourable outcomes, as well as what not to do, to avoid punishing ones. In this way expectancies about outcomes are built up, as well as beliefs about how events are connected and what consequences are likely to follow specific actions. As judgement is exercised about these outcome-expectancies and beliefs, capability levels are established, constituting efficacy. Moreover, Bandura (1977) thought individuals then learn to estimate whether the exercise of selected behaviours, in order to bring about specific outcomes, lies within their personal competence or not: *'The strength of a person's conviction about their own capacity, is likely to affect how far they are successful in that form of behaviour.'* This personal interpretation of expectancy outcomes, incentives and competency levels he termed *self-efficacy*.

Applied to older people, self-efficacy is built up over many years and is generally high. However, low self-efficacy, is thought to be demonstrated when older adults lose confidence in their performance after a setback, such as illness or accident. Doubting their ability to bring about a favourable outcome, they may give up attempting behaviour which previously may have been well within their capability. Learning must then be structured for them, so that through demonstration, opportunity for repeated practice, and several small successes, confidence and competence can be restored. Health visitors will readily appreciate that this is the notion which underlies rehabilitation and assertion-education, which Doty

(1987) and others have used with older people. A derivation of this theory is the Health Belief Model, which also has relevance in later life (Becker 1974, Rosenstock et al 1988). (See also Ch. 5, p. 90 and Ch. 8, p. 179.)

Learned helplessness

An extension of the concept of low self-efficacy, thought to be pertinent to some older persons, is 'learned helplessness', propounded by Maier & Seligman (1976). They postulated that persons tend to behave resignedly if their personal competency levels have been eroded and they feel that, whatever behaviour they produce, they cannot produce desired outcomes:

> A person, or animal, is helpless with regard to some outcome, when the outcome occurs independently of all their voluntary responses.

It was considered by Maier and Seligman that the only way to change such futility is to change the environment. Where this cannot be done, apathy and depression are likely to result.

It has been argued that while learned helplessness can be applied to any age group, it is demonstrated by elderly people when they feel themselves powerless to control their own lives. Such behaviour may be noticed when reluctant old people are admitted to residential care, or are moved to live with others whose lifestyles and social rules prevail.

The implications for practice

The implications for health visiting practice of these various psychological theories of ageing include:

- recognising the richness and validity of older adults' experiences and building on them whenever possible
- assisting older individuals to preserve strong links with their past, while moving positively into the present
- strengthening confidence and competence levels and encouraging older people to utilise well-developed coping mechanisms, in new circumstances
- modifying environmental situations so that they facilitate independence and enable older adults to retain control of their lives for as long as possible.

SOCIOLOGICAL THEORIES OF AGEING

Disengagement theory

One of the earliest theories in this field, the notion of disengagement, was propounded by Cumming & Henry (1961). They developed their ideas, following a 5-year study of 275 fit, financially secure persons aged 50–90, living in Kansas City, USA. They contended that, as individuals age, they relinquish certain roles, either on their own initiative, or through pressures from society. Inevitably and universally, mutual withdrawal or disengagement occurs between ageing persons and the social systems to which they belong. This disengagement varies within groups, paving the way for the ultimate withdrawal — death. Societies retract because of the need for continuity, with younger persons filling the roles vacated by older persons, while ageing individuals retreat because of awareness of diminishing capacities. Problems may arise if societies force withdrawal when individuals are not ready for such disengagement.

Later, Cumming amended some of her earlier views. She acknowledged the effects of individual differences, although still claiming her research supported the likelihood of earlier disengagement in those older persons who customarily react to stress by turning inwards and insulating themselves from society (Cumming 1975).

Critics say testing of the theory has led to contradictory findings. According to Crandall (1980), consensus supports it as *only one of several lifestyles* manifested in later maturity; while Fisk (1986) suggests that its existence

> provides professionals working with elderly clients with a means of rationalising their own, often negative stereotypes.

Disengagement theory is considered by Victor (1987) to have led to age-segregation policies, which have enabled barriers to be erected between older people and other social groups, or the professionals working with them.

Alerted health visitors, cognisant of such criticisms, would recognise the right of older individuals to disengage if they so wish, and would support them in their decision. However, they would recognise those vulnerable persons and would discourage blatant withdrawal and consequent social isolation. Encouraging re-engagement at different levels and within new social roles and networks, especially with persons of varying ages, would also seem to be indicated.

Activity theory

The opposite of Disengagement theory is Activity theory, as advocated by Maddox (1963), Havinghurst (1968), Neugarten (1972) and Bromley (1976). It asserts that older people institute compensatory activities to offset role loss, narrowing of their social radius and threats to their self-esteem. By developing alternative role options, as well as maintaining an active lifestyle, they sustain their morale and hence well-being. However, merely busying oneself with meaningless activities is not thought to contribute to adjustment. Both longitudinal and cross-cultural studies have shown a positive, though not incontrovertible, association between personal adjustment, morale and activity levels in later maturity.

The social policy implications of activity theory are considered by Victor (1987) to be considerably more positive than those of disengagement theory, in that they provide for the integration of older people as full society members. However, she questions the value judgements inherent in the theory that 'activity in old age is a good thing'. She asks, 'in the light of this perspective, what happens to those who lose the battle to remain middle-aged?'. No doubt Ellard (1988) utilised activity theory when he advocated that older clients need to be prepared 'not for retreat, but for a regrouping of their forces!'.

Subculture theory

This theory, proposed by Rose (1965), asserts that older persons interact within a group composed of persons of the same age, or social background. Sharing similar interests, values, jokes and friendships, they tend to develop strong group identity, which may then be linked to recreational or political activity, e.g. Pensioners' Link in the UK or The Gray Panthers in the USA, multi-purpose senior citizen clubs, or holiday schemes for the over 60s. Such peer groups are compared somewhat unfavourably by Harris (1983) with the extension of social relationships which can be brought about by grounds other than age.

Nevertheless, the importance of encouraging communication and sharing between older persons is emphasised by both Butler & Lewis (1982) and Lewis (1985), the latter also stressing that older clients may sometimes respond to older staff members if they do not seem to be relating quite so well to younger ones.

However, Walker (1980) and Victor (1987) consider the theory has limited utility. While accepting that shared problems like dependency, housing needs, health status or income may increase peer-group interaction, they highlight the dangers of marginalisation which such interaction may bring. Furthermore they stress that not all older people live within age-segregated communities, nor would wish to do so. Nor do they confine themselves to activities with their own age group. Grasping the principle of heterogeneity, as applied to the elderly population, enables practitioners to perceive some of the flaws in the subculture perspective, while recognising and building on the mutual support that peer group activity affords.

Social exchange theory

Under this idea, successful ageing is perceived as involving a rebalancing of exchange relationships. The theory assumes that individuals offer certain inputs to society, in order to gain certain rewards. The level of social interaction is determined by the benefits received, in relation to the costs involved. However, with less influence over their environment, together with shrinking social networks, older people have fewer commodities with which to bargain. In consequence, it is asserted, some use compliance as a means of winning support and acceptance from others. An example of social exchange theory in action is seen where older people have been used as sources of local history for school children. The children are then encouraged to contact senior citizens and ask them questions relating to their earlier lives. Tape-recordings of such interviews enhance the children's learning, while older people are able to barter their knowledge and experience in exchange for increased social contact and prestige-rating. At present, society possibly undervalues its older citizens, and hence does not exploit this theory sufficiently.

Social breakdown theory

Linked to the notion of social exchange, the proponents of social breakdown theory systematically underline the inter-dependence between older people and their social world. They argue that older persons, affected by unfamiliar circumstances, role loss, or dramatic change in lifestyle, reach out for clues to guide their actions. However, this very act of reaching out for help is regarded as evidence of incompetence. Concern is then generated in those around them, which gives negative feedback to the older individual. In turn, somewhat bewildered, they adopt the negative characteristics ascribed to them, thus deepening their dependent status (Kuypers & Bengtston 1973). These researchers thus describe this process as 'the social breakdown cycle of old age'. It has much in common with the concept of 'labelling', which has been seen to apply to other age groups, as well as some similarity to the notion of 'learned helplessness' discussed earlier. Enabling persons to function competently within more structured environments, and emphasising their personal strengths, can help to replace the cycle of breakdown with one of reconstruction — an approach advocated by Clarke (1984).

Age stratification theory

This theory is based on the belief that all societies arrange themselves in age strata, with rights and obligations linked to the social roles considered appropriate to each age band. The matching role behaviours are, however, influenced by a number of factors. One major interpreting force is thought to be the unique social conditions with which history presents each biological cohort. Prevailing social and economic conditions produce overriding values, which dominate outlook and shape social roles. Thus behaviour is related to sociohistoric context. (This cohort differential is supported by Svanborg et al 1986, from their Longitudinal Research.)

This theory was likened, by Riley et al (1972), to persons stepping onto an escalator at birth and moving up in a collective, though not an identical, manner. Various external factors influence their ride, determining the manner and point at which they get off. However, as successive cohorts move up, they alter the conditions to such a degree that subsequent cohorts never experience the same ride. Thus the general reaction towards ageing of those now aged 85 years in our society might be expected to differ considerably from those now aged 60 years. This is because they grew up before the First World War, when the work ethic predominated, and the welfare state did not exist. Their thinking was often dominated by fear of the workhouse, and their reactions led to values of frugality, thrift, self-sufficiency and mutual aid. Similarly one might expect that the reactions of those who grew up in the more affluent 1960s, when more permissive values prevailed, would differ considerably, when they become old, from those persons who experienced the grinding poverty of the economic depression in the 1930s.

Biographical theory

Biographical theory developed from the work of Townsend (1981) and Phillipson & Walker (1986), who highlighted older persons' experiences of welfare policies and examined inequalities in ageing. Thus attention was directed towards life and work histories, the meanings attached to retirement and their relationship to subsequent ageing. Further impetus was given to the development of this perspective (which has strong links with symbolic interactionist and continuity theories) by the work of Marshall (1986) and Johnson (1988). Life histories are of course individual and unique. They contain a record not only of the events experienced, but of the ways in which different individuals have reacted and coped with them. They can be used both to build up the self-esteem of older people, and to generate further hypotheses about the subsequent experiences of old age (see di Gregorio (1986, 1987), Kohli (1986), Matthews (1986) and Coleman (1988)). This theory complements age stratification theory, which adopts a collective approach, whereas biographical theory is more individualistic.

Political economy theory

Located within a Marxist framework, and adopting a global stance, this theory views old people as an integral part of society, set within socially constructed roles, rules and institutions, which define old age. Like biographical theory, it stresses the need to examine the differential experience of ageing, between various subgroups, but then relates these to social and economic policies. Thus it considers such factors as

- gender
- social class
- age divisions of society
- the means of production
- retirement policies set in the context of national and international economics.

Under its proposals the status, resources and experiences of old people are regarded as conditioned by their place in the social structure. In turn this social structure is seen to be shaped by global socio-economic forces and by political decisions. Retirement policies are deemed to be related to differential labour needs, rather than being determined by biological or psychosocial factors.

Thus, it is argued, in times of recession and high unemployment, early retirement is encouraged. Conversely in times of labour shortage, older people are no longer regarded as expendable but urged to remain in, or return to, employment.

Retirement is officially regarded as synonymous with exclusion from employment. Hence to preserve the work ethic and to differentiate the status, proponents of this theory argue, retirement benefits are deliberately kept well below the average national manual wage. At times when any return to employment is being actively discouraged, an earnings rule is imposed upon retired persons, who lose benefit if they earn more than a limited amount. Should the demographic or social situation change, and it be perceived as politically expedient for older workers to be retained, the earnings rule may be abolished.

The consequences of such policies, it is claimed, force those who have to retire, cannot work and have limited savings, to rely entirely on state benefits. Since these are low, political economy theorists argue, recipients are thrown into *socially constructed dependency*. It is currently estimated that some two-thirds of pensioners may fall into this category (Victor & Vetter 1986).

This perspective also highlights issues such as gender differences in the experience of ageing (as does the biographical theory), and the tendency to engage in 'victim blaming' of elderly people. One question it asks is: how far do professionals contribute to the experience of old age as socially constructed dependency?.

These and other issues are debated in several works, including Phillipson (1982), Minkler & Estes (1984), Guillemard (1986), Phillipson & Walker (1986, 1987) and Victor (1987).

The significance for practice

The significance for health visiting practice is seen in that these various theories can help to clarify issues related to pyschosocial ageing and so assist practitioners to decide their own particular views.

Adopting an eclectic stance, it is important for professional workers to recognise and respect individual differences, especially related to the personality characteristics, value systems and cultural motivations of elderly people. Account needs to be taken of socio-historic contexts when assessing and interpreting client behaviour, as well as culture, class and gender differences related to the experience of ageing.

Practitioners will recognise the right of older persons to disengage, if they so wish, but will encourage older people to identify and make the best use of their abilities, take up new interests, keep mentally active and foster independence and competence.

Furthermore, workers will be aware of the risks of apathy and resignation in those older people who feel they are no longer in control, and hence will take action to prevent their social breakdown. Moreover, they will encourage communities to recognise and utilise the contribution which older persons can offer. Pressing for improved social, economic, environmental and educational provisions for older persons could facilitate their development and participation; hence practitioners will wish to take account of the ways in which they can help to influence policies favourably (Phillipson & Strang 1984).

PSYCHOLOGICAL ASPECTS OF AGEING

Distinct from the many *theories* of ageing, which are at times tentative and debatable, the psychological and social aspects of ageing have been relatively well documented. The psychological components are both cognitive and emotional. Cognitive elements include: intelligence; perception; memory; reasoning; the capacity to assess, analyse and interpret situations; to process, store, recall and utilise information; to orient oneself in time and space; to respond to stimuli and to organise complex data.

As with biological ageing, chronological age is a poor indicator of cognitive state. Some old people are alert, mentally active, and successfully hold down positions of great financial or political responsibility, while others become less able at a much earlier age.

In contrast to age changes, which are largely biologically determined, age differences stem mainly from complex and interwoven environmental influences. Educational experiences, nutrition, health status and stress situations in earlier life are, therefore, some of the components found to be associated with cognitive development in old age (Woods & Britton 1988).

Intelligence

Current concern about intellectual capacity and performance is indicative of cultural values and often reflects individual and societal fears. In Western society there is an almost obsessive preoccupation with this, and Ebersole & Hess (1985) question what differences might arise in the assessment of adequacy in older people if our dominant cultural values were based on a capacity for coping, caring, on survival strategies, or character strength!

Questions too are raised about the appropriateness and validity of the tests used for elderly people (see Miller (1977), Kendrick (1982) and Volans & Woods (1983)). For some years research indicated that maximal intellectual performance was attained around 30 years. Older persons mainly demonstrated some 75% of the intellectual acuity of younger persons. However, the rate of deterioration varied, depending upon intellectual performance in earlier years and the absence of disease. However, more recent evidence suggests that the research methods used impeded a proper understanding of the relationship between ageing and cognitive competence.

Using 'sequential designs' (a combination of cross-sectional and longitudinal studies, rather than the cross-sectional studies used formerly), Schaie (1976) and Labouvie-Vief (1977) showed a very different trajectory for the course of intellectual development in later life. They advocated a 'plasticity model' for studying the relationship between chronological ageing and intellectual performance, but Botwinick (1978) and Woods & Britton (1988) point out that not even this sophisticated method provides all the answers.

A study by Huppert (1982) supported the view that those elderly people who remain in good health and keep active may be just as efficient in carrying out mental tasks as younger persons. This appears to be a significant point for health visitors to note, since if mental creativity enables one to cope more effectively with the cognitive aspects of ageing, a case would seem to be made out for mental stimulation of older people. Support for such action is found in the work of Garfunkel &

Landau (1979), Zivian & Myers (1983) and Slater (1988).

Crystallised and fluid intelligence

The potential cognitive capacity of older adults is seen in research studies to be related to both crystallised and fluid intelligence (Hayslip & Sterns 1979, Ebersole & Hess 1985).

Crystallised intelligence, which is considered to arise from the dominant cerebral hemisphere, increases throughout adult years. Using prior experience as a criterion for problem-solving, its presence indicates that the ability to resolve problems is well retained in normal ageing. Furthermore, crystallised intelligence relates positively to educational levels, income and the number and frequency of cognitive activities in later life (Zivian & Myers 1983).

Fluid intelligence on the other hand emanates from the non-dominant hemisphere, is strongly related to spatial perception and to creative thought, hence it produces aesthetic appreciation and innovative behaviour. It has been argued that non-dominant function has been underdeveloped in Western culture, although some modern educational philosophies encourage exploratory and creative learning styles and lateral thinking (Cory 1979, Ebersole & Hess 1985).

Such underdevelopment may account for the belief that fluid intelligence either declines somewhat after childhood, or lies dormant. Some researchers claim a resurgence occurs in later life, when a more contemplative approach is possible. Certainly, creative works such as compositions by Handel, Haydn, Verdi and Goethe were produced after the age of 70. Titian completed his last picture at 99 years of age, while Grandmother Moses, the American folk painter, is an example of latent ability surfacing in old age.

The value of intelligence for older people

Intelligence is of particular importance for older people. It assists them in assessing, manipulating, and organising their environment, thus helping them to retain control over their lives. Where measurable cognitive decline exists, there is a tendency for response patterns to be rigid, especially if there is also some sensory deficit. However, routine and experience may provide some compensation. While spatial perception and decoding ability may decline with advanced age, intelligence decreases appear to be mostly associated with loneliness, poor social relationships and isolation. Thus, encouraging older people to be involved with, and accepted by, others would seem to be a very worthwhile health visiting activity.

Reaction time *does* slow in later life. This is due to diminished conduction time, alterations in the perceived strength of neural signals, and sometimes lower levels of interest and motivation. It is exacerbated in those suffering from cerebral ischaemia, or depressive states.

Speed is sacrificed to greater accuracy, but comprehension and verbal fluency are preserved into extreme old age, particularly among women.

Memory

Short-term memory is generally thought to be somewhat blunted in old age, though Craik (1977) disputes this. Some loss of brain cells in the hippocampal region, which is associated with memory, may account for this. It may also arise partly from a lack of concentration, or limited interest in recent events. How far long-term memory is affected in later life is a controversial issue, with research producing some contradictory findings (Dye 1989).

It is pointed out by Slater (1988) that memory is an exceedingly complex construct, making any delineation of normal age changes quite problematic. He therefore concludes, like Baddeley (1986) and Schaie & Willis (1986), that there are wide individual differences in memory performance. He thus reinforces the continuing principle of heterogeneity in later life, and highlights the need to avoid prejudicial stereotyping.

Nevertheless, it is pertinent to appreciate that an individual's subjective perception of memory changes can be negatively clouded by depression

(Kermis 1984, Ebersole & Hess 1985). Health visitors will realise that self-reports of memory impairment are notoriously unreliable. They will also appreciate that when clinical depresssion is diagnosed and treated, some older clients respond favourably, increasing both their motor speed and memory tasks.

Facilitating memory in later life

It is possible to facilitate memory, by encouraging older clients to rehearse material so that it can be laid down in longer-term memory. This requires time, and concentration, so clients and their carers should keep disruption to a minimum when material is being presented. Reducing memory load through the use of aids such as notes, diaries, calendars, or bulletin boards and adopting systematic routines, can also prove helpful. Some older persons find mnemonics useful, and in group settings memory games can be entertaining, although their longer-term value is not proven (Welford 1985, Dye 1989).

Learning

Contrary to popular belief, older persons do continue to learn and to respond to new situations, given time and motivation. This indicates the value of educational opportunity at all stages of the life-span.

> If our ultimate aims are to increase the quality of life in the later years, and to eradicate our negative social construction of ageing, then we must seek to make learning as visible a vocation of older people as gardening or grandparenting currently are. This goal will never be realised if education continues to be defined in terms which are irrelevant to the vast majority of people.
>
> Allman (1983)

Consequently it is worth noting that a group called FREE (Forum for the Rights of Elderly people in Education), has been set up in association with Age Concern, to encourage more educational facilities for retired people (Manthorpe 1986). Already older individuals respond well to a range of classes offered by Local Education Authorities, or by such voluntary organisations as The Workers' Educational Association. Some take up correspondence courses, while others attend weekend seminars, study tours, or summer schools run by Adult Residential Colleges. These courses cover a variety of academic, creative and artistic topics.

Researchers such as Gearing et al (1988) contend that older people can continue to learn, remember information and successfully reproduce it. They cite as evidence those nine thousand older persons finally registered with the Open University. Furthermore, students over 60 tend to have a slightly lower drop-out rate than do younger students, and they perform slightly better in continuous assessment; however, they perform rather less well in examination settings, which call for increased speed and reactions (Clennell et al 1984).

There is also a considerable response to the University of the Third Age (U3A). This is an organisation run for, and by, older people, which, while it does not offer degrees, provides a range of activities, summer schools and courses (Midwinter 1984).

Health visitors should note that fear of failure, or lessened concern with success, may inhibit learning responses in some older persons. They should also consider the significant features of learning in later life:

- material presented should be relevant to the needs of older clients
- should preferably meet with any expressed requests
- should relate to the educational background of the person or group
- should take account of the health state of older clients
- learning situations should be anxiety free.

Material given must therefore be strong, logical and meaningful. It should be presented in well-defined stages, with opportunity for spaced repetition. Time should be allowed for assimilation, and, most of all, older persons should be encouraged to discuss freely and relate the material to their own experience (Strehlow 1983).

Cognitive dysfunction

Exercising judgement and making decisions about their lives are also crucial activities for the elderly. Thus all that is known about these complex mental activities can be related to persons in later maturity. Nevertheless, it must be recognised that impairment from organic brain syndrome is not uncommon, and can affect memory, comprehension, judgement, orientation and affect. Functional disorders arising from loss, bereavement and/or social isolation may lead to apparent cognitive deterioration, which is usually reversible. Thus, as with biological ageing, it is important to distinguish pathology from the inevitable developmental age changes. In this way what can be prevented, treated, possibly reversed, or at least controlled and ameliorated, can be identified.

EMOTIONAL ASPECTS OF AGEING

The personality structure and characteristics displayed in earlier life become crucial to emotional well-being in later maturity. There is a tendency for individuals to become more what they are: e.g. their personality traits are exaggerated. Nevertheless, sound self-esteem in earlier years, together with well-practised coping strategies, can help individuals to weather the stresses of ageing.

Positive influences include a realistic appreciation of body image changes; identification with various groups; and unobtrusive support from family, friends, lay and professional carers.

A range of mental defence mechanisms, which are familiar to health visitors and which may be used by individuals from earlier years, may be utilised in later maturity. These defences help to counteract the anxieties and frustrations which may accompany bodily changes and limitations (Ebersole & Hess 1985). However, because psychological resilience and energy levels may lessen, there may be greater dependence on a narrower range of defences. Thus some older persons may appear rigid and over-defensive in their approaches to situations. Examples of adaptive mechanisms which may be shown include the following.

- Denial — some older persons may use this selectively, as in disregarding age changes, disabilities or deprivations, thus enabling them to maintain a more positive self-view
- Detachment — this may sometimes be utilised when the older person wishes to avoid further inter-personal loss
- Projection — this mechanism may be used when dissatisfaction is present and the older person needs to be assertive or to display strong feelings. It may become disruptive if an older client persistently blames others and complains
- Regression — some level of regression may be helpful, in allowing an older person to tolerate increasing dependency and accept help
- Somatisation — some elderly persons convert their emotional reactions into physical symptoms
- Sublimation — this may sometimes be used by older adults to divert strong drives, which otherwise cannot find expression, into socially approved and personally satisfying activities. These may be, for example, showing great interest in, and associating strongly with, the activities of younger people (vicarious satisfaction).

Health visitors will appreciate that these unconscious defences help to ward off the anxiety and insecurity some older persons feel, and so preserve ego-functioning. However, at times, emotional reactions can be so intense that their habitual use may be insufficient to protect against anxiety. Such events call for skilled identification and added support, so that emotional equilibrium may be restored.

SOCIAL ASPECTS OF AGEING

As has already been seen, ageing is to a certain extent socio-culturally determined. Although there are some universal institutions and values, there may be considerable variation in their expressions. Thus the customs and conventions associated with growing old vary.

Culture is a learned way of thinking, acting and communicating. It embodies formulations about the nature of man and the universe, as well as cognitive and emotional elements of living. The language unique to a group, and the values, beliefs, concepts and patterns of behaviour inherent in a specific culture, are transmitted from generation to generation. There will of course be some modifications in the process. Because these socialisation processes go deep, it is hard to generalise about social manifestations of ageing.

There are, for instance, long-settled rural and urban elderly; there are those who have travelled widely, often gaining experience in different working environments, and those who have remained home-based. Some come from differing racial and ethnic backgrounds, with varying histories accounting for their migration, including those with refugee status. Hence it is important for professional workers to try to understand the cultural background of their older clients, so that interventions may be tailored more appropriately (see Ch. 10, pp. 254–259).

There is a sense, however, in which such understanding is not conceptually fully possible. Once accepted, a more culture-general approach is possible, with respect for the validity of others' assumptions and values, while appreciating the tenacity of one's own (Ebersole & Hess 1985, Norman 1985, Spector 1985, Dobson 1989).

Transcultural aspects of ageing

Ethnicity reflects culture, and race, as well as other influences, including social support subsystems. Thus in a pluralist society, such as now exists in the UK, the elderly from ethnic minority groups may show very diverse reactions to ageing, even though they may be categorised together. It is imperative that health visitors recognise such heterogeneity, and avoid stereotypic expectations. However, some factors may have general applicability. For example, elderly immigrants may feel particularly lonely and isolated. There may be language barriers, or a history of discriminations, compounded by role uncertainties. Sometimes ethnic minority elderly find themselves living with their families, who may have assimilated much of the host culture. In such circumstances they may feel bewildered and may experience a profound sense of loss (Fenton 1987) (see also Ch. 10, pp. 257–258).

The social aspects of ageing and ethno-cultural diversity of older people are reflected in the health practices and attitudes shown towards health services. Examples include the methods used to prevent or treat illness and maintain health (Qureshi 1989). These remedies may employ folk medicine or require the involvement of 'natural healers'. They form a rich reservoir of data, which Spector (1989) considers should be annotated, using her Heritage Tool, before it is too late.

Socio-environmental factors and successful ageing

A key element in deciding whether ageing can be termed socially successful is the interaction between the individual and his or her environment. Health visitors should note the threats to self-identity and coping behaviour, which can arise from unsuitable, intrusive, demanding, or limited environments.

Social relationships and ageing

Since humans are fundamentally socially interdependent beings, older persons will interact with family, friends, neighbours, or informal carers. Health visitors may sometimes find there are three or four generations to consider when planning the care of an elderly person, although they may not be living together. Taking account of mutual responsibilities and role-reciprocity can be helpful in such circumstances, as older persons in many cultures participate in caring for children, the sick or disabled, domestic and community activities, and in providing family counsel and stability. Conversely, older persons may be the direct recipients of assistance.

Geographic mobility may sometimes pose considerable problems for families, and it is not uncommon to find couples in late middle-age or early elderlihood who have two sets of older parents to care for, as well as other aged relatives. It is in such circumstances that the 'family visitor' role of the health visitor is so relevant and where the belief in continuity of care applies.

While the important part played by informal carers in the help and support of older persons is increasingly being recognised (see Ch. 8, pp. 183–186 and Ch. 10, p. 234), there are those without families or supportive social networks. The particular needs of elderly vagrants have been emphasised by Blacher (1983), and others, especially the uncertainties of their health care. Furthermore the affluent elderly may sometimes be ruthlessly exploited (Alford 1978).

MORAL AND SPIRITUAL ASPECTS OF AGEING

Just as people develop and change in other dimensions with ageing, so do they morally and spiritually. Older persons may cling even more firmly to personal values, and principles, discovered through life experiences. Especially is this so if their biophysical or psychosocial world is shifting. Although spirituality is not necessarily synonymous with religious observance, many older people derive considerable strength and comfort from identification with a church group. They are often also helped by following through the practices and rituals of their specific religious body.

Assessment over a period of time will enable a health visitor to determine the level of spiritual interest displayed by an aged person, so that liaison with appropriate carers, such as ministers, can be made. Recognising the value of prayer, meditation, and worship, and accepting one's own spiritual needs, will help health visitors to see that the spiritual needs of their older clients are appropriately met. It will also help to ensure that prescribed regimes do not infringe client beliefs.

Spiritual care widens the definition of caring, since it introduces the concept of love, into what may be a technical service (Coleman & Coleman 1983). Thus the spiritually aware practitioner may be able to introduce that spiritual quality into work with older persons, which is the vital element in caring (Simsen 1988).

SUMMARY

This chapter had as its focus the psychological, social and spiritual aspects of ageing, and stressed the important influence of culture and environment. This was in direct contrast to the biophysical aspects of ageing, which were the subject of Chapter 2. However, the separation of the different aspects of ageing is at best artificial and undesirable, and at worst dangerous. In real-life situations these life-components are inextricably interlinked and influence each other. They must be respected accordingly. The case study of Miss Martha Brown is intended to demonstrate this close inter-relationship, as it so often presents itself.

CASE STUDY

Miss Martha Brown is 90 years old and still enjoys life to the full. Her personal history has spanned the early years of the internal combustion engine up to the space age. She has learned to adapt from an era of oil lamps to one of micro-technology, and, as she works in her kitchen or listens to her transistor radio, her seamed face and gnarled hands tell their own story.

Miss Brown regularly surprises her visitors by her quick insights, fund of anecdotes, rich humour and remarkable perspective. The eldest of seven children, she grew up in a Scottish city, where she knew poverty and deprivation throughout her childhood. Impelled by the need to help support her family, she emigrated to the USA before she was 20. Here she quickly found work, although she passed through a difficult time when tuberculosis was diagnosed and she required treatment.

Her fiancé was killed in the First World War and subsequently she never married. Her social status as a domestic servant, although valued at a personal level, never allowed her to become affluent. However, habits of thrift and frugality, together with a strong sense of filial duty, enabled her to provide financially for the care of her ageing parents, during the economic depression of the 1930s.

Returning to Britain for the first time, after the Second World War, to care for a recently widowed brother, she faced a culture from which she had grown away. The subsequent deaths of four of her younger siblings, and the years she spent caring for her brother with an organic brain syndrome, added to her personal stresses. However, her strong faith in God, and the belief that she should solve her problems without undue reliance on others, carried her through these various vicissitudes.

5 years ago Miss Brown was reluctantly transferred to sheltered accommodation, since her general frailty rendered her vulnerable. However, she maintains a fierce pride in her personal and domestic independence, only accepting limited help since she became a nonogenarian. Partially sighted for the past six years, her outings outside the home have lessened, as have her social networks, through the loss of many of her contemporaries. Nevertheless she views television and reads large-print books, as much as her vision permits.

Not for her the peer group activities of the nearby over-60s club, although she acknowledges the benefits this may provide for others. Miss Brown has strong views on life; she is self-contained, monitors her own health assiduously, and is sometimes intolerant of weakness in others! Her dry, often philosophical manner endears her to her relatives and her friends. They admire the fortitude with which she has coped with cataract removal, major abdominal surgery and the sequelae of a mild 'stroke'.

Which theory of ageing best applies to her? Her biological decline is apparent in almost every system — is her 'biological clock' running down? Age stratification theory might serve to explain her interpretation of social roles, rights, responsibilities and behaviour. Or biographical theory might account for her fierce determination to remain 'in control'. Does she demonstrate activity theory, as she keeps abreast of current affairs, and pushes her frail body to its limits in the management of her home? Or does disengagement theory explain her ability to tolerate social restriction and apparent community withdrawal?

Genetic and environmental influences have played their part in her longevity and present health status. Personality characteristics, present since childhood, have enabled Miss Brown to face old age with dignity and equanimity. Nevertheless she remains assertive, inquisitive and tenacious. She has seemingly accomplished many of the developmental tasks outlined by Erikson and others. Has she achieved ego-integrity? Like Jung, she has searched for meaning in her life and her beliefs and sense of purpose now sustain her. Does this support Hall's contentions? At times her psychological outlook is dominated by her biological needs, bur mostly she over-rides such frailty, considering it 'weakness to give way'.

Miss Brown derives much comfort from the regular weekly visits from her minister, and from taking communion. She shares her wisdom with those who care to listen, yet never assumes she has a monopoly on this commodity. In the matter of daily coping and living Miss Martha Brown triumphs; to that extent she transcends all theories.

REFERENCES

Abrahams J P 1983 The search for forgiveness: a theme in geriatric psycho-therapy. Paper published by Department of Psychiatry and Biobehavioural Sciences, University of California, Los Angeles

Alford D 1978 The affluent elderly: problems in nursing care. Journal of Gerontological Nursing 4 (44) (March/April): 44–47

Allman P 1983 The potential for learning in later life. In: Jerome D (ed) Ageing in modern society. Croom Helm, London

Baddeley A 1986 Working memory. Clarendon Press, Oxford

Bandura A 1977 Self-efficacy: towards a unifying theory of behavioural change. Psychological Review 84: 191–215

Bandura A 1986 Social foundations of thought and action. Prentice Hall, Englewood Cliffs, New Jersey

Becker M H (ed) 1974 The health belief model and personal behaviour. Health Education Monographs p 324–473 (published for the society for Public Health Education by Wiley, New York)

Blacher M 1983 Elderly vagrants. In: Ageing in modern society. Croom Helm, London

Botwinick J 1977 Intellectual abilities. In: Birren J E and Schaei K W (eds) Handbook of psychology of aging. Van Nostrand Reinhold, New York

Botwinick J 1978 Aging and behaviour, 2nd edn. Springer, New York

Bromley D B 1976 Research in social and behavioural gerontology: problems and prospects. British Council for Ageing, London

Buhler C 1964 The human course of life: its goal aspects. Journal of Humanistic Psychology 4: 1

Burbank P M 1986 Psycho-social theories of aging: a critical evaluation. Nursing Science 9 (1): 73–86

Butler R 1963 The Life Review: an interpretation of reminiscence in the aged. Psychiatry 26: 65–76

Butler R N, Lewis M I 1982 Aging and mental health: positive psycho-social approaches, 3rd edn. Mosby, St Louis

Clarke L 1984 Domiciliary services for the elderly. Croom Helm, London

Clayton V 1975 Erikson's theory of human development as it applies to the aged: wisdom as a contra-indicative cognition. Human Development 18: 119–28

Clennell S et al 1984 Older students in the Open University. Regional Academic Services, Milton Keynes

Coleman P 1988 Issues in the therapeutic use of reminiscence with elderly people. In: Gearing B, Johnson M, Heller T (eds) Mental health problems in old age. Wiley, Chichester

Coleman P, Coleman M 1983 Spiritual care. In: Clark J, Henderson J (eds) Community health. Churchill Livingstone, Edinburgh

Cory C 1979 Newline: the right hemisphere awakens during trances and ages faster. Psychology Today 13 (30th October)

Craik F I M 1977 Age differences in human memory. In: Birren J E, Schaie K W (eds) Handbook of the psychology of aging. Van Nostrand Reinhold, New York

Crandall R C 1980 Gerontology: a behavioural science approach. Readings. Addison Wesley, Massachusetts

Cumming E 1975 Engagement with an old theory. Aging and Human Development 1(3): 187–191

Cumming E, Henry W 1961 Growing old: the process of disengagement. Basic Books, New York

di Gregorio S 1986 Growing old in twentieth century Leeds: an exploratory study based on the life-histories of people aged 75 years and over. PhD Thesis, London School of Economics, London

di Gregorio S 1987 (ed) Social gerontology: new directions. Croom Helm, London

Dobson S 1989 Conceptualising for transcultural health visiting: the concept of transcultural reciprocity. Journal of Advanced Nursing 14: 97–102

Doty L 1987 Communication and assertion skills for older people. Hemisphere, New York

Dye C A 1989 Memory and aging: a nursing responsibility. In: Dye C (ed) Nursing elderly people. Recent advances in nursing series, No 23: 53–65

Ebersole P, Hess P 1985 Towards healthy aging: human needs and nursing response, 2nd edn. Mosby, St Louis

Ellard J 1988 Growing old: what it is and what it is not. Geriatric Medicine 18 (6): 71–77

Erikson E 1963 Childhood and society, 2nd edn. Norton, New York

Erikson E H, Erikson J M, Kivnick H Q 1986 Vital involvement in old age: the experience of old age in our time. Norton, New York

Fenton S 1987 Ageing minorities: black people as they grow old in Britain. Commission for Racial Equality, London

Fisk M J 1986 Independence and the elderly. Croom Helm, London

Garfunkel F, Landau G 1979 Short term memory course for the well older adult. Perspectives in Aging 8 (Jan/Feb): 19

Gearing B, Johnson M, Heller T 1988 Mental health problems in old age. Open University Press, Milton Keynes

Guillemard A M 1986 Social policy and ageing in France. In: Phillipson C, Walker A (eds) Ageing and social policy: a critical assessment. Gower, Aldershot

Hall E G 1983 Spirituality during ageing. Gerontologist 23: 210 (Special issue)

Harris C 1983 Associational participation in old age. In: Ageing in modern society. Croom Helm, London

Havighurst R H 1968 Personality and patterns of ageing. The Gerontologist 8: 20–23

Hayslip B, Sterns H 1979 Age differences in relationships between crystallized and fluid intelligence in problem-solving. Journal of Gerontology 34: 404

Huppert F 1982 Does mental function decline with age? Geriatric Medicine (January): 32–37

Johnson M L 1988 Biographical influences on mental health in old age. In: Gearing B, Johnson M L, Heller T (eds) Mental health problems in old age. Wiley, Chichester

Joyce S 1989 Reminiscent groups in Islington. Personal communication

Jung C 1971 The stages of life. In: Campbell J (ed) The portable Jung. (Translated by R F C Hull). Viking Press, New York

Kendrick 1982 Why assess the aged? British Journal of Clinical Psychology 2: 47–54

Kermis M D 1984 The psychology of human ageing: theory, research and practice. Allyn and Bacon, London

Kohli M 1986 The world we forgot: a historical review of the life-course. In: Marshall V (ed) Later life. Sage, London

Kuypers J A, Bengtston V L 1973 Social breakdown and competence: a model of normal ageing. Human Development 16: 181–201

Labouvie-Vief G 1977 Adult cognitive development: in search of alternative interpretations. Merill-Palmer Quarterly 23(4): 227–263

Lewis C B 1985 Ageing: the health care challenge. An inter-disciplinary approach to assessment and rehabilitation. F A Davis, Philadelphia

Maddox G L A 1963 A longitudinal study of selected elderly subjects: activity and morale. Social Forces 42: 195–204

Maier S F, Seligman M E 1976 Learned helplessness: theory and evidence. Journal of experimental psychology 105: 3–46

Manthorpe J 1986 Elderly people: rights and opportunities. Logman Self-Help Gindes. Longman, Harlow

Marshall V (ed) 1986 Later life. Sage Publications, London

Maslow A H 1962 Towards a psychology of being. Harpes & Row, New York

Maslow A H 1987 motivation and personality. Revised by Frager R, Fadiman J, McReynolds C, Coxr. Harper & Row, New York

Matthews S M 1986 Friendships through the life course; oral biographies in old age. Sage Publications London

Midwinter E 1984 Mutual aid universities. Croom Helm, London

Minkler M, Estes C (eds) 1984 Readings in the political economy of ageing. Baywood Press, New York

Miller E 1977 Abnormal ageing. The psychology of senile and pre-senile dementia. Wiley, Chichester

Neugarten B L 1972 Personality and the ageing process. The Gerontologist 12: 9–15

Norman A 1985 Triple jeopardy: growing old in a second homeland. Centre for Policy on Ageing, London

Peck R 1968 Psychological developments in the second half

of life: In: Neugarten B (ed) Middle age and aging. University of Chicago Press, Chicago

Phillipson C 1982 Capitalism and the construction of old age. Methuen, London

Phillipson C, Strang P 1984 Health education and older people: the role of paid carers. Health Education Council in association with Department of Adult Education, University of Keele, Keele

Phillipson C, Walker A 1986 Ageing and social policy. Gower, Aldershot

Phillipson C, Walker A 1987 The case for a critical gerontology. In: di Gregorio S (ed) Social gerontology: new directions. Croom Helm, London

Qureshi B 1989 Transcultural medicine. Kluwer, Dordrecht

Riley M W, Johnson M, Foner A 1972 Sociology of age stratification. Ageing and Society 3: 9

Rose A M 1965 The subcultures of the ageing. In: Rose A M, Peterson W A (eds) Older people and their social world. F A Davis, Philadelphia

Rosenstock I M, Strecher V J, Becker M H 1988 Social learning theory and the health belief model. Health Education Quarterly 15 (2): 175–183

Ruff C 1982 Successful ageing: a developmental approach. The Gerontologist 21: 209–214

Schaie K W 1976 Quasi-experimental research designs in the psychology of ageing. Van Nostrand, New York

Schaie K W, Willis S L 1986 Can decline in adult intellectual functioning be reversed? Developmental Psychology 22: 223–232

Simsen B 1988 Nursing the spirit. Nursing Times 84 (37) (14th Sept): 31–33

Slater R 1988 Memory in later life: an introduction to the basics of theory and practice. In: Gearing B, Johnson M, Heller T (eds) Mental health problems in old age. Wiley, Chichester

Spector R E 1985 Cultural diversity in health and illness, 2nd edn. Appleton-Century-Crofts, Norwalk, Connecticut

Spector R E 1989 Heritage consistency. In: Dye C A (ed) Nursing elderly people. Recent advances in nursing series, No 23. Churchill Livingstone, Edinburgh

Strehlow M S 1983 Education for health. Lippincott nursing series. Harper and Row, Cambridge

Svanborg A, Berg S, Mellström D, Nilsson L, Persson G 1986 Possibilities of preserving physical and mental fitness and autonomy in old age. In: Häfner H, Moschel G, Sartorius N (eds) Mental health in the elderly. Springer-Verlag, Berlin

Townsend P 1981 The structured dependency of the elderly: creation of social policy in the 20th century. Ageing and Society 1 (1) (March): 5–28

Victor C 1987 Old age in modern society: a textbook of social gerontology. Croom Helm, London

Victor C, Vetter N J 1986 Poverty, disability and the use of services by the elderly: an analysis of the 1980 General Household Survey. Social Science and Medicine 22: 1087–1092

Volans P J, Woods R T 1983 Why do we assess the aged? British Journal of Clinical Psychology 2: 47–54

Walker A 1980 The social creation of poverty and dependency in old age. Journal of Social Policy 9: 49–75

Welford A T 1985 Changes of performance with age: an overview. In: Charness N (ed) Ageing and human performance. Wiley, London

Woods R T, Britton P G 1988 Cognitive loss in old age — myth or fact? In: Gearing B, Johnson M, Heller T (eds) Mental health problems in old age. Wiley, Chichester

Zivian M T, Myers 1983 Memory performance in the elderly: a function of daily activities. Gerontologist 23: 154 (Special issue)

CHAPTER CONTENTS

4

Health visiting and the elderly client

Health visitor students often raise questions about the care of persons in later life. Animated discussions are provoked by questions such as:

Many professions offer their services to elderly people; what does health visiting offer which is unique?

and

Does health visiting care offered to older persons, differ from that offered to persons in other age groups; if so, how does it differ?

The issues that lie behind these questions are complex, since they are concerned with defining a specific and possibly unique contribution to care on the one hand, yet raise ethical points about discrimination on grounds of age on the other. Many students recognise, also, that what health visiting can offer persons in later maturity depends on a blend of factors, not all of which lie within professional jurisdiction. Thus care is influenced not only by practitioner competence, but by the timing of the intervention, the expectation of clients, their particular needs and circumstances and the policies of employing authorities.

Some students and practitioners argue strongly that the particular developmental needs arising from the process of ageing justify a modification of practice with older people. This stance is reinforced by those who feel that recognising individual and developmental differences, and exercising more positive discrimination in favour of vulnerable groups, allows resources to be concentrated on those in greatest need. The extension of such thinking is therefore seen in policies of 'targeting'. A counter-view, however, is that labelling any group as 'different' increases the risk of stigma — in this case leads to agcism. Furthermore, others claim that as the strength of health visiting lies in its universal application, selectivity undermines the essence of the service.

While each of these viewpoints appears relevant, answers to the questions posed above can only really be found if one examines, *what health visiting is, what it seeks to be, and what it aims to achieve*. Then, through a comprehensive and rigorous research programme, process and outcome must be examined, to evaluate whether professional practice attains its goals.

In this chapter we can only concern ourselves with the intent of the professional activity, and so we discuss the matter under the following headings:

- the nature of health visiting
- the nature of the professional commitment
- the nature of the professional relationship

The frameworks and processes of health visiting care are then considered in Chapter 5.

THE NATURE OF HEALTH VISITING

The nature of any human service is constantly challenged and changed by the goals of the social mileu in which it operates, and by the varying capabilities and commitment of those who provide the service.

Freeman & Heinrich 1981

Clearly health visiting is no exception, since some of its distinctive features have arisen from earlier stages of professional development, having been moulded by the social and political influences then prevailing. Other characteristics stem from current definitions of the service. These not only indicate reality, but contain idealised elements, representing the service not only as it is, but what and how practitioners perceive it, or intend it, to be. Nevertheless the real situation may differ considerably from these perceptions and intentions. This is a significant point to note when considering the care of elderly people, because the health visiting role with this age group is currently underdeveloped.

FEATURES OF EARLIER HEALTH VISITING PRACTICE

Traditional features indicate that early health visiting aimed to stimulate self-respect and personal–social responsibility, through education, encouragement and participation. As agents of social change, the early practitioners offered an unsolicited, non-coercive and non-stigmatising service. These characteristics still mark present day practice. Such features appear relevant to the care of older people, who need to maintain their dignity, self-competence and independence, for as long as possible.

A pro-active service

Offering an unsolicited service meant that health visitors did not depend on referral before contacting potential clients; they *actively* sought out those who needed preventive or remedial help and proffered this.

However, proffering an unsought service might be considered by some people as an intrusive act, hence some older persons may perceive it as an invasion of privacy. This calls for great tact and sensitivity when making initial contact. Visiting by appointment, inviting older persons to express their views on the type of health care they require, and respecting their contribution and their idiosyncrasies, are ways of recognising rights and upholding dignity. Nevertheless, this nurturing of tenuous relationships until clients are ready and able to utilise care is not confined to elderly people.

A non-coercive service

Balancing the offer of an unsolicited, yet comprehensive, service must be the assurance that it is non-coercive. Care is therefore needed to ensure that the health visiting role is presented as enabling and non-authoritarian, with emphasis on client participation and self-determination.

Because health visiting generally operates on a universal basis, without qualification of need, it is usually perceived as non-stigmatising. Hence it emphasises self-respect and personal responsibility, as noted by Beatrice and Sidney Webb (see Ch. 1, p. 16).

OTHER EARLIER CHARACTERISTICS OF THE SERVICE

These features of earlier health visiting were enhanced by other characteristics. Whereas early practitioners came from several differing backgrounds, including medicine, the Council for the Education and Training of Health Visitors, soon after its inception, stipulated *nursing* as an essential pre-requisite for entry to health visitor training (CETHV 1969). This meant that, although many professional workers shared the perceptual, relational, teaching and planning skills used in practice, the particular combination derived from basic nursing, additional post-registration experience and the health visitor course, constituted a unique blend (RCN 1972, 1983).

Another characteristic, stressed by the Health Visitors' Association, was *the independent nature of the activity*, since practitioners initiated most of their care (HVA 1970, 1980). This did not mean that health visitors did not accept referrals, neither did it mean that they operated a solo practice without recourse to others. Rather it meant that, as qualified practitioners, they had the right to make their own judgements about health visiting needs, and to arrive at decisions about how best to meet these. Of course professional awareness, education, competence, attitudes and values clearly affected such discretionary decisions. This led to accountability for practice becoming a major professional issue (RCN 1983, 1984, UKCC 1984, 1989).

Furthermore the position of health visiting within the constellation of caring professions indicated another important characteristic: namely, *inter-dependence*. This was because the profession occupied the interface between medicine, nursing, midwifery, social work and teaching, having much in common with each of these disciplines.

A further definition of practice, which incorporated hallmarks of the service, was made following an intra-disciplinary participative exercise, which was held to re-appraise health visiting principles, in 1975–1977. The statement is reproduced in full here, because it encapsulates much that is believed about the nature of health visiting and hence much of what it is thought can be offered to clients.

> The professional practice of health visiting consists of planned activities, aimed at the promotion of health and the prevention of ill-health. It thereby contributes substantially to individual and social well-being, by focusing attention at various times, on either an individual, a social group, or a community. It has three unique functions:
>
> 1. Identifying and fulfilling self-declared and recognised, as well as unacknowledged and/or unrecognised health needs of individuals and groups.
> 2. Providing a generalist health service in an era of increasing specialization, in the health care available to individuals and communities.
> 3. Contributing to the fulfilment of these needs and facilitating appropriate care and service, by other professional groups.
>
> CETHV 1977

Similarities in this and other world-wide definitions of community health nursing can be noted (RCN 1983).

In addition to the definition above, four reformulated principles were agreed, which have since guided health visiting practice. Each of these has an application to the older client:

- the search for health needs
- the stimulation of awareness of health needs
- the influence on policies affecting health
- the facilitation of health-enhancing activities.

It is necessary at this point to extrapolate, from these various features, those which have particular relevance for present-day practice.

The value of an unsolicited service still prevails. Such a service is particularly useful for older people, who are less likely to seek help in the early stages of need, perhaps because they do not always recognise the significance or severity of events. Furthermore some older people are less articulate than others. They may lack knowledge concerning sources of available help, or have greater difficulty contacting these services. They may have a cultural tradition of self-sufficiency, and toleration of circumstances, even when these are adverse, yet remediable. They therefore frequently benefit from unobtrusive surveillance.

The non-coercive and non-authoritarian nature of the service is also still required. Especially is this so in the case of those fewer older persons who may regard practitioners as representatives of a threatening bureaucracy, causing them to react negatively to overtures of care. Such reactions may be heightened if older persons are striving to retain independence in the face of declining capacity.

An enabling, non-stigmatising service, which emphasises client autonomy, also remains highly relevant. However, Luker's study (1982) showed a small number of elderly women who perceived the health visiting service as 'intended for the ailing, the lonely or the disabled'. Consequently, when they became the recipients of the service they felt demoralised, their coping skills were undermined and they were not helped by the intervention. Recognising the relevance of such findings is important, as workers are frequently unaware of their client's perceptions of the service, or of the *unintended consequences* of health visiting intervention.

CONTEMPORARY CHARACTERISTICS OF THE SERVICE

These various characteristics, the definition and the principles, are embodied within:

- planned activities
- multi-focused practice
- comprehensive, co-ordinating and facilitating service.

Planned activities

The health visiting service for the elderly is, as for any other age group, designed to be systematic and purposive, rather than random or reactive. Thus, desirably, it is seen as planned and continuing, even when contact is intermittent. It operates on a long-term basis, from conception throughout life, on the premise that all activities designed to promote health and prevent ill-health in earlier years, contribute to a healthier old age. Given opportunity, it is intensified at periods of greater vulnerability. Most particularly it should direct its attention to those in young adulthood and in middle age, where its educative thrust can enable people to control those behaviour patterns and environmental hazards which build up problems for later life. It uses logical processes, identified conceptual frameworks, and models of care. It aims to:

- maximise independence
- promote optimum well-being within the limits of ageing
- improve the quality of life
- assist in the achievement of a dignified and peaceful death.

Multi-focused practice

To be effective, health visiting must be multi-focused, operating at individual, group and community levels. This means practitioners are not only interested in caring for individual elderly people, their families and the many groups in which older persons share experiences, but that they also consider the general population as well. Particularly this applies to aggregates of elderly persons within the practice area. This enables an epidemiological perspective to be adopted.

Epidemiology is defined as that field of science which examines the factors affecting the distribution and determinants of health and disease within populations. It includes the occurrence of deprivation, defect, disability and death, but focuses on the positive factors affecting health status as much as on the negative ones. Thus health visitors using an epidemiological approach are interested as much in discovering the reasons why a particular condition is *not* present among one aggregate of older people, as they are in determining why it exists in another similar aggregate.

For example, health visitors may find, through astute observation and scrutiny of statistics and patterns of consultation, that a certain segment of the elderly population appears exceptionally fit. Further study may show an association with certain behaviour patterns, calling for deeper investigation, so that all may benefit. Such rigorous assessment of the status of the elderly within the community, which utilises the search principle, can equally well discover poverty, loneliness, contentment or fulfilment. It is an essential prelude to informing the community about their elderly members, so that more imaginative participation can improve their care.

Through stimulating awareness of the health needs of elderly people, based upon epidemiological findings and community appraisal, health visitors can play their part more effectively in enhancing health (Fawcett-Henessy 1987). Unless clear statements about local needs and progress are regularly made to the public, health visitors will have little opportunity to influence policies affecting health. At a time when the wise utilisation of resources is uppermost in everyone's mind, community health initiative must also be cost-effective. This calls for further skilled and sophisticated communication and participation.

Comprehensive, co-ordinating and facilitating service

The health visiting service for the elderly should also be seen as comprehensive, co-ordinating and facilitating. Because of its generalist nature, across all age groups, and within a variety of settings, practitioners adopting an holistic approach are well placed to note family and community interrelationships. Thus they can also observe the multifactorial influences which operate on older clients.

Comprehensive health visiting care includes the dissemination of relevant findings to clients, carers and, where appropriate, to other team members. A pointed example is the observation of the effects of prescribed regimes upon older persons and their families. Where these effects are noted to be beneficial, the decisions of prescribing specialists are confirmed. Detrimental effects can probably be altered. An interpreting and advocacy role may therefore have to be assumed by health visitors, when visiting older clients or client groups, especially when such older persons are too nervous or overawed to tell 'experts' that they are not benefiting from their treatment. Such advocacy calls for courage and humility from practitioners. It should be undertaken only with client consent and in conjunction with client empowerment whenever possible.

Co-ordinating care becomes a particular challenge when older persons, with their multipathology, receive multi-specialist care. Discovering the ramifications of such care, and maintaining contact with all the agencies involved, can be very time-consuming, but is necessary to reduce the risk of a fragmented or depersonalising service. Elderly people often become confused, anxious or frustrated about prescribed treatments. They may therefore require help to decipher prescribed regimes, or to understand multiple drug therapy. The educational nature of health visiting means that practitioners can offer such help. They can also contribute to discussions on ethical prescribing for elderly people, make prompt referral of elderly persons to other workers, whenever their particular skills are required, thus reducing avoidably deteriorating situations, and can participate in case-conferences. Other co-ordinating activities include attending intra- and inter-disciplinary meetings, consultations, and the provision of informative, succinct reports.

Another aspect of facilitating activity lies in building up clients' confidence in the care they are receiving from other workers. A case study, involving an elderly widower, serves to illustrate this.

> CASE STUDY
>
> An elderly widower was receiving care from a district dietician as part treatment for his diabetes. When visited by an health visitor he expressed some anxiety about the inclusion in his diet of items he found unpalatable. He was assured the dietician would welcome a discussion. Contact was arranged and the client received a modified programme which enabled him to comply with therapy, yet enjoy his meals. He thus became aware that his wishes were regarded as important and his regard for those treating him was enhanced.

Contributive, facilitating service is also shown when health visitors work with students from different disciplines. During fieldwork practice they can help such students identify the needs of older persons and their families. They can emphasise the importance of shared care between client and various practitioners, and can enable students to differentiate the roles of other workers, whereby they can correctly select agencies for referral purposes. Presenting learning experiences which enable students to appreciate the intricacies of effective follow-up care, and encouraging students to liaise with other workers, can foster respect for particular roles and so enhance multi-disciplinary service.

Thus the role of health visitors with elderly clients can be seen to be both multi-faceted and dynamic. However, as already hinted, although these characteristics describe the nature of health visiting activity, the extent to which they are actually demonstrated in practice varies considerably. Influencing factors which may foster or constrain development include:

- the pattern of health needs presented by the elderly population in a given locality
- public expectations of the health visiting service and the attitudes shown by members of the public towards those health visitors caring for older people
- the size of the available workforce and the extent of the demand upon the health visiting service from competing vulnerable groups
- the organisational and administrative structures within which health visitors work
- the type and extent of health visitor education, and the attitudes of tutorial and managerial staff concerning health visitor involvement with older people
- the number and types of other workers with older people, operating in a locality, and the scope, format and aims of their care
- the expectations of the health visiting service held by these various other workers, as well as their attitudes towards the health visiting role
- national and local policies affecting the care of older people, especially those operating within the NHS.

The degree of financial and moral support afforded elderly people can also profoundly enhance or hinder their care.

Ensuring quality of care

The challenge of offering quality care to vulnerable groups such as elderly people, in spite of the constraints and influences just outlined, calls for flexibility, adaptability and professional courage. The RCN's Health Visiting Forum has addressed this task as a high priority. They recommend the utilisation of the three dimensions of quality identified by Donabedian (1966): namely, structure, process and outcome.

- *Structure* refers to the environmental, physical and organisational characteristics required in the service
- *Process* refers to the actions and behaviour which the professional worker is required to perform
- *Outcome* refers to the effect of the actions on patient or client.

Through small local groups of health visitors, working together with a facilitator, to set standards relevant to their own area of practice, standardised formats based on these three dimensions may be produced. An indexing system will then enable standards set in one domain of practice, to be related to similar ones set elsewhere. These standards can then be used to test and improve the quality of the service offered. They should be regularly reviewed (RCN 1988).

The need for greater flexibility and increasing attention to efficiency, effectiveness and quality of care, has also been recognised by Goodwin (1988). In an important Keynote speech, she stated

> health visiting is trapped in a tradition of routine home visits, child-centred models of practice and with few stated targets or specific objectives, which can be monitored. Professional credibility is being undermined by an inability to respond to other client groups, or to the changing pattern of health and disease. Heavy work loads and inadequate staffing levels, for now and the forseeable future, compound the situation. Consequently health visiting is at a cross-roads.

The way forward, Goodwin argued, is for health visitors to take the lead, and adequately to foster user-participation — targeting their services to specific client groups.

These factors suggest a more political dimension to the role. It is no longer sufficient, if indeed it ever was, for health visitors to concern themselves only with the provision of a personal service to clients and carers, important as this is. Research has to be initiated to more fully identify the health visiting needs of client groups such as older people and the best ways of meeting these. The role expectations held by health visitors, clients and other workers, have to be clarified, and congruence sought. Such expectations will then require to be tested against actual performance, so that valid, acceptable indicators can be determined. At times of fierce competition for scarce resources, claims for shares have to be justified. This requires that health visitors, in concert with their older clients and managers, clarify what constitutes an appropriate, accessible and available service. It entails practitioners being prepared to:

- increase their own professional monitoring
- develop assertiveness in arguing their case
- stimulate public interest in, and recognition of, their role with elderly people
- improve their knowledge-based practice through continuing education, training and research.

All these activities are embodied in the professional commitment.

THE NATURE OF THE PROFESSIONAL COMMITMENT

In discussing the rights and responsibilities of nurses and patients, Chapman (1980) emphasised the reciprocal nature of their contract. This reciprocity has been further discussed by Thorne & Robinson (1988), although they researched the issue in the context of chronic illness. This reciprocal perspective is in contrast to the traditional expectation, that clients and patients place absolute trust in their health care professionals, and embodies an element of client/patient trust in their own competence as well.

In health visiting elderly clients, health visitors may pledge themselves to offer safe, competent and accountable service. However, the extent to which clients can fulfil their side of the contract, by co-operating and undertaking agreed or recommended actions, is likely to vary. Although practitioners believe in the principle of client self-determination, (whereby each client exercises the right to decide what shall be done to help him or her, and how much care shall be carried out), the client's cognitive state may sometimes prevent this principle being fully implemented. It is then that client-carers are placed in the position of having to trust that actions taken will be in the client's best interests. Workers may have to accept a greater share of decision-making, and occasionally may have to take action for others as well as the client's safety. In such situations the worker may be cast in the role of *social control agent*.

Such situations increase the need for ethical and prudent behaviour, emphasising the importance of full consultation and collaboration with families, colleagues, and health visiting managers. Conversely, at times it may be necessary to champion the individual's cause, in the face of others' opinions. Elderly clients are often extremely vulnerable; they may on occasions need a skilled advocate, or even a protector. When confronting such issues, all aspects should be fully examined, and hasty decisions are inadvisable.

Professional confidence

Having studied the many facets thus far discussed in this chapter, and after examining the many reports which stress the need for increasing involvement with elderly clients, students may consider the work exacting and rather demanding. This may make them question their readiness for such tasks. This is a thoughtful and mature response, injecting realism and showing an awareness of accountability. However, although it is a commendable reaction, it is one that should provoke further thought and action to increase confidence.

Professional confidence stems from professional ability. In turn, ability rests on adequate professional education, the acquisition and maintenance of a valid knowledge base, appropriate professional values and traits, and a constantly updated repertoire of professional skills and techniques.

Steps were taken, soon after the inception of the United Kingdom Central Council for Nurses, Midwives and Health Visitors, to determine the competencies to be achieved at Registration (UKCC Statutory Instrument No 873, 1983). More recently, expected learning outcomes have been laid down for Project 2000, and the various National Boards have issued circulars for guidance (e.g. ENB 1989). Similarly, each National Board has laid down the competencies to be acquired by health visitors in their qualifying examinations. These will be modified shortly to take account of the new preparation for practice, at basic level. Moves are also afoot to determine standards for continuing professional education. Thus it is anticipated that professional standards will be maintained and improved.

Even so, it is important to appreciate that *professional ability* means more than high-level professional knowledge and technical competence. It includes being able to wield matching resources, such as equipment, space, information, access, and time. Only when this level is achieved is care more likely to be commensurate with knowledge and competence (Bergman 1981).

What does this mean for health visitors working with older people? The ability to care adequately for the older population rests largely on the capacity of health visitors to have access to *all* the elderly persons within their locality or practice population. Only in this way can they identify priorities, determine the health promotion needs of different groups, and hence offer appropriate contracts of service. For this access to be possible, some administrative device is required. This must be broad enough for representative measurement, but sharp enough to enable practitioners to detect susceptibility.

In the case of young children this need has long been recognised: it has been met through the national system of notification and registration of births. There is no similar national system of notification or registration of older persons. Indeed the desirability of instituting one is highly debatable. Some local systems exist, but, in the absence of a standard procedure, health visitors have been forced to find alternative ways of discovering their older clients. Relying entirely on methods of referral would be to negate the universal health-promoting and disease-preventing nature of their work. Such alternatives include age–sex registers, mainly in use within general practice settings; vulnerability indices; and/or computerised records of geographic or practice populations.

Nevertheless this situation is gradually changing. Since April 1987 every District Health Authority has been required to comply with central demands for minimum data, as outlined in the Körner Report (DHSS 1984) and Memoranda (DHSS 1987). This capturing of data on computer should enable health visitor managers to supply maps giving details of relative need across a community. It should enable priorities to be determined, staff time to be directed where it is most needed, and the relative dependencies of clients to be evaluated for case-load purposes.

Further impetus to the identification of need and resources management should also be given when Family Practitioner Committees are obliged to ensure the introduction of computerised information systems in every general medical practice. To date it has been estimated that fewer than 40% of those health visitors working in general practice settings have had access to age–sex registers of the practice population. Fewer than 10% have an efficient cross-referencing system.

Additionally there are other examples of under-resourcing which affect the ability of health visitors to care effectively and creatively for older persons. They include:

- inadequate supplies of equipment
- unsuitable premises
- insufficient time and space in which to conduct health advisory consultations
- a paucity of appropriate tests for determining levels of dependence.

Furthermore, deficits in supportive social services often render meaningless the detection of need and referral for help. However, this may change when the new recommendations on Community Care are implemented, and if they are adequately resourced as to make them a reality (DSS 1989).

Another factor affecting professional ability concerns the low staff–population ratios. These have been very arbitrarily determined: the standards so set have not been fully realised, and this often means that within busy generic case-loads there are too few health visitors to meet the needs of older people.

Part of the professional task is to point out such deficits and to call for remedial action. This may be particularly difficult in times of financial stringency, and calls for professional courage. In the past, practitioners may have accepted under-resourcing as almost inevitable and so may not have pressed firmly enough for redress. It is now clear that such behaviour constitutes a negation of the professional commitment, and does gross disservice to clients. It also infringes the UKCC code of conduct (UKCC 1989).

PROFESSIONAL RESPONSIBILITY

Closely linked to professional confidence and professional ability, is professional responsibility. This is defined as *'a mandate, or charge; a trust, for which, if accepted, one becomes answerable'* (Batey & Lewis 1982a). Responsibility as a charge, should not be confused with *being responsible*. This latter term refers to a personal attribute, which all professional practitioners should demonstrate.

Responsibility for the care of elderly persons can only be accorded to health visitors when practitioners have recognised the content and implications of the charges being assigned them, and have signified their willingness to accept these. Sometimes health visitors have accepted roles and functions assigned to them, without necessarily questioning whether or not these fell legitimately within their professional province. Moreover, they have not always considered whether they have the professional ability (in the broad sense in which it was discussed earlier) to fully implement these duties. Now there is a growing realisation that it is *not* a negation of the spirit of vocation, to submit roles and functions to the 'reality test'. Neither clients nor communities can benefit, and they may in fact even be harmed, if duties assigned are accepted and then cannot be fulfilled.

Moreover, effective responsibility requires *authority*. Such authority may be derived from the power of position, from professional knowledge, or from the situation (Batey & Lewis 1982b). Responsibility without authority undermines professional confidence. It reduces professional autonomy, and creates intense frustration, as many health visitors ruefully discover when they find themselves powerless to implement assignments. An incident of this nature, all too common, is described in the case study of Miss T.

CASE STUDY

Miss T, aged 70 years and severely arthritic, was sent home late one Friday afternoon from the local casualty department, having been treated for a fractured right wrist and severe bruising of shoulders and legs. Follow-up care was requested and the health visitor asked to assess the situation and mobilise appropriate services.

Miss T lived alone. She was clearly only marginally independent in normal circumstances, so it was apparent that domestic assistance and facilitating aids were urgently required. Additionally she needed nursing care. This last was quickly arranged, but authority to provide domestic assistance and aids is vested in another administrative department — the Local Authority Social Services Department. Because of timing, help could not be obtained immediately. Miss T had thus to depend on the goodwill and services of her neighbours, until alternative arrangements could be made, several days later. Although such community help is to be encouraged, it is not always available, or appropriate.

ACCOUNTABILITY: MEANINGS AND MEASUREMENT

Another facet of the professional commitment concerns accountability, to which we have already made some reference. There are several definitions, including those of Bergman (1981), Batey & Lewis (1982a), RCN (1984) and the UKCC (1984, 1989). We have chosen the definition given by Murray & Zentner (1975):

> Accountability is being responsible for one's own acts, and being able to explain, define, or measure in some way, the results of one's own decision-making.

Accountability thus includes notions of purpose, disclosure, justification, evaluation and reckoning.

It refers to acts of commission (what *is* done) and to acts of omission (what is *not* done). Accountability may be direct or indirect. Where delegation occurs, there is no abdication of responsibility or accountability.

Accountability is also multiple. In health visiting older persons, while the primary focus is towards the client, account must also be rendered to other carers, to peers and colleagues, to employing authorities and eventually to society. Self-accountability is also important. Moreover, although practitioners may pledge themselves to provide safe, efficient and appropriate care for older persons, it must be appreciated *that this must be seen to be done*. By contrast with hospital settings, where work is mainly publicly observed, the interactions between older clients and health visitors are often conducted in the mostly unobserved privacy of homes. Consequently accountability can only be indirectly demonstrated. This is done mainly through the the record of the visit, the documented health care plans and the stated, pre-determined criteria for evaluation.

Documentation raises many issues. These include the authenticity of records; practitioner integrity, objectivity and perceptual ability; standardisation and comparibility of records; and confidentiality (UKCC 1987). The comprehensiveness and ready availability of health visitor records are thus central to accountability. They should be:

- accurate
- relevant
- contemporaneous
- legible
- concise
- fulfilling legal requirements.

Records should contain a written declaration of the purpose of each visit, making health visiting activity explicit to any reader. Aims, objectives, plans, interventions and outcomes of care should be clearly stated, having been decided upon in partnership with clients and client-carers. Sharing records in this way reduces misconceptions and facilitates continuity of care. Some health visitors find that documentation based on the health visiting process assists systematic recording (see Ch. 5 pp. 99–111). For some practitioners the sharing of records with clients is an innovation. Others may be uncertain about implementing the idea, because they fear the negative aspects of accountability, or the potential risk of managerial censure, sanctions or control. This calls for discussion and managerial support.

At present most health visitor records for older people contain biographic data, medical-social history, brief details of personal and situational progress, and practitioner's assessment. Process recordings of action taken, details of interactions, subjective perceptions and evaluations are rather less common. This could be a serious drawback to health visitors if the system of peer review were to be implemented. Already, medical audit is being introduced. It is highly likely that this could be extended to other professional health care staff. If a small group of independent but professional peers, checking retrospectively for evidence of quality care, had insufficient data on which to base their evaluations, then inadequate or false judgements might be made. At a time when computerisation is being implemented, an urgent review is required of documentary standards, record formats, storage, retrieval facilities, and the time required to correctly and adequately complete necessary documentation.

Meantime, health visitors need to give careful attention to the way they explain, disclose and report their assessments, plans, interventions and outcomes of care. Such safeguards may be even more important when dealing with older clients, who are so often over-tolerant, or uncritical of their care, or who may, at times, experience distortions of reality (RCN 1989).

THE NATURE OF THE PROFESSIONAL RELATIONSHIP

Closely linked to the professional commitment, is the quality of the professional relationship. This is one of the most sensitive aspects of the care of older clients. Through such relationships clients present their needs and expectations and practitioners demonstrate their knowledge, skills and attitudes. By exchanging information, ideas and feelings, both parties can learn and develop. Such a relationship, however, depends on the extent to which both persons feel comfortable within it, can trust each other, act freely and show respect for each other. In order to achieve this, honesty, integrity and reliability must prevail.

Older people come to these relationships with a different, and sometimes much wider, frame of reference than do practitioners. By virtue of their age they have long histories, clear identities and much life experience. They have filled many different roles, often very competently. They have encountered various status transitions and developed different coping strategies, which they can bring to bear on current situations. Some of their attitudes towards old age will have derived from their perceptions of it in others. However, their experiential learning will depend upon their circumstances, their personality attributes, cognitive abilities, physical and mental health and the rate and form of their ageing. Sometimes, therefore, elderly people may be interested, tolerant, upset, or puzzled about either their ageing or their state. They may also exhibit marked differences in their reactions between the 'young elderly' and 'the very old'.

Not all older people grow old gracefully. Some become rebellious, cantankerous, hostile or aggressive. Others may be dejected, apathetic or confused. A few may project their feelings onto practitioners. While many are likely to show indomitable spirit and, having spent many years developing independence, will be reluctant to lose it, a few may become over-dependent. Others will have developed a philosophical manner and some show marked humour. They may frequently indulge in light-hearted banter, gentle teasing, or use jokes to ease their tension, increase rapport, test out practitioners, or demarcate the boundaries of the relationship. Recognising the value of humour, and using it at times to motivate clients, may therefore be an important health visiting technique (Armour 1974, Ebersole & Hess 1985).

Ethnic and cultural influences also affect the behaviour of older people, sometime explaining the somewhat strong reactions they may show towards others' dress, speech or manner. Recognising and allowing for these differences, perceptions and language; addressing older people in terms which afford them dignity; and taking account of their value systems, are, therefore, essential courtesies.

At times in the professional–client relationship, older persons may associate professional workers with authority-figures from their past. This can sometimes evoke reactions which appear incongruent in present circumstances. Conversely, they may sometimes over-identify with the parental or grandparental role, regarding practitioners as 'children', and becoming over-solicitous, over-protective, or even dominating in their manner towards them. Awareness of this phenomenon of transference can help health visitors to deal with emotional reactions from clients, which seem inappropriate. They can also try to use the particular mechanism to help propel older clients towards mutually desired goals.

Another point is that sometimes older people feel they 'should have all the answers', because they have lived so long. In such circumstances they may feel ashamed to reveal their needs, admit weaknesses, or ask for help. They may then display bravado, tend to over-compensate for problems, or adopt such stances as 'what can you teach me?'. Such responses, especially the latter, may prove disconcerting to an inexperienced health visitor. Under such circumstances it is helpful to realise that it is the professional knowledge, derived from education and experience, which enables workers to contribute effectively.

Occasionally, older clients react by listening politely and concurring with all suggestions-only to ignore them afterwards! When this happens health visitors need to search for interest and relevance in what they are recommending, since this is often the key to motivation. However, many older people are outgoing and co-operative, eager to relate and appreciative of help given. They therefore bring very positive contributions to the relationship, and can often teach practitioners much. The research findings of Käppelli (1987) and Thorne & Robinson (1988) extend thinking on this matter.

Nevertheless, the relationship is *not* one-sided.

Like clients, practitioners are also constrained by their personality attributes, life experiences and attitudes (Käppelli 1987). Their frames of reference, drawn from personal and professional life, may clash with those of clients, thus creating potential misunderstanding. Sometimes health visitors unconsciously react to older clients on the basis of former relationships with their own parents or grandparents. They then demonstrate countertransference. One student found that she was virtually unable to implement professional-type care, because she cast herself into the role of 'daughter' to a particular elderly client. Prior awareness of such risks can help practitioners guard against them, but, if such situations do arise, they should be discussed with a senior professional colleague, in order to allow effective work to continue with the client.

Occasionally anger, or fear, may enter into the relationship, because workers have not resolved their own reactions to ageing. They may have difficulty handling the dependency–independency conflicts which clients sometimes exhibit. If practitioners have hitherto regarded all older people as 'near-omnipotent beings', they may sometimes experience revulsion at the helplessness of some frail old people. Additionally there may sometimes be over-attachment to, or over-possessiveness of, some older clients, especially if they have appealing attributes.

Recognising the gamut of possible reactions evoked in work with the elderly can enable health visitors to develop the disciplined and objective approach which is needed to care effectively, so that they maintain professional rather than social relationships. This may be facilitated if the team approach is adopted, with joint responsibility for case-loads being held.

The basic ingredients of professional relationships between clients and practitioners include acceptance, empathy and purposive communication. These apply equally to contact with any age group.

Acceptance

Although sometimes used rather glibly, conveying an impression of resignation, or weakness, acceptance is, in fact, a very active concept, meaning a ready acknowledgement of client uniqueness and worth. It does not mean agreeing with inappropriate behaviour, but it does include the belief that elderly clients, as all others, have the right to continuing professional attention, regardless of their behaviour. It includes responding to older persons in a positive and non-judgemental manner, without either altering one's own standards or imposing these on others.

Not everyone is easy to accept. Nevertheless, reaching out to older clients, even when they show negative reactions, can enable practitioners to gain insight into the reasons for their behaviour. Caring for clients is thus displayed through the sustaining of helping contact with the less attractive, as well as with more gracious and responsive older people.

One of the many interesting examples of acceptance, demonstrated by a student assigned to study the care of an older person, is described in the case study of Miss E.

CASE STUDY

Miss E, aged 79 years, was a former nursing sister, now partially disabled after a cerebrovascular accident. The client lived alone in a ground-floor flat, and her querulous and demanding manner had alienated many of her neighbours and most of her relatives, so that she became isolated and depressed. The health visitor student initiated and maintained an openness of contact, refusing to be daunted by the client's carping comments. Focusing on their shared experiences, the student elicited accounts about the client's earlier rigorous nursing training. This helped her to understand Miss E's high expectations of care, and explained some of her exacting behaviour. Over several weeks the student led the client on to express and explore some of her fears about total dependency, discussing the hurt she had experienced when the image of herself as 'one in command' had been forced to change to 'one needing help from others'.

Frequently Miss E reverted to acid comment; often she compared her own treatment, unfavourably, with the care she felt she had given to others. At times she abruptly terminated visits, or scorned suggested interventions. Each time the student pointed out the inappropriateness of such behaviour, but maintained the open relationship, until the client, somewhat grudgingly at first, allowed her to mobilise much-needed services. Eventually a small cadre of caring workers were able to assist Miss E to maintain optimal functioning, within her own home and within the limitations of her own lifestyle.

Empathy

Empathy is the ability to see the problems and needs of others, as it were through their eyes, in order to appreciate their reactions and attitudes. It differs from sympathy, in that objectivity is retained, in order to offer non-emotive help. Because older people are often the victims of pity, they look to professional practitioners to offer them deeper understanding and more practical help. Practitioners display their empathy through the medium of verbal and non-verbal communication, and in the marshalling of resources to meet need.

Empathy can be developed, provided that workers have warm, flexible personalities, the capacity for imaginative thought, perceptual and social skills and a readiness to listen. Interpretation and insight can also be fostered, especially if practitioners maintain sound physical, mental and emotional health and can control their personal stresses, freeing themselves from undue anxiety and negative emotions, which distort perception.

Communication

Communication forms an essential part of all health visiting. It requires special skills and has been studied and discussed by many practitioners and researchers, including Raymond (1983), Montgomery-Robinson (1986) and Fisher (1988). In the care of elderly people, however, communication is not only particularly important, it is also extremely complex. It is important because it is a vital ingredient in maintaining relationships, thus enabling mutual understanding to be developed between elderly clients, practitioners and others. It serves to prevent the client's social isolation, affording scope for client participation. It is through communication that assessment can be made, goals be mutually determined, plans developed and explanations given.

Nevertheless, it is complex, because communication in elderly people is often hampered by sensory or neural deficits which result from the ageing process. For example, there is generally slower word-association and word-retrieval with advanced age, greater dysfluencies, more frequent interjections, word repetitions and dysrhythmic phonations. In addition, presbycousis (auditory deterioration associated with ageing) leads to some loss of hearing acuity, especially for higher-pitched tones. Consequently, older people often have more difficulty in hearing women's and children's voices, and may miss certain consonants, so that speech intelligibility is affected. Furthermore some 60% or more of older persons have specific hearing impairments, while the majority of those with visual disabilities are also elderly (see Ch. 10, pp. 247–251).

Thus while all the rules for successful communication on verbal and non-verbal levels apply equally to the elderly client, special attention must be given to those older people who experience difficulties. This includes those with sensory deprivation; speech impairments arising from stroke or other neurological disorders; perceptual difficulties; disturbances of affect, such as depression or emotional illness; or suspicious elderly people. Those who are non-English-speaking also need special consideration. Deliberate techniques may have to be selected; hence close liaison with speech therapists is recommended.

A useful tabulated list of techniques, modified for application with elderly clients, is given by Leitch & Tinker (1978). A summary of important helping functions for communication-disordered older persons, is also given by Ebersole & Hess (1985). This important issue is further addressed by MacLeod Clark et al (1987), Fisher (1988) and MacLeod Clark (1989).

One helpful maxim, often quoted concerning communication, is that professional workers should be noted for their large ears, wide eyes and small mouths! (Schulman 1974, Beaver 1983).

SUMMARY

This chapter began with two questions: one concerning what health visiting could offer to older persons, the other regarding what differences, if any, such care might involve. By exploring the nature of the professional activity and examining the earlier and contemporary characteristics of health visiting, together with the principles, values and goals of the profession, some inferences have been drawn about the forms and directions of future care. There are, however, many issues about the nature of the service, which demand further discussion.

The professional commitment was examined, because the service which health visitors can render elderly persons rests on practitioner ability, responsibility, accountability and sense of vocation. The professional relationship has been discussed in some depth, because it constitutes the medium through which care is given, although principles, rather than detail, have been emphasised.

That there are differences sometimes in the way health visitors offer care to older clients, compared with other age groups, has been indicated. However, these have been seen to be related to individual differences, heterogeneity within patterns of ageing, specific developmental needs, levels of functional ability and client uniqueness. Throughout the discussion the emphasis has been directed towards stimulating thought about what underlies health visiting activity for any age group, but chiefly, in this context, for older people. In this way we hope readers will have derived answers for themselves, to the questions asked.

At a time when existing health visiting work with older clients is considerably under-rehearsed, it is our contention that the profession has much to offer the older client — given that practitioners resolve some of their equivocalness, and given that essential resources are forthcoming to allow professional claims to be fully demonstrated.

REFERENCES

Armour R 1974 Going like 60: a light-hearted look at the later years. McGraw Hill, New York

Batey M V 1982a Clarifying autonomy and accountability in nursing service. Part 1. The Journal of Nursing Administration(Sept): 13–18

Batey M V 1982b Clarifying autonomy and accountability in nursing service. Part 2. The Journal of Nursing Administration(Sept): 10–15

Beaver M L 1983 Human service practice with the elderly. Prentice Hall, Englewood Cliffs, New Jersey, p 75

Bergman R 1981 Accountability: definition and dimensions. International Nursing Review 28 (2): 53–59

CETHV (Council for the Education and Training of Health Visitors) 1969 Fourth Report. CETHV, London

CETHV (Council for the Education and Training of Health Visitors) 1977 An investigation into the principles of health visiting. CETHV, London

Chapman C M 1980 The rights and responsibilities of nurses and patients. Journal of Advanced Nursing 5: 127–136

DHSS 1984 5th Report of the Steering Group on Health Services Information, Chairperson: Mrs E Körner. HMSO, London

DHSS 1987 First edition of Körner implementation statement of central requirements for aggregated returns on Community Health Services. Ref No 36, DHSS, London

Donabedian A 1966 Evaluating the quality of medical care. Millbank Memorial Fund Quarterly 44 (Pt 2): 166–206

DSS 1989 Caring for people: community care in the next decade and beyond. White Paper, November. HMSO, London

Ebersole P, Hess P 1985 Towards healthy aging, 2nd edn. Mosby, St Louis

ENB (English National Board for Nursing, Midwifery and Health Visiting 1989 Circular): Project 2000 'A new preparation for practice. Guidelines and criteria for course development and the formation of collaborative links between approved training institutions with the NHS and centres of Higher Education'. ENB, London

Fawcett-Henessy A 1987 The future. In: Recent Advances in Nursing series, No 15, Littlewood J (ed) Community nursing. Churchill Livingstone, Edinburgh, p 170–194

Fisher V 1988 Toil and trouble: the work of health visitors versus the trouble telling of elderly clients. MSc Dissertation, University of Surrey, Guildford

Freeman R B, Heinrich J C 1981 Community health nursing practice, 2nd edn. W B Saunders, Philadelphia, p 36

Goodwin S 1988 Whither health visiting? Health Visitor 61 (December): 379–382

HVA (Health Visitor Association) 1970 Health visiting manifesto. HVA, London

HVA (Health Visitor Association) 1980 Health visiting in the 80's. HVA, London

Käpelli S 1987 A matter of definition. Nursing Times 83 (44): 67–69

Leitch C, Tinker R 1978 Primary care. F A Davis, Philadelphia, p 475–480

Luker K 1982 Evaluating health visiting. RCN, London

MacLeod Clark J 1989 Nurse–patient interaction. In: MacLeod Clark J, Hockey L (eds) Further research for nursing: a new guide for the enquiring nurse. Education for Care series. Scutari Press , London, Ch 11, p 113–121

MacLeod Clark J, Kendall S, Haverty S 1987 Helping nurses develop their health education role. Nurse Education Today 7: 63–68

Montgomery-Robinson K 1986 Accounts of health visiting. In: While A (ed) Research in preventive community care. Wiley, Chichester

Murray R B, Zentner J 1975 Nursing concepts for health

promotion. Prentice Hall, Englewood Cliffs, New Jersey, p 123

Raymond E 1983 The skills of health visiting. In: Owen G (ed) Health visiting, 2nd edn. Bailliere Tindall, London, p 221–231

RCN (Royal College of Nursing) 1972 The role of the health visitor. RCN, London

RCN (Royal College of Nursing) Health Visitor Advisory Group, The Society of Primary Health Care Nursing 1983 Thinking about health visiting. RCN, London

RCN (Royal College of Nursing) Health Visitor Advisory Group, The Society of Primary Health Care Nursing 1984 Further thinking about health visiting: accountability in health visiting. RCN, London

RCN (Royal College of Nursing) 1988 Standards of care: health visiting. RCN, London

RCN (Royal College of Nursing) 1989 Standards of care: health visiting. Published for the RCN by Scutari Press, Harrow, Middlesex

Schulman E D 1974 Intervention in human services. Mosby, St Louis

Thorne S E, Robinson C A 1988 Reciprocal trust in health care relationships. Journal of Advanced Nursing 13: 782–789

UKCC (United Kingdom Central Council for Nurses, Midwives and Health Visitors) 1983 Statutory Instrument No 873, Sections 18–24: Rules concerning competencies to be achieved at Registration. UKCC, London

UKCC (United Kingdom Central Council for Nurses, Midwives and Health Visitors) 1984 Code of professional conduct for the nurse, midwife and health visitor, 2nd edn. UKCC, London

UKCC (United Kingdom Central Council for Nurses, Midwives and Health Visitors) 1987 Confidentiality — an elaboration of clause 9 of the 2nd edition UKCC's code of professional conduct for the nurse, midwife and health visitor. UKCC, London

UKCC (United Kingdom Central Council for Nurses, Midwives and Health Visitors) 1989 Exercising accountability: a framework to assist nurses, midwives and health visitors to consider ethical aspects of professional practice. UKCC, London

FURTHER READING

National Standing Conference of Representatives of Health Visitor Education & Training Centres 1989

Health visitor education and training: the way forward. Report of a Study Conference Weekend. National Standing Conference of Representatives of Health Visitor Education & Training Centres

CHAPTER CONTENTS

5

Frameworks, models and processes of health visiting care

Chapter 4 took as its theme what health visiting is or seeks to be, and therefore what it can offer the elderly client. This chapter is related, in that it discusses *how* health visiting the elderly may be carried out. It uses a conceptual approach, rather than a firm recipe for practice, on two main counts. First, there are as many differing health visiting situations as there are clients; hence practitioners need to be flexible in their response. Understanding the theoretical ideas and principles which underlie practice helps health visitors to adapt and apply these to differing circumstances. Second, although health visiting is essentially a practical activity, its practitioners require a body of knowledge which is constantly reviewed and updated, a matching range of skills and techniques, appropriate attitudes and traits and carefully considered professional and personal values.

Examining these various components can help one draw inferences about how this particular professional activity might best be demonstrated. In the space of one chapter it is clear that the scope for exploration of theory is limited. However, we offer some notions in the hope that they may provoke thought and discussion, and stimulate students and practising health visitors to explore them further.

KNOWLEDGE

Knowledge is acquired in two ways. The first way is to seek out theories which are held by others, examine these and then draw inferences which can be applied to one's own practice. A plumber does this, for instance, when he makes use of theory from the science of physics and the associated laws of hydrodynamics, to enable him to repair a leaking pipe. This deductive approach — reasoning and inferring from the general to the particular — was adopted in Chapters 2 and 3, when we studied the ageing process. It is also the method much used in nursing and health visitor research (e.g. McClymont 1982, Copp 1987, Goodwin 1987, Walker & Campbell 1989) and in education, where curricula are based on theories from various disciplines. This approach is helpful, especially if one constantly challenges the presented theories and if the deductions made and inferences drawn for practice are regularly reappraised and tested (see Fawcett & Downs 1986, Jennings 1987, Holter 1988).

The second way of acquiring knowledge is through the inductive method, inferring general laws from particular instances. Events encountered in practice are carefully observed, then defined, described and classified, before being used to generate hypotheses which can then be tested. Rigorous evaluation of empirical ideas in this way means the theory is then grounded in practice. Health visitors are increasingly employing this method, either by carrying out investigations themselves, or by studying other practitioners' work and then testing out their ideas within their own practice. Examples from nursing and health visiting are given by Benner (1983), Benoliel (1983), Clark (1983, 1985), Hunt & Montgomery-Robinson (1987), Leininger (1987), Chao (1989). Such action is a necessary process, because if health visiting is to establish itself as a scientifically credible and socially useful discipline, it must collectively identify and refine its concepts and test its theories and principles (CETHV 1977, 1979).

CONCEPTS: THE FIRST STAGE IN THEORY BUILDING

Some readers may wonder why a chapter about how elderly people may be cared for within health visiting practice should begin so theoretically. The answer is that it is the concepts, or global ideas or constructs which workers hold, which largely determine how they operate. Therefore, concepts may be regarded as the first stage in theory building, and such knowledge will eventually underpin practice.

Health visiting employs many intricate concepts, but all too often they are taken for granted, being held and used implicitly, in the mistaken belief that everyone else acknowledges and understands them. Unfortunately this belief can sometimes lead practitioners into conflict, because different meanings are attributed to words and ideas. Therefore, differing frameworks underlie care — causing variation in practice. Since practice rests on knowledge, theory development consists partly in making concepts explicit, and then analysing them. This is an issue stressed by many writers, including Dickoff & James (1968), McFarlane (1977), Riehl & Roy (1983), Parse (1987), Falco (1989) and Kim (1989).

The concept of holistic care

Fundamental to the way health visitors relate to, and care for, elderly clients are the ideas and beliefs they hold about people. Believing that they are biological, psychological, social and spiritual beings, who live in matching environments, health visitors claim to adopt an integrated approach, based on the assessment of the whole person. This notion has given rise to the concept of '*holistic care*', a term increasingly used in nursing practice generally (Passant 1990). Of course this does not mean that health visitors regard themselves as responsible for the entire and sole care of clients; rather that they see the client as the prime determiner of his or her needs, and workers as seeking to provide complementary help in order to meet these needs, in each of these different dimensions. Although the idea is sound, full implementation may sometimes be very difficult. Nevertheless, practitioners strive towards this goal as part of their role as one of the major caring professions.

The concept of health

Another concept basic to health visiting care is the concept of health, since the aim of all practice is to promote optimum well-being. However, although most practitioners have strong ideas about what health means, a precise definition is difficult, so consensus is lacking. Nevertheless, the way health is perceived, and the way in which health visitors consider elderly persons to be healthy, or not healthy, affects the ways in which they deliver care. Thus the frameworks and models used for health visiting action rest upon fundamental beliefs.

Five different conceptions of health are now considered. Each gives rise to particular models of care, which are relevant to health visiting practice with elderly people. These five conceptual ideas are:

- health as the absence of disease
- health as a positive state
- health as a fluctuant experience
- health as independence in living
- health as adaptation.

Health as the absence of disease

Traditionally health was perceived as freedom from disease. Logically, therefore, the model of care which followed was the medical one. Using this framework, disease must first be identified and then differentiated, so that a diagnosis can be made. However, diagnosis rests upon knowing and recognising the unique course which each disease follows, as well as the specific signs and symptoms which are exhibited. For this reason a knowledge of aetio-pathology and the natural history of diseases becomes necessary. Once diagnosis has been correctly established, specific remedies can be applied, which hopefully will lead to cure or control of the disorder. Thus a knowledge of therapeutics and the principles of evaluation applied to follow-up, in order to determine outcomes, are other necessary components. Of course, where natural resistance, or specific therapy, are ineffective, deterioration and/or death may follow.

Like all nurses, health visitors are very familiar with this conceptual framework. Much of their basic nursing education currently rests on it, and the prescribed elements of their role frequently stem from it. Practitioners adopting this concept and its derived model can, therefore, engage in secondary prevention. They act on the assumption that if disease can be detected early, preferably at the pre-symptomatic stage, it may be more amenable to treatment. It is for this reason that screening and surveillance, together with case-finding, form part of health visiting functions with elderly people (see Ch. 6).

Similarly, tertiary prevention can also be justified. By accepting referrals, and carrying out surveillance and follow-up of those elderly persons with established disorders, or prone to disease and/or disability, health visitors can help to ameliorate their effects.

Community application of this concept allows for an epidemiological approach to be adopted. It aims at identifying health and disease states in aggregates of elderly people, and the causal environmental influences and stressor agents which act upon older hosts. In this way health visitors play their part in the control of community disease.

However, the limitation of the concept of health as the absence of disease, is that it focuses on the pathological process, rather than on the person and is therefore rather negative in approach. If health visitors were confined only to the medical model of care, which this concept generates, they would be less likely to engage in health promotion activities, or undertake primary prevention. This would of course negate their professional values. It might also give less job satisfaction, since fewer older clients may achieve complete freedom from disease. For these reasons most health visitors adopt alternative frameworks on which to base their care, although they use this concept and its derived model as an adjunct (see also van Maanen 1988).

Health as a positive state

This framework, established by the World Health Organization, defines health as

> a state of physical, mental and social well-being and not merely the absence of disease or infirmity.

This positive concept lays emphasis on *potential* — with total well-being as the goal for which to aim. Thus health visitors using the developmental

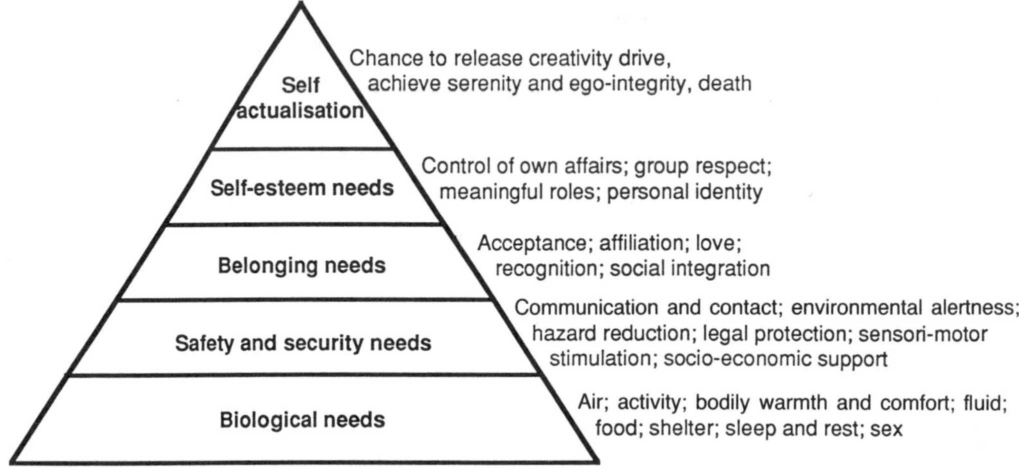

Fig. 5.1 Maslow's pyramidal model of human needs, adapted for use with older people (after Maslow 1954, Ebersole & Hess 1985).

model which derives from this concept, direct their efforts, not to finding out what is wrong, but rather towards improving optimum performance in all three realms. Major activities are therefore concerned with personal and community development, health education and health promotion.

The hierarchy of needs model, adopted by Maslow (1962, 1987) (see Fig. 5.1), is based on similar notions, and Ebersole & Hess (1985) have usefully applied it to the older client. Using this concept at the level of individual client care, efforts are first directed towards discovering and meeting basic biological and safety needs, so that attention can be next directed towards increasing client self-esteem and sense of belonging, and thence self-realisation. Such an approach has much to commend it, and many health visitors make use of the concept, or of Maslow's model, albeit implicitly. Nevertheless, many practitioners are aware that it is much easier to identify and meet clients' lower-order survival needs than it is to help older people feel loved, protected and fulfilled. However, it is in endeavouring to achieve these higher-order levels of well-being, that the main challenge to high-quality health visiting care lies (Houldin et al 1987).

Health as a fluctuant experience

The positive state described above has been criticised by some as being unrealistic, hard to achieve and almost impossible to measure. One such critic, Dubos (1959) regarded health as a mirage: *not a state, but rather a dynamic process*, with the organism striving constantly against a changing environment, in an effort to achieve homeostasis.

This striving towards well-being and balance underlies Dunn's approach (1959). He perceived health as a fluctuant but dynamic experience, rather than a constant state. Consequently he depicted health as a continuum, ranging from high-level wellness at one end, to imminent death at the other (Fig. 5.2). Individuals were then seen as occupying positions at different points within

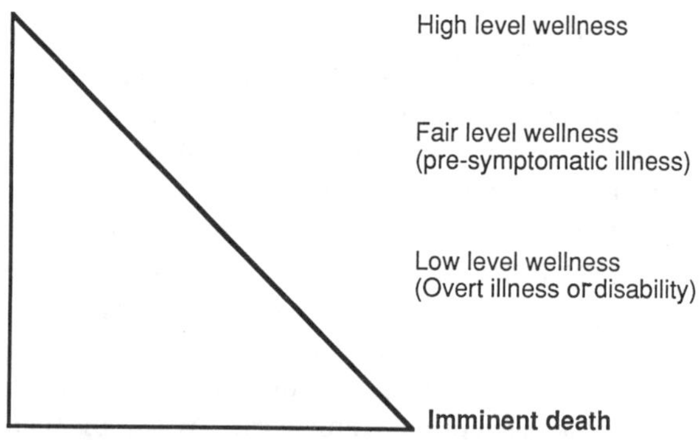

Fig. 5.2 The health-illness continuum-health conceptualised as a fluctuant experience (after Dunn 1959).

these two poles, depending on the degree of environmental threat they faced and their levels of personal resistance at any one time. This notion of health status as differing from day to day, is one which seems highly pertinent to elderly people, who so often have a very tenuous grasp on well-being and may shift their hold very readily.

Health visitors adopting this concept require data to enable them to estimate and plot the position of their elderly clients along the health continuum. They can then determine the amount and direction of care needed to bring these older persons as near as possible to high-level wellness.

A version of this model was used by Hobson & Pemberton as far back as 1956, when they coined the phrase 'effective health levels', to help study functional ability in elderly people. 'Good effective health' they applied to those functionally independent elderly people who were maintaining reasonably high levels of well-being. 'Fair effective health' denoted those who were housebound and somewhat functionally restricted, but nevertheless were coping, in spite of medium-to-low levels of well-being. 'Poor effective health' was used to describe those who were physically and mentally unwell and dependent.

A later example of the use of this concept of health as a fluctuant experience is shown by one general practitioner (Williams 1979). He used a modified version to help him categorise elderly people in his practice. In this way he identified 4% as being at the lowest point of the health continuum, thus allowing him to deploy scarce medical resources more effectively. He was then able to identify 36%, whom he considered in 'fair effective health'. Although they were coping, they were in danger of being overwhelmed, and thus slipping further down the health scale. Thus he considered they required more medical surveillance than the 60% whom he graded as being in 'good effective health'. Health visitors can learn much from these examples. For instance they can be caused to think about devising criteria for recognising levels of well-being among their elderly clients, as a prelude to priority-setting in caseload management. The concept can also remind them of the precarious balance some older people experience, in health terms, and hence alert them to the need for constant vigilance. It is a particularly useful concept for practitioners working within team settings, where doctors and district nurses can direct their main efforts towards secondary and tertiary prevention and health visitors can concentrate on promoting and maintaining the health of the apparently well majority of older people.

Health as independence in living

Closely allied to the concept of health as a fluctuant experience, with the derived notions of health levels, is that of health as independence in living. The strength of this idea is that it focuses, not so much on an individual's limitations, but rather more on how well he or she can manage within these. Thus even those who are experiencing illness or disability are regarded as achieving some level of health, commensurate with their levels of independence. For many older people, health is often subjectively equated with their level of functional ability and independence.

This idea is somewhat similar to that propounded by Roper et al (1980, 1983, 1985, 1990). For over two decades the ideas underlying their 'Activities of Living' model have been worked on and refined. From this thinking, a model specifically for nursing has been derived. These writer–researchers regard individuals as holistic beings, constantly active and uniquely striving towards independence and self-fulfilment, throughout their lifetime. This individuality and independence is demonstrated through 12 common activities of living, which are in turn strongly affected by five main influencing factors: physical, psychological, sociocultural, environmental and politico-economic (Fig. 5.3).

Under this model individuals are perceived as moving unidirectionally and inevitably along their life-span, while at the same time occupying fluctuating positions on an independence–dependence continuum, for each activity of living. Clearly the various activities are closely related to one another. Together they constitute a complex global concept. At certain periods of life, when individuals undergo developmental or role transitions, such as in retirement, or when illness or accident occur,

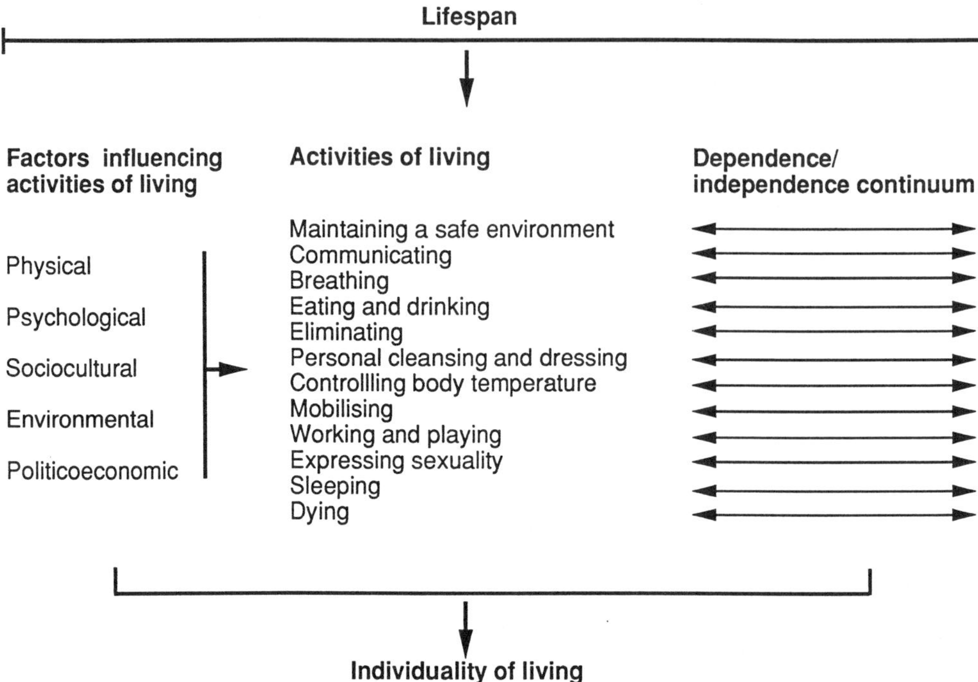

Fig. 5.3 The Activities of Living Model (after Roper et al 1990; reproduced by kind permission of the authors).

independence may be threatened. The level achieved may then be altered. Plotting the person's position on the independence–dependence continuum can provide a profile and hence pinpoint the action which may be required to help them achieve greater independence.

Health visitors, like nurses, are therefore regarded as having an enabling role. They may enable persons to *retain* their independence by preventing or alleviating threats to their functioning, or they may facilitate the *regaining* of independence if it has been lost. One health visitor/researcher considers this model is well suited to the care of older people.

> It would provide a frame of reference which would make assessments or surveillance by health visitors meaningful, in giving quality of life for the elderly its due recognition.
>
> (Luker 1982a)

An example of one way in which this model might be applied to the care of a very old client, thus demonstrating the concept of health as independence, is given at the end of this chapter, in Tables 5.1 to 5.3 and Figures 5.4 and 5.5.

Health as adaptation to stress

This last concept perceives health as synonymous with adaptation. The theory, which is based on ideas propounded by Selye (1956), postulates that throughout life individuals are constantly bombarded with stimuli from changing internal and external environments. They respond to these stress-stimuli by a series of inherent and learned behaviour patterns, which are designed to maintain or restore equilibrium, comfort and stability. Sometimes, however, stimuli are overwhelming; then balance is lost. In such circumstances individuals need help to regain homeostasis.

According to this concept, therefore, health visiting intervention is logically directed in two ways: one directed towards manipulating the stimuli, so as to minimise their harmful effects; the other focused towards strengthening the coping abilities of individuals, groups and/or communities, so that they can adapt and achieve balance. This idea appears relevant to the care of elderly people, who have had long experience in adapting to different types of stress situations, and who have developed coping abilities in consequence. Furthermore, older people are often susceptible to upsets in their circumstances, because their adaptive processes become more delicately poised. Whereas a younger person might easily shrug off a simple infection, in the frail elderly person it may constitute a crisis. Changing house; modifying life-style, as in retirement; losing supportive networks such as a helpful neighbour leaving the district; coping with a chronic disorder; or the loss of a loved person or pet, may prove devastating to an older person.

Health visitors make use of this concept of health as adaptation when they use anticipatory guidance techniques; advocate prophylaxis; develop systems to predict potential crisis events and then institute 'early warning measures'; or mobilise resources to meet needs and so strengthen and support vulnerable elderly persons. Four main nursing models currently make use of this concept:

- The Neuman Health Care Systems Model (Neuman & Young 1972, Neuman 1980)
- The crisis intervention model (Caplan 1964, 1974)
- Roy's adaptation model (Roy 1970, Riehl & Roy 1983)
- The stress adaptation model (Saxton & Hyland 1979).

Within the constraints of this chapter, only the first model is discussed here. A summary of the other three together with some additional models used in nursing generally, and which may have some application to health visiting, plus one specific health visiting model, is given in Appendix 3.

The Neuman Health Care Systems model depicts individuals as unique beings who constantly face stresses, to counter which they have certain *lines of defence*. These are conceptualised as:

- an outer or *'flexible line of defence'*, which is constantly utilised to maintain equilibrium
- a second or *'normal line of defence'* which is brought into action when stressors breach the flexible line of defence and disturb host equilibrium.
- still deeper *'lines of resistance'* which help to stabilise people and return them to equilibrium, when stresses are overwhelming and have overcome normal and flexible lines of resistance.

One health visiting practitioner considers that the Neuman model fits well into the nature and purpose of health visiting, because it sees the individual as being mostly in balance, and the practitioner's job as being to maintain that steady state (Clark 1982a, 1982b). When this model is used in practice, it fits well into the framework of primary, secondary and tertiary prevention, which characterises health visiting care. For example, primary preventive care is directed both towards reducing the possibility of individuals' encountering stresses, and strengthening their *'flexible lines of defence'*, through raising their general and specific resistance and improving their coping abilities. Secondary preventive care, recognising that deviation from normal balance has occurred, seeks to repair the breach quickly, through early detection and prompt treatment. In this way the *'normal line of defence'* is strengthened, so that balance can quickly be restored. Tertiary preventive care is employed when balance has been lost in physical, mental, emotional, social or spiritual realms, and the client needs help to enable him, or her, to readapt, and thereafter maintain stability. Thus the *'deeper lines of resistance'* are restored and the client re-educated to help prevent further stress-reactions.

An example of how the Neuman Health Care Systems model might be used in health visiting practice is given in the case study of Mrs Rosina Black, and in Tables 5.4–5.7 at the end of the chapter.

The significance of models

Models therefore provide a way of thinking about professional activity and offer some guidance for practice. They are made up of a number of concepts, and they serve to assist practitioners in organising their thoughts and justifying how and what they do. However, Chalmers (1989) points out that their present level of sophistication calls for further evaluation and the refinement of concepts. In this way they act as precursors of nursing and health visiting theory.

Links between concepts, models and behaviour

By now readers will probably have perceived some linking of ideas between the various concepts of health, as just discussed. They will have noted some similarities, as well as differences, in the models associated with them and seen some overlap in the inferences drawn for practice.

However, it is not only health professionals who formulate frameworks to help them think about health, people and environments, and so plan and implement their activities. Clients also have their notions about what constitutes health; beliefs about the causes of ill-health; and ideas concerning prevention and treatment. The entrenchment of such health perceptions, and the strong cultural and class beliefs influencing them, are reflected in the health behaviour of older people, as Dunnell & Cartwright (1972) have shown.

This variation in conceptualisation between clients and health visitors, or other workers, can mean that each may pursue very different approaches and therefore set different goals in care. This is one reason why it is so important to make ideas *explicit* and to seek to find some congruence in perceptions (Lau et al 1982, van Maanen 1988, Thorne & Robinson 1988b, Allen & Hayes 1989).

This is of particular relevance in relation to health education, which is designed to effect change in behaviour. In this latter context the *Health Belief Model* (HBM) may be pertinent. This postulates that health-related actions depend upon the simultaneous occurrence of three facts:

1. That an individual is sufficiently motivated or concerned about his/her health as to give it priority
2. That the individual believes that he/she is personally susceptible to a serious health problem, or the sequelae of same (i.e. there is a perceived health threat)
3. That the individual believes that if he/she follows a particular health recommendation, the perceived health threat will be reduced. The cost of the action involved in both personal–social and economic terms must not exceed the benefits to be derived, or this will constitute a perceived barrier to action (Becker 1974, Janz & Becker 1984, Rosenstock et al 1988).

Endeavouring to discover client health beliefs and concepts, bearing in mind the HBM, assists practitioners in selecting health care goals in line with such beliefs (see also Ch. 8, p. 179–181).

Another way to reduce the possibility of 'clashes of ideas' concerning health and health care, is to adopt one particular model for all staff to follow. This is a mode in some hospitals, or educational establishments, but is less common in community settings. It has certain merits, since all involved are aware of the concept-base and are hence more likely to adopt similar viewpoints in organising care. However, it may prove restrictive; so retaining an eclectic stance may be preferred. Those who wish to explore these various issues further are referred to Binnie et al (1984), Clark (1985), Parse (1987), Akinsanya (1989).

SKILLS IN HEALTH VISITING PRACTICE

In concurrence with Argyris & Schon (1974), we believe that

> learning a theory of action, so as to become competent in professional practice, does not consist of learning to recite the theory: the theory of action has not been learned in the most important sense, unless it can be put into practice.

Hence, for this reason, the concepts discussed above, which form an important part of an health visitor's knowledge base, must be accompanied by commensurate skills and appropriate attitudes, traits and values. These various components are then welded together in the process of delivering care — in this context, to older people. Thus health visiting may be regarded both as *a science and an art.* Possibly no other client group needs this special blend more than do older persons.

The dictionary defines skill as 'adroitness, dexterity, expertness, ingenuity, or practised ability'. Thus an idea is conveyed of smoothness in execution of a task, procedure or technique.

Skills may be practical or intellectual, and those used in health visiting are as diverse as the clients and their settings. The CETHV (1967), Raymond (1983) and Luker & Orr (1985) have discussed these skills in some detail, relating them to health visiting knowledge and the practitioner role. The various National Boards have also defined the competencies required at qualification. However, in the care of the elderly client, certain skills assume even greater importance. They are briefly considered below, under the following headings, even though in practice it is difficult to separate them:

- perceptual skills
- inter-relational or social skills
- teaching and counselling skills
- skills in organisation, planning and decision making.

Perceptual skills

Because old people are often reticent about their state, are sometimes unaware of the significance of events, and frequently display non-specificity in illness, with atypical symptoms, the *observational* and *interpretive* skills of the practitioner must be highly developed (see Chs 2, 3, 4, 9, 10).

Astute observation includes learning to read body language as it is displayed through posture, facial expression, gesture and dress. Often the relaxed attentive position, or the blank uncomprehending stare, the covert twinkle in the eye, the nervous movements of the fingers, or the vague responses in conversation, tell their own story. Similarly, so do gross or subtle changes in personal appearance, or surroundings. Study of the environment helps practitioners to note the presence or absence of artefacts, such as books, photographs, pictures, ornaments, radios, television sets, or of pets. All of these may give some clues to personality and lifestyle; to interests, mood or status. Particular resources, or specific problems, may be discovered through an unobtrusive examination of the environmental layout.

Of course nursing education will have helped to develop skills in observation, listening, and interpretation, while health visitor preparation should enhance awareness and insight. However, each practitioner has the ongoing responsibility to sharpen and refine these abilities. The perceptual skills of the health visitor will also be extended to any family or group members with whom the older client may have contact, as well as to the community of which they form part. Identifying community needs and perceiving levels of community support for, and involvement with, elderly clients, are important adjuncts to personal client care.

Inter-relational and social skills

Closely allied to perceptual skills are those used in developing inter-personal relationships. These include the techniques of verbal and non-verbal communication already touched on in Chapter 4. *Interviewing skills* are particularly relevant to elderly people, since it is within the context of purposeful conversation that rapport and confidence are developed and information is elicited which is pertinent to care. The importance of relationships with older people has already been stressed, and the point made that full reciprocity may not always be possible with older clients. These various issues have been discussed by Wahl (1980), Dobson (1987, 1989) and Thorne & Robinson (1988a).

However, modification of these inter-relational skills is related to the slower reaction time which may be present, the constraints of sensory ageing, sometimes the narrowing of the client's social networks so that suspicion and hesitancy initially characterise contact, or the limitations of physical illness and/or disability. Whenever possible, contact should be made in a quiet environment, with few auditory or visual distractions. Health visitors should sit reasonably near to, and facing, clients, in a good light to facilitate lip-reading if necessary. Sometimes it may be helpful to kneel beside less mobile elderly persons. Enunciation should be distinct, with rate slightly slower, pitch rather lower, and volume rather stronger than for younger persons, although shouting and elaborate speech mechanisms should be avoided.

While *'leading'* is a technique frequently adopted by health visitors, it must be used selectively with elderly people. Closed-ended questions, which are used to elicit specific data, usually of a factual or biographic nature, can sometimes give an impression of catechisation. They should be introduced in awareness and with care. Similarly, while open-ended questions are usually preferable, since they promote understanding and help communication flow, they can lead to irrelevancies, clouding of original issues, or confusion.

Teaching and counselling skills

Mention has been made in several places of the teaching skills of the health visitor. For older people these skills are frequently employed on a one-to-one basis, or in small groups. Contact may be in the home, or in clubs, day centres, clinics, residential homes, or similar settings. Teaching may involve work with larger groups, not always composed of elderly persons themselves, but of those seeking to understand the needs of older people. Teaching skills include information-giving, demonstrations, conducting discussion groups, lecturing, participation in exhibitions, the mounting of displays, and participation in special programmes including festivals, health fairs, radio or television. Socio-drama is a technique much enjoyed by some older people, so health visitors may make use of this during health education sessions (see also Ch. 8, p. 175).

Each of these activities requires different skills, as well as a wide knowledge about educational and group processes. When applied to older people, practitioners require to take account of *relevance, motivation, the constraints of ageing, differences in learning styles, the need for spaced repetition and the time required to consolidate learning* (see also Ch. 3, p. 59).

Counselling differs from teaching in that it encourages clients to become more aware of alternative courses of action, inviting them to take the lead in problem solving and decision making. In work with older people, such counselling may often relate to decisions about the type and settings of future care. Counselling is also a skill much used with carers of elderly persons. Some practitioners say they have found it useful to take additional study in the techniques of counselling, after they have gained initial health visiting experience.

Skills in organisation, planning and decision making

Closely linked to, and utilising, the previous skills, are those affecting the organisation and management of a caseload. The ability to identify need and determine priorities, especially from a welter of competing demands, is clearly of relevance to elderly clients. They do not always recognise their own needs and may play down, or ignore, the severity of some difficulties. Skill in *exercising judgment, weighing up the relative merits of alternative strategies, as well as the timing and execution of tasks*, also fall under this heading. Similarly health visitors may head up a team of other workers, so they need to be able to exercise skills in appraisal, delegation, supervision and control. They require skills in leadership, the motivation of others, in the wise deployment of resources, especially personpower, and in facilitating job enrichment.

Planning must also take place at the community level. Strategies frequently have to be developed with different groups who are involved with elderly people, so that collaborative programmes can be undertaken. Sometimes such plans may be longer-term, in which case practitioners may find themselves fostering and stimulating interest and motivation, so that persons, especially volunteers, do not grow 'weary in their well-doing'.

ATTITUDES, TRAITS AND VALUES

What nurses and health visitors *do* depends not only on their educational and professional ability, but also on the type of people *they are* — the attitudes and

expectations they bring to their work, as well as the organisational frameworks within which they operate.
(Hockey 1979)

These organisational frameworks are discussed in Chapter 6, while some of the attitudes which practitioners need to display are mentioned in Chapter 4. They include positive attitudes towards accountability, commitment, acceptance and empathy. However, with elderly people, *approachability* is a much-valued trait, since little can be achieved if older clients feel practitioners are remote from them. Flexibility, tolerance, a high degree of self-knowledge and awareness, adaptive capacity, resourcefulness and initiative are also required. Other necessary traits include humour, practicality, a spirit of co-operation and willingness, and an appreciation of professional values. Perhaps tenacity in the face of difficulties is one of the most valuable assets, since frustration is common in health visiting activity! Additionally creativity and a readiness to innovate and act as an agent of social change is important.

It is easy to depict an 'ideal type' of practitioner; such a paragon rarely exists. However, warm and insightful workers with a variety of different traits and an enthusiasm for their work, can learn to develop attitudes appropriate to the care of older clients, provided they are patient and willing to do so. Most of all, practitioners will find they can learn much from their older clients, so that they can benefit from the contact as well. This is most likely to happen when practitioners are prepared to make the effort to work within the clients' value systems, and develop respect for their culture (Dobson 1989).

PROCESSES OF CARE

Processes of care involve not only the knowledge, skills, attitudes and values held by practitioners, but also the service received by clients. Health visitors use several different processes in the course of their work, including those involving research, communication and team-building. Sometimes these may be used concurrently, although their foci and goals may vary. Only the health visiting process is discussed here.

THE HEALTH VISITING PROCESS

More recently there has been an effort to make explicit the process by which practitioners systematically identify, describe, define and classify initial events, situations or problems. Additionally attention has focused on *how* they plan and implement care. This sequence has become known as the health visiting process. It has similar elements to the nursing process, with which practitioners may also be familiar.

A number of students and practitioners find this systematic approach helpful as a means of co-ordinating their knowledge and skills and enabling them to structure their work, so that they can clearly see what they are doing, and where they aim to go. Furthermore, when such data are adequately recorded, other persons, including clients and client-carers, can see how decisions have been reached, which goals are to be attained, and how outcomes are to be evaluated. Thus they are informed about the rationale of care. Such records need not have complicated formats, although their initial completion is likely to be rather more time-consuming. They should eventually save time, when practitioners and others can see at a glance exactly what is intended for a particular client, and can quickly pick up the threads from a previous visit, or take over from a colleague. Of course no recording system should ever be allowed to become a ritualistic performance, but kept flexible enough to follow, rather than dictate care.

Some practitioners find the mnemonic *SOAPIER* helps them to check out the sequences of the process. These are ordered as follows:

S subjective data gathering — or what is said, stated as perceived
O objective data gathering — or what is observed
A analysis and interpretation of data – in order to assess total situation and set aims
P planning — immediate, intermediate and longer term
I implementation — the action taken to put plans into operation

E evaluation — judging results against goals set and relevant pre-determined criteria
R review and re-organisation — re-assessing and revising plans as necessary.

Subjective data gathering

Gathering subjective data is of paramount importance when working with older people, because practitioners are often unaware of their clients' perceptions of problems, or their expectations of care. This activity should not be confused with the *issue of subjectivity*, to which of course everyone is prone. An example of subjective data gathering is given in the case study.

CASE STUDY

An elderly female, living alone, with limited social support. Has severe varicose veins, arthritis and general circulatory problems.

Aim of visit: to encourage greater activity and independence.

Subjective data: 'I cannot follow your advice to increase my walking, because I cannot put on the (prescribed) support stockings.' 'I have tried stocking appliers but I do not have the strength to manipulate them, because of pain and stiffness in my hands and weak muscles. I suppose it is the arthritis.' In response to a question regarding client perception of her needs: 'Someone from the health or social services should visit me daily to help me put on these stockings. How else am I going to prevent my condition from worsening?'.

Because such help was not forthcoming, nor had any alternative measures been proposed, the client was frustrated, upset and critical of services.

Subjective data give scope at individual level for estimating congruence between health visitor and client perspectives. It can equally be applied at group and community levels of care. The possibility of effectively stimulating an awareness of health needs, facilitating self-help and encouraging people to take positive steps to help control their own ageing, will not occur unless one has a clear grasp of *their* views and goals.

Objective data gathering

Practitioners will realise that this must be as comprehensive and factual as possible; hence observation and measurement must be widely employed and validated. The risk of subjectivity should be borne in mind.

Sight can point out incongruities in the client's view of his or her domestic state, food supplies, general amenities, or coping ability. Smell reveals the presence of soiled linen, stale food, damp housing, inadequate personal or domestic hygiene, the presence of animals, or the characteristic odour of specific diseases. Touch indicates temperature, skin texture, muscle tone, and may reveal problems. Cognitive analysis and assessment can be made through listening to the client's answers to questions, which involve thinking, memory, judgement, problem-solving, or the carrying out of simple instructions.

However, whenever possible, these observations should be supplemented by the use of valid measurements. These include not only the recording of vital signs, such as temperature, pulse, respiration, blood pressure, weight, height, and skin folds, but blood tests, urine analysis, and screening tests for vision and hearing as applicable. The measurement of pain levels and the use of health questionnaires and life satisfaction indexes, such as those used by Neugarten et al (1961), Luker (1982a) and Salmon & Hodkinson (1989) are other examples. These forms of measurement are relevant to health visiting practice, even though the practitioner may not obtain them all herself, and is not engaged in clinical nursing duties.

Analysis and assessment

Analysis

Analysis refers to the interpretations that the health visitor undertakes when studying the collected subjective and objective data. It enables the practitioner to make 'an health visiting diagnosis', concerning the nature of actual and potential problems (Dobson 1988). The term *'problems'* in this context refers to any aspect on which it is necessary to take action or potential action, especially related to preventive functions and health promotion.

Assessment

This term refers to the practitioner's estimation concerning the total client situation. It uses prior history and current subjective and objective data concerning client and client-family, as related to the potential for positive health functioning.

The development of an appropriate operational assessment tool for each model, when there are so many models from which to choose, might prove an area of consternation for those health visitors who seek a framework for their care. In the constraints of this chapter it is not possible for us to give detailed examples of suggested operational tools for each of the models we have described earlier. This would, however, be a useful exercise for students and practitioners to undertake, and one that fieldwork teachers might find helpful. Instead, mention is made below of some operational frameworks, with more detail being given for two of the models at the end of the chapter. These are 'The Activities of Living' model and the 'Neuman's Health Care Systems' model. In presenting these two illustrations, it should be noted that care needs have been met at the individual level only. Each illustration deals with an 'oldest old person', receiving mainly tertiary preventive care. This in no way negates our contention that the major role of the health visitor lies in primary prevention. The examples are intended to complement examples of primary and secondary prevention discussed in other chapters (particularly Chapters 6 and 8). Furthermore, the illustrative use of these two models does not imply superior merit.

Some operational tools for assessment

Those who advocate the use of the *medical model*, and conceptualise health as mainly the absence of disease, are most likely to use the *body-systems framework* for their assessment. Headings will then be adopted such as:

- sensorimotor state
- mental–emotional state
- nutritional state
- circulatory and respiratory state
- elimination and skin state
- sleep and bodily comfort state
- economic and environmental state.

This approach was used by Price (1981) 'to assess from head-to-toe'; it is also advocated by Ebersole & Hess (1985) and by Houldin et al (1987). The advantages and disadvantages of this model and its associated operational framework are discussed by Smith (1983).

Those who conceptualise health as a positive state and therefore adopt *a developmental approach*, are more likely to use a human needs framework. They may use Maslow's example and formulate headings such as:

- physiological needs
- safety needs
- belonging needs
- self-esteem needs
- self-actualisation needs.

Others may use Bradshaw's taxonomy (Bradshaw 1972), with the framework of normative needs, felt needs, expressed needs, and comparative needs. A framework more commonly adopted by health visitors using this concept and associated model employs such headings as physical needs, mental and emotional needs, social needs, spiritual needs, financial and environmental needs.

When health is viewed as a fluctuant experience, the operational assessment tool used is likely to reflect functional ability related to levels of wellness. This approach adopts the method used by Houldin et al (1987). Their headings included 'functional health patterns' as follows:

- Health management — health perception
- Nutrition — metabolic
- Elimination
- Activity — exercise
- Sleep — rest
- Cognitive — perceptual
- Self-perception — adaptive response
- Role — relationships
- Sexuality — reproductive

- Coping — stress tolerance
- Spiritual support.

The idea that health is synonymous with independence in living is a *combination of the developmental approach, a systems approach and the functional ability framework*. Here the assessment tool determines client ability in a number of common activities. The 'Activities of Living' model is one such framework, illustrated in Fig. 5.3. It is used as an example at the end of this chapter (Tables 5.1–5.3 and Fig. 5.4 apply).

Lastly, when health is regarded as adaptation, the operational assessment tool logically takes account of the stresses which clients encounter and their response patterns. Thus headings might include

- stress agents
- client perceptions of stress stimuli
- adaptive/maladaptive behaviour patterns
- client coping mechanisms
- client expectations.

This approach is illustrated in the second case study, which involves the assessment of an elderly female client and uses the Neuman model (Tables 5.4–5.7 apply). For illustrative purposes these details have been elaborated rather more than might be possible to record in practice; however, they may serve as a guide to the data required, the cues and inferences. Readers will note a detailed care plan is *not* given in this case. Furthermore the possible use of such an assessment tool, as with the others, is open to debate.

Nevertheless, students and practitioners will recognise that whichever frameworks and headings are operationalised for assessment purposes, the approach *must always be systematic*. Data collected should relate to each dimension of client need, even though the ageing process may modify the techniques which can be used to gather information. In order to ensure comprehensive care, health visitors should try to obtain as much family and community data as they can (see Appendices 1 and 2). Such data act as background information, reducing the risk of inaccuracies and consequent skewing of care. They also help to set the client into context and so enable the health visitor to work with and help families and communities (see Chapters 4 and 6).

Planning care

Once subjective and objective data have been obtained, cues noted, inferences drawn and analyses and assessment made, the major needs/problems can be identified and the problem-solving process begun. This also utilises 'health visiting diagnosis'. This term means 'a professional decision, or opinion, formed after careful consideration of all relevant material'. If it is not a familiar term, this formulation should not be confused with a medical diagnosis. The differences lie in the nature of the problem investigated, and the assessment made reflects those needs which can best be dealt with by health visiting interventions.

The goals or care will therefore be mutually determined, and will reflect the client and family behaviour patterns, and their culture. Immediate goals will shape short-term health care plans. Likewise, longer-term goals will cover broader activities and will include the overall aim of health visiting intervention.

Whenever possible, these goal statements should be given in behavioural terms. Goals should always be concise, feasible, relevant, and realistic. Plans derived from them should be personalised, comprehensive yet succinct, so that others can quickly detect purposes and proposed action. Where possible the time-scale expected for the accomplishment of the specific activity should be given. However, this is sometimes more problematic when visiting elderly clients, whose reactions may be less predictable. Every participant in the planning process, including other team members, must be clear about their own and others' responsibilities.

Implementation

This is an highly active phase of the process. It constitutes a record of all the activities involved in endeavouring to reach the set goals. It therefore includes all that clients, carers and significant others, as well as practitioners, *do* to accomplish the goals. Active participation is the keynote of this phase; hence each step should be monitored to check that it fulfils part of the overall plan.

Evaluation

Health visiting practice should be evaluated with respect to both client outcomes and the process or care. Without measuring outcomes against desired goals it is not possible to identify or compare client progress. Without measuring the care process it is not possible to demonstrate how far the health visitor practitioner has contributed to care (Luker 1982b). The secret of effective evaluation lies in determining relevant and clear criteria. Client outcomes can then be assessed against these predetermined criteria and related to the goals set. The criteria for determining process, however, and hence health visitor contribution, must relate to *effort, efficiency* and *effectiveness*. Negative as well as positive evaluation should be encouraged, since setbacks as well as successes can indicate which courses of action should continue and which must be changed.

Review and reorganisation

As a result of the evaluation against set goals, plans should be reviewed and reorganised. Reassessment may well be needed. New goals may have to be mutually established, new actions considered. The whole activity is thus seen as a dynamic, interactive and continuing process, which operates throughout a client's life.

For further reading on the application of the health visiting process readers are referred to Clark (1982b), Burgess & Ragland (1983) and Luker & Orr (1985). The application of the process to care of elderly clients is covered quite extensively by Ebersole & Hess (1985).

SUMMARY

This chapter has examined the practice of health visiting the elderly, within the context of knowledge, skills, attitudes, traits and values. It has looked at how health visiting may be undertaken with elderly clients, using a conceptual approach rather than a detailed account of procedures. It has particularly explored ideas of holistic care and health, seeing these as basic to health visiting practice. Attention has been directed towards the various models which may be used as frameworks for care. The assumption is that an explicit model of care is likely to assist the practitioner to structure her diverse observations and to reach a knowledge-based assessment, so that this judgment can then be explained in a written record for others to follow. The need for a systematic approach to the delivery of care has been stressed at a time when the unstructured nature or some health visiting is a controversial issue.

Two case studies have been given to illustrate possible ways of applying these specific models to the assessment and care of older people. However, it has not been possible to discuss the application of appropriate models to group and community level care. This is undertaken to some extent in Chapter 8.

Underlying the chapter has been the belief that a major part or the health visiting role with the elderly is to encourage older people to take a lively interest in the preservation and enhancement of their own well-being, as a means of controlling some of the problems associated with ageing. Emphasis has also been laid on the priority to be given to improving the quality of life for older clients, through a consideration of their views and expectations.

If some readers are disappointed that they have not been given more detail about specific procedures related to practice, we can only point out that the strength of a professional preparation is that it provides its members with principles, concepts and theories, in order that professional judgement may be exercised in their application.

If the reality of practice is thought to fall short of the intent and potential of the service, as discussed here, it may be that this indicates a need for professional re-examination of the professional activity. This re-examination we suggest should include role performance, service priorities, cost-effectiveness of activities, and an exploration of how best to render quantifiable the qualitative data relating to prevention. It is only by measuring outcomes against specific objectives, that health visitors will have the performance indicators needed to justify their present and continuing role.

If one reason for any incongruence between professional intent and professional performance is gross under-resourcing and underdevelopment of the health visiting service, could it be that the time has come for a corporate posing of the question 'Can society afford to ignore the preventive care and health promoting role which health visitors, given the resources, could offer its middle-aged and elderly members?'

CASE STUDY
Mrs M L Davison, an elderly woman, living alone

Mrs M L Davison, aged 88 years, normally lives alone and copes well. She sustained a fall while gardening, twisting her left ankle and causing extensive bruising to her left leg and both arms. She was relatively shocked. Medical aid was summoned by a neighbour. After initial examination and diagnosis, Mrs Davison was prescribed Ponstan 100 mg tds and advised to rest with her left leg elevated. Cold compresses were advised tds and a supportive Tubigrip bandage was applied to her left foot and ankle. Because she had difficulty weight-bearing and could not easily manage personal dressing or washing, nor cope with domestic duties, she was invited to stay with her daughter, Mrs Penelope Charger.

Mrs Charger is a retired teacher, married and living with her husband in another district of the same town as her mother. Mrs Davison and her daughter and son-in-law do not get on well. Nevertheless Mrs Charger signified her willingness to care temporarily for her mother, during the post-trauma period.

At a short meeting of members of the primary health care team, decisions were made that clinical nursing care was not required. However, it was agreed that Miss Brand, the health visitor, who had been paying surveillance visits to the client, at 4-monthly intervals, should visit Mrs Davison at Mrs Charger's address, to maintain continuity. Miss Brand arranged to pay an assessment visit and subsequently maintained a supportive and teaching role to the client and her family.

Table 5.1 Example of health visiting history, for Mrs Margaret Davison

SURNAME	*FORENAMES*	*MARITAL STATUS*	*DATE OF BIRTH*
Davison	Margaret Louisa	Widowed 1974	21.2.1901
ADDRESS	*TEL. NO.*	*FORMER OCCUPATION*	*RETIREMENT DATE*
1 Lower Street Old Town Boldsworth	223344	Biology Teacher	1961
NEXT OF KIN	*ADDRESS*	*RELATIONSHIP*	
Mrs Penelope Charger	6 Brook Street New Town Boldsworth	Daughter	
PRESENT RESIDENCE AND COMPOSITION OF HOUSEHOLD			
Staying with daughter at 6 Brook Street, New Town, Boldsworth Self (Client) Mrs P Charger — Daughter — Retired Teacher (62 years) Mr F Charger — Son-in-Law — Engineer (64 years)			
SIGNIFICANT OTHERS			
Name	*Address*	*Relationship*	
Mrs Barbara Thomas Mr David Thomas Paul Thomas	6 West Street, Taunton S/A S/A	Granddaughter Grandson-in-law Great Grandson (8 years)	
HEALTH CARE TEAM			
Mrs V Jones Miss J Brand Dr B Quick	District Nursing Sister Health Visitor General Practitioner		
ADDRESS	*TEL. NO.*		
Health Centre, Old Town, Boldsworth	556677		
CLIENT'S HEALTH HISTORY			
Prolapsed uterus, treated by pessary insertion 1974. Cataract operation, lens extraction Rt eye 1972; Lt eye 1974. Fractured lt wrist 1977. Has osteo-arthritis; occasional vertigo. 2-yearly medical appraisal carried out by General Practitioner. 4-monthly health surveillance carried out by Health Visitor.			
SIGNIFICANT SOCIAL HISTORY			
Husband died Jan 1974 (former solicitor) Son Killed 1975 (road traffic accident)			
DETAILS OF PRESENT EVENT			
Twisted/sprained left ankle due to fall while gardening. Unable to weight-bear at present. Has extensive bruising of left leg and both arms. Complains of pain; was initially shocked. Neighbour called GP who prescribed Ponstan 100 mg tds for pain relief; elevation of left leg with application of cold compresses tds × 2 days. Tubigrip support applied. District nursing help not sought, as client temporarily transferred to care of her daughter who 'feels she can manage for a time'. Referral from Dr Quick to health visitor, requesting visit and maintenance of continuity of care.			

Table 5.1 Continued

IMPACT OF PRECIPITATING EVENT ON CLIENT
Subjective account (client)
'I am in pain and feel very shaky. Because I cannot stand or walk at present, nor manage to look after myself, I have to go and stay with my daughter. I am grateful but do not think her husband will really like this.'
PERCEPTION OF SIGNIFICANCE OF EVENT
Subjective account (client)
'This fall indicates I am at risk. It means I must re-plan my future. I do not wish to go into care, but fear my daughter may make me do so. I need help to sort things out quietly.'
Objective account (HV) (what was observed)
Client appears distressed. Has obvious pain, which is eased by medication. Left ankle swollen, cannot weight-bear. Daughter offering help, but relationships are strained.
Perception of significance of event (HV)
Temporary incapacity, but indicative of increasing vulnerability. Needs immediate care and rehabilitation. Will need to consider future, but no haste; family pressure may well need countering. It appears important to client to make her own decisions.
AVAILABLE RESOURCES
Self (client) resources
Physical: Has limited capacity; increasing frailty (octogenarian). *Mental:* Has good cognitive ability; is aware of her circumstances and need to make plans for future. *Emotional:* Has a strong will and keen sense of independence. Well-motivated towards self-help. Normally cheerful and resilient. *Socio-cultural:* Generally exhibits middle-class values, Traditional lifestyle. Good rapport with neighbours. Supportive network from friends and church members. Attends one O.P. Club regularly. *Spiritual:* Is a member of St John's Church, Old Town. In regular contact with Minister, participates in church activities. *Environmental:* Owns own home: house in good repair; Close to shops and amenities; large garden, but has help. Also has domestic assistance 2 × weekly. Has some difficulty coping with own housework but cooks for self. *Political-economic:* Formerly an active member of local branch of Age Concern. Still supports organisation. Has retirement pension and teacher's pension; some savings but finds upkeep of house a drain on financial resources.
USUAL COPING STRATEGIES
Client's view
'I usually size up situations, then do my best to soldier on.'
Health Visitor's view
A practical person. Usually seeks help early and follows advice. Rather stoic manner. Tenacious.
FAMILY RESOURCES
Daughter: retired teacher, very capable person. Homeowner, with good facilities. Has never been close to mother. Unemotional manner. Son-in-law: presently in full-time work, but planning to retire at 65 years. Does not get on with client. Couple are not willing to have client to live with them permanently. Are 'prepared to do their duty by her, as far as possible, without this'.
CLIENT'S USE OF HEALTH SERVICES
Infrequent to date. 2-yearly medical check; 4-monthly health visitor surveillance. Chiropody at 6-weekly intervals. Ophthalmic examination 2-yearly: bifocal spectacles worn (cataract lens). Use of social services: No contact so far. May need aids and/or adaptations later.

Table 5.1 Continued

CLIENT'S CAPACITY TO MEET PRESENT BASIC NEEDS
Unable to move freely; cannot prepare own food, manage housework, personal washing or laundry. Has some difficulty getting to toilet, will require use of a commode. Must rely on temporary care from her daughter.
ABILITY TO IDENTIFY AND DEAL WITH PROBLEMS.
Has knowledge of biology, simple home nursing and much life-experience. Perceives threat to independence from increasing physical frailty. Anxious about dependence on her daughter. Heeds teaching and tries to adapt to changing circumstances. Does not want to go into care, at present.
DESIRED DIRECTION OF HEALTH VISITING CARE
Client seeks pain relief, restoration of function and regaining of independence. Maintenance of future independence and functional capacity for as long as possible. Requires help to examine alternatives for future care. Hopes to effect improvement in relationships with daughter and son-in-law; welcomes help in improving communication with them.

Table 5.2 Health visitor's initial assessment of independence in activities of living for Mrs Davison

ACTIVITIES OF LIVING	USUAL ROUTINES — WHAT CLIENT CAN/CANNOT DO INDEPENDENTLY	CLIENT NEEDS AND PROBLEMS	(a = actual, p = potential)
Maintaining a safe environment	Independent until now. Owing to accident requires help to recover. Also needs help to assess hazards/guard against future accidents.	Has some instability of balance. Takes some risks. Requires help to balance own drives/wishes against risks.	(a) (a) (p)
Communicating	Cognitively clear. Speech good. Experiencing some pain and discomfort. Distressed over present dependency. Some relationship problems with her daughter and son-in-law	Fears a deterioration of relationships if she remains for any length of time with daughter and son-in-law. Depressed about poor rapport. Wants to improve future relationships.	(a) (a) (a)
Breathing	Normal.	Runs risk of respiratory infection if immobility is prolonged.	(p)
Eating and drinking	Has small appetite. Normally cooks and shops for herself. Temporarily unable to do so.	Nutritional impairment might occur if not well fed after this injury. Requires high fibre intake to combat risk of constipation. Also extra fluids; extra vitamin B complex and vitamin C.	(p)
Eliminating	Normally independent. Occasional stress incontinence. Occasional constipation. Temporarily unable to get self to WC.	Requires a commode. Requires help to combat risk of incontinence. Requires mobilisation ASAP to reduce risk of constipation.	(a) (a) (p)

Table 5.2 Continued

ACTIVITIES OF LIVING	USUAL ROUTINES — WHAT CLIENT CAN/CANNOT DO INDEPENDENTLY	CLIENT NEEDS AND PROBLEMS	(a = actual, p = potential)
Personal washing and dressing	Usually well groomed. Has temporary difficulties.	Requires help from daughter/family to assist her to wash; get dressed. To avoid skin soreness and avoid pressure	(a) (a)
Controlling body temperature	Normally has no difficulty.	Suffered initially from shock; complained of being cold and shivery. Could be at risk of infection.	(a) (p)
Mobilising	Normally very active. Temporarily cannot weight-bear due to injured ankle.	Has pain and stiffness. At risk of venous thrombosis if prolonged immobility. Needs help to become mobile.	(a) (a) (a)
Working/playing	Cannot manage own housework at present. Temporarily unable to attend church/clubs and other usual activities.	Requires temporary care. Risk of boredom and strained family relationships.	(a) (p)
Sleeping	Usually sleeps well. Sleep pattern may now be fitful due to sequelae of accident and changed environment.	Insomnia Fatigue Reduced resistance to infection Need to ensure adequate pain relief Simple means for meeting body comfort Need to promote total relaxation	(p) (p) (p) (a) (a) (a)
Expressing sexuality	Widowed. Has good social relationships with friends of both sexes. Very feminine client.	Strained relationship with son-in-law. Likely to miss her friends during temporary stay with daughter. Requires help to notify friends of whereabouts and to resume contacts.	(a) (p) (a)
Dying	Death does not appear imminent. Is likely within next 2 decades. Client awareness of survival risks now heightened.	Client requires help to confront her own dying and to prepare herself for eventual event; to encourage a healthy attitude to eventual death.	(a)

SUMMARY: Presenting problem is post-traumatic immobility and dependence. Family giving temporary support. Are well able to give adequate care if they receive appropriate guidance and information. Need to ascertain that they understand and can meet client's need for pain relief and gradual return to mobility and independence. More significant and underlying problems: increasing frailty; increased accident risk; need to seek longer-term solution for care while maintaining optimum independence. Major difficulty strained family relationships: need to explore sources of tension, reduce same if possible. Encourage increased rapport. Try to build up a more stable and caring relationship for the future. Help client and family relax with one another; to discover the practitioner's role and function and utilise it appropriately. Ensure family feel free to discuss problems and call directly for help if needed in the future.

Table 5.3 Health visitor's plan for the case of Mrs Davison, based on Activities of Living Model

ACTIVITIES OF LIVING	NEED OR PROBLEM (a = actual, p = potential)	GOAL OF CARE (s = short-term, l = longer-term)	HEALTH VISITING INTERVENTION (s = short-term, l = longer term)	EVALUATION CRITERIA STATED AS EXPECTED OUTCOMES (s = short-term, l = longer-term)
Maintaining a safe environment	Need to remain accident free.	Maintain safety (s) (l) Identify risks compatible with quality of life.	Check safety of client in own and daughter's home; alert family to hazards: invite improvements.	Client and family will each value safety and will remove hazards (s) (l) Maintain vigilance.
	Problem: 1. Instability (a)	Discover cause: Remove/reduce if possible.	Arrange medical check; explain any subsequent treatment.	Doctor will give check to see reason for instability. If treatment is prescribed this will be followed correctly.
	2. Failing vision (a)	Maintenance of optimum sight.	Visual check encouraged; advise on low vision aids if needed (s) (l)	Visual checks will be arranged and any prescribed aids will be worn (s) (l)
	3. Risk of further falls (p)	Restore client confidence.	Encourage client to move freely as improves; to act confidently (s) (l)	Client will regain confidence and will balance care with confidence on return home (l)
	4. Risk of incorrect handling of medication (p)	Safe administration of drugs.	Check client and family understand use of medication and can handle same safely.	Medication will be taken and stored correctly. Client will note/report any adverse reactions. Client will retain respect for care of drugs.
Communicating	Client needs: 1. To release feelings about accident (a)	Appropriate release of emotions: positive adaptation towards restoration.	Encourage verbalisation, interpret behavioural needs to family. Help family adapt to situation and behave restoratively (s) (l)	Client will talk out feelings. Family will demonstrate their awareness of client's feelings and will meet her care needs in a helpful manner (s) (l) Client will act positively and will discuss ways of restoring normal function (s) (l)
	2. Client needs to understand reaction to dependency state.	Reduction of adverse dependency reactions (s) (l)	Carefully explain dependency reactions to family; explore appropriate family actions with them (s) (l); encourage caring within a rehabilitative approach (s) (l)	Client and family will learn to understand her dependency needs and reactions; will accept these but encourage moves towards restoration of independence compatible with physical potential. Family will be positive towards rehabilitation

Table 5.3 Continued

ACTIVITIES OF LIVING	NEED OR PROBLEM (a = actual, (p = potential)	GOAL OF CARE (s = short-term, l = longer-term)	HEALTH VISITING INTERVENTION (s = short-term, l = longer term)	EVALUATION CRITERIA STATED AS EXPECTED OUTCOMES (s = short-term, l = longer-term)
	3. Client needs to obtain relief from pain.	Pain relief and restoration of normal functions (s)	Check family understand simple pain relief measures and can/will use them to help client obtain comfort/restoration (s)	Family will act appropriately to relieve pain, e.g. will apply cold compresses as prescribed. Client will be relieved of major discomfort & pain within one week (s). Function will be gradually restored.
	4. To recognise source of family tensions and modify own behaviour which helps create same.	Tension reduction (s) (l)	Elicit behaviour which creates tension. Identify family flash points (s)	Client will relax; both parties will try to modify behaviour and so reduce tension.
			Explore with family more appropriate alternatives (s) (l)	Family will learn HV role in care (s) (l) and will use the contact to discuss their own health needs also (l)
	5. Improve rapport.	Build warmer relationships (s) (l) Promote care actions (s) (l)	Encourage interaction: study needs of each member; monitor progress (s) (l)	Family will discuss more freely with one another. Rapport will be improved (l)
Breathing	Needs to maintain normality. Runs risk of infection (p)	Respiratory health, freedom from infections (s) (l)	Demonstrate/encourage breathing exercises. Advise on measures for preventing infections following trauma.	Client will carry out breathing exercises. Respiration will remain normal. Client will be infection free (s) (l)
Eating and drinking	Small appetite (a) Temporarily unable to obtain/prepare own food (a)	Maintain adequate nutrition and promote healing (s) (l)	Review diet with client/and carers; advise on content; ensure vitamin intake (s) (l) Restore independence but monitor future plans.	Client will maintain weight within appropriate limits. Family will give client healthy diet and will arrange a suitable intake to be maintained after her return home (s) (l)
Personal washing and dressing	Requires help from family to wash and dress (a)	Facilitate personal grooming (s) (l) Restore independence (s)	Encourage carers to help. Institute measures for early return to self-care (s)	Family will assist client to maintain personal toilet. Full independence will be restored within one month.

Table 5.3 Continued

ACTIVITIES OF LIVING	NEED OR PROBLEM (a = actual, p = potential)	GOAL OF CARE (s = short-term, l = longer-term)	HEALTH VISITING INTERVENTION (s = short-term, l = longer term)	EVALUATION CRITERIA STATED AS EXPECTED OUTCOMES (s = short-term, l = longer-term)
Mobilising	Temporarily unable to weight-bear (a) Ankle swollen.	Maintain flexibility (s) Avoid stiffness. Restore independence.	Advise/teach leg exercises. Check client and family can understand use of walking frame (s) Encourage gradual mobility.	Family will monitor client exercises. Client will gradually resume weight-bearing. Client will improve mobility in 3 weeks.
Eliminating	Temporarily unable to get to WC (a)	Interpret needs to family and teach to use alternative methods safely.	Explain problems to family. Help them to obtain a commode (s) Advise on use (2-hourly by day) (s)	Client and carers will appreciate needs and will obtain a suitable commode; and site it safely (s) Client will manage to use the commode safely (s)
	Has stress incontinence (a)	Maintain continence; improve same.	Teach pelvic exercises.	Toilet needs will be monitored.
	Fears lapses; falls (p) Fears daughter's displeasure	Improve pelvic tone; increase confidence	Explore fears and reduce risk of falls	Patterns of continue will be established (s) (l) Client will continue pelvic exercises Client fear of falls will be reduced.
	Constipated (a)	Avoid constipation	Review diet; Increase fibre/fluid.	Diet will include extra fluid and 30 g. fibre daily.
	Anxious (a)	Restore independence	Encourage early return to full independence	Client will regain full independence in toilet matters
Sleeping	Usually sleeps well. Currently fitful (a) Fatigue (p)	Restore normal sleeping pattern (s) (l)	Teach natural sleep measures. Monitor sleep levels.	Client's sleep will improve. No undue fatigue will be present (s) (l)
Working and playing	Cannot manage own housework at present (a) May need domestic help on return home.	Daughter cares without undue stress. Client considers her future needs (s) Plans for the longer term.	Discuss domestic help. Maintain client self help in future. Outline alternative courses of action, including need to plan for longer-term.	Client will accept help from daughter with good grace (g) Client will regain contact with friends and resume leisure interests within 6 weeks. Client will examine her future circumstances and will reach own decision about type of care required (l)

Table 5.3 Continued

ACTIVITIES OF LIVING	NEED OR PROBLEM (a = actual, p = potential)	GOAL OF CARE (s = short-term, l = longer-term)	HEALTH VISITING INTERVENTION (s = short-term, l = longer term)	EVALUATION CRITERIA STATED AS EXPECTED OUTCOMES (s = short-term, l = longer-term)
	Unable to socialise (a)	Client resumes contact with friends in 2 weeks. Returns to clubs in 6 weeks.	Discuss need to keep up interests. Encourage contact with friends. Check client has notified club leader and encourage return to normal activities ASAP.	Client will find diversionary short-term interests. Will keep in touch with club leader/members. Will resume church activities as she wishes within 6–8 weeks.
Expressing sexuality	Maintain contact with both sexes (a)	As above	As above	Client will retain heterosexual relationships.
Dying	Need to consider eventual death.	Approach future death with equanimity.	Encourage client to meet spiritual needs as indicated by client.	Client will adopt a healthy attitude to her future death and will seek own form of spiritual support.

It should be appreciated that the above health visitor care plan is very detailed. The information contained therein would have been collected over several visits. It is expected that adaptations will be made to reflect individual record keeping and that priorities will be identified at each contact as indicated. A blank summary sheet is therefore shown in Figures 5.5(a) and (b).

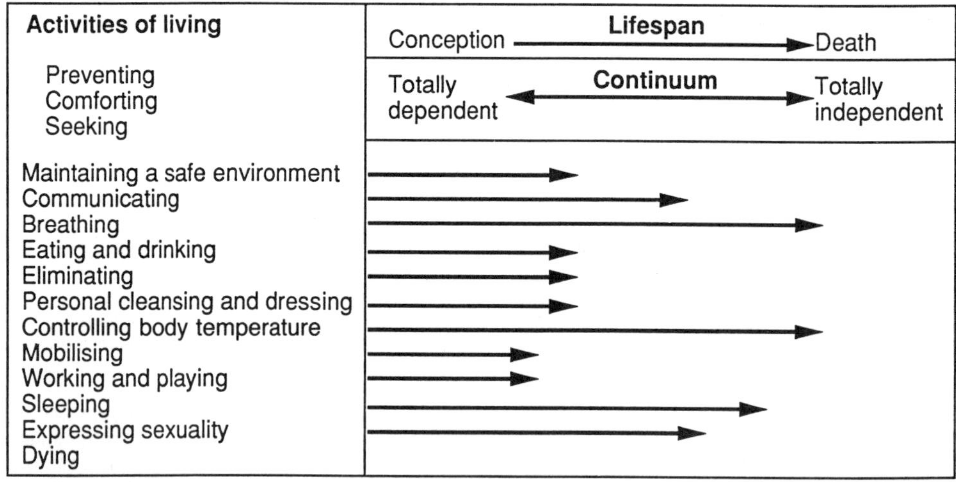

Fig. 5.4 The assessment of an elderly client, Mrs Margaret L. Davison, in relation to health as independence, using the Activities of Living Model (after Roper et al 1980–1990; reproduced by kind permission of the authors).

Health visiting care plan: related to ALs

Goals	Interventions related to ALs	Evaluation

Fig. 5.5(a) Health Visiting Care Plan form, related to health as independence, using the Activities of Living Model (after Roper et al 1980–1990; reproduced by kind permission of the authors).

Health visiting care plan: derived from medical/other prescription

Interventions	Goals	Evaluation
Other notes		

Fig. 5.5(b) Health Visiting Care Plan Form, derived from medical or other prescription, as related to health as independence, using the Activities of Living Model (after Roper et al; reproduced by kind permission of the authors).

CASE STUDY

Mrs R Black, an elderly woman living in warden-supervised, sheltered housing

Mrs Rose Black, aged 85 years, was referred by the Warden to the Health Visitor, Mrs East, during the latter's regularly weekly liaison visit. The client moved to her new home 3 weeks ago, but now appears very anxious and unsettled. Previously she had lived in another area of the town, for 20 years. She was widowed 2 years ago.

6 months ago Mrs Black was an inpatient for 4 weeks at North Town District General Hospital, suffering from 'jaundice'. Treated successfully by medical means, but incorrectly assumed surgery was contemplated. Refused same. Since discharge has been rather apathetic, reluctant to resume earlier activities and functionally less able. Transfer to sheltered accommodation was therefore expedited, because of lessened coping ability.

Client has a history of mild maturity-onset diabetes, first noted in 1981. Now attends Diabetic Clinic North Town District General Hospital. Is seen 6-monthly; under supervision of Dr Stewart (Consultant). A 2000 kcal diet is prescribed and client's condition is generally stable. Cataract operation (lens extraction) performed in 1978; spectacles prescribed and worn.

Client lives alone but is visited weekly by her only daughter, who lives in a neighbouring town, is married and has four young children. There are two sons: one living in Canada, and one in Norwich (England). The client was very attached to one helpful neighbour in her former location. Mrs Black is a member of several Elderly Persons' Clubs.

Has recently registered with Dr Green; medical records being transferred.

Table 5.4 An assessment/intervention tool adapted from the Neuman Health Care Systems Model, showing the content of the model

1. *Client details*
2. *Stressors and responses to same*
3. *Client views*
   Subjective data (what is stated)
a. Client's view of his/her major difficulties.
b. Client's perception of present circumstances and whether these differ from the usual pattern of living.
c. Client's view of whether he/she has experienced similar problems, needs, or concerns, before. If so, how these were dealt with.
d. Client's anticipations/expectations for the future, as a consequence of present situation, (and whether these are feasible and reality-based).
e. Client's views on what he/she is doing to help self.
f. Client's expectations from friends/family, practitioner and others.
4. *Stressors encountered and responses to same*
   Objective data; practitioner-derived, supplemented by information from records, colleagues, other carers
a. Major needs, problems, stress areas, or concerns, (degree of congruence with client's perceptions).
b. Client's present circumstances, compared with usual lifestyle.
c. Client's experience of similar situation and an objective evaluation of client response in such similar situations; outcomes on these similar/previous occasions.
d. Practitioner anticipations for the future, re the consequences of the present situation.
e. Practitioner views on client's actual and potential levels of self-help.
f. Practitioner views of client's expectations, (degree of congruence perceived between client and practitioner views).

Summary of impressions

(1) Intra-personal aspects
(2) Inter-personal aspects
(3) Extra-personal aspects.
Formulation of problems, needs, concerns, ranking same in priority order.

Table 5.5 An assessment of an older client, Mrs Rosina Black, using the Neuman Health Care Systems Model, giving client's views

1. *CLIENT DETAILS*

Name	*Date of birth*	*Marital status*
Mrs Rose Black 2 Gayler Terrace North Town	19th April 1904 Socio-economic status Social Class 5 (by Registrar General's classification of former occupation of husband)	Widow
Newly transferred to General Practice team based at North Town Health Centre. Formerly cared for by General Practice Team at Merryfield Surgery, North Town	Dr Green Mrs Fox Mrs East	— General Practitioner — District Nursing Sister — Health Visitor
Referred by:	Mrs Ann Jones, Warden, Gayler Housing Association. Concerned at client's anxiety level and general lack of coping ability, since transfer to sheltered accommodation.	

2. *STRESSORS AND RESPONSES TO SAME*

A. Client's view of her major difficulties/stresses/concerns

'My worst problem is diabetes, but it's not very bad. If I keep to my diet I'll be all right. I want to do this because I lost a sister from gangrene of her feet. Six months ago I spent a month in hospital and still feel weak. I went in because my legs were like jelly and I was yellow all over and felt bad. I think they wanted to operate but I refused as it's my flesh and I wish to keep it.'

Table 5.5 Continued

'I've been waiting to move here for 2 years but I don't know if I'll like it; the move has been a nightmare. I miss my old home and neighbour. I've not been out much since I came here. It worries me to do my washing in this machine with everyone else.'

'My legs will not go like they used to; but I manage.'

'This move has cost me a lot of money and I'm very worried about this.'

B. Client's perception of how her present circumstances differ from her usual pattern of living

Usual lifestyle	*Present lifestyle*
I used to do everything for myself.	I don't seem to have the same interest here.
I looked after my husband before he died.	I can't be bothered about anything now.
You have to get on with it.	I feel too weak and wobbly to get on with it now.
I usually get up at 7 a.m. and go to bed at 11.30 p.m.	I don't want to get up before 9 a.m./go to bed any time after 7 p.m.
I used to sleep well	I wake a lot now.
I tried to follow my diet — meat and 2 veg every day.	I don't feel hungry now but I force something down.
I visited my daughter and her family on Sundays.	I don't go out now. My daughter cooks for me for Sundays.
I used to do my own laundry.	I worry about washing. I don't like this machine.
I went to my club on Mondays and collected my Pension after.	I think it is too far to go to my clubs now. The warden collects my pension.
I get the Income Support and they pay my rent. It's not much but I managed with care.	I don't know how I will afford this central heating. It worries me so.

C. Client's view of whether she has experienced similar needs or problems before

Previous perspective	*Present perspective*
I've never been 'yellow' before, but I have felt weak.	I worry if the yellow will come back.
I worked it off: you see I knew everybody round me and it helped.	I have no strength to work it off: they are all strangers here.

D. Client's anticipations for the future as a consequence of her present situation

'I can't see things will ever be right for me again. I can't seem to tackle this place like I did my old one.'

E. Client's perceptions of what she is doing to help herself

'I'm very busy getting myself straight. I've no time to go shopping even if I wanted to, because I've all this housework and washing which I do.'
'I do as I am told from the diabetic clinic.'
'I'm quite independent now.'
'I manage although I feel tired and miserable.'

F. Client's expectations of family, friends, practitioner and others

'My family will do all I need, my daughter will come and help and my eldest grandchild especially. The diabetic clinic will stop me getting gangrene. I don't suppose I will need to bother this new Dr Green very much, because the yellow has gone away, but I expect he'll help me if I need him. He will come and see me here.'
'I don't expect to need the hospital again.'
'I know you will come and see me, but I shan't need much.'
'I do wish the Income Support would give me a bit more for the heating.'
'Perhaps some of my friends in my old area will move here when they close those old houses. I known they will visit me a lot here.'

Table 5.6 Assessment of Mrs Black, using the Neuman Health Care Systems Model, giving practitioner's observed data

A. MAJOR NEEDS, PROBLEMS, STRESS AREAS OR CONCERNS

Octogenarian with history of increasing frailty, some instability and vague abdominal discomfort, increasing over past year. Familial history of diabetes/1 sister died from it. Diagnosed maturity-onset diabetes 3 years ago, well controlled by diet alone. Widowed 2 years ago after a 4-year period of caring for sick husband in very poor environmental circumstances.

Health visiting support given by colleague intermittently following bereavement. Planned move to sheltered accommodation expedited as a result of hospital admission for jaundice 6 months ago. Diagnosis not fully established; treated medically although client incorrectly assumed surgery was contemplated, and refused this. Became very distressed. Otherwise independent. Moved here by Local Housing Authority 3 weeks ago. Has found experience threatening and seems overwhelmed. ? slightly disoriented. Has registered with Dr Green but not yet consulted; will need immediate referral and full check-up. Is mobile but rather unsteady, has a walking frame for use in home.

History of strict personal and domestic cleanliness but is now untidy in home and rather dishevelled in appearance. Sleeping and eating routines disturbed, stability of diabetes state potentially threatened.

Clearly grieving for loss of old home and security of known neighbourhood. Highly anxious, tension habits present, emotionally labile. Flattened responses, depressive manner. Previous account of resilience now incongruent. Own perceptions of coping ability are rather unrealistic.

B. CLIENT'S PRESENT CIRCUMSTANCES COMPARED WITH USUAL LIFESTYLE

Usual lifestyle	*Present lifestyle*
Independent	Becoming dependent Functionally restricted
Coping with diabetic diet	Dietary intake uncertain
Managing full domestic duties	Domestic care poor Unable to establish routine
Budgeted well	Anxious about finances
Socialised well	Withdrawing

C. PRACTITIONER VIEW OF CLIENT EXPERIENCE OF SIMILAR SITUATION

Has not moved for many years. Clearly uncertain of how to adapt. Limited experience of illness and hospitalisation, very disturbed by recent experiences, fearful of repetition and eventual outcome.

Health visitor colleague reports 'Colourful character; usually very resilient, adamant manner and decided views.' Clearly, present reaction is out of character.

D. PRACTITIONER'S ANTICIPATION FOR FUTURE AS A CONSEQUENCE OF PRESENT STATE

Client deterioration likely unless prompt action taken. Will likely need intensive rehabilitative measures, possibly short-term, but depends on establishing diagnosis/prognosis of medical condition.

Will require greater involvement of family.

Anticipate programme of social support/restoration, mobilising home help: (at least short-term).

Increased input from health visiting service.

Possible use of luncheon club/voluntary visiting service.

Increased liaison with social services department, hospital staff, and general practice team.

Likely treatment for ? depressive state.

E. PRACTITIONER VIEW ON CLIENT LEVELS OF SELF-HELP

Potentially sound in short-term, given intensive help now. Likely need for increasing involvement of caring services in longer-term.

F. PRACTITIONER'S VIEW OF CLIENT'S EXPECTATIONS OF CARE-GIVERS

'Low level of fit'. Client generally rather unrealistic. Daughter burdened with family responsibilities and some transport difficulties. Relationships caring.

Old friends interested but circumscribed by age from giving much practical help. Diabetic clinic will supervise but cannot guarantee her condition. Will likely need more help from social services than she envisages.

Table 5.7 Summary of impressions formed by practitioner assessing Mrs Black, using the Neuman Health Care Systems Model

(i) *Intra-personal factors*
Biology. Client's functional ability and nutritional status fair, but under threat. Sleep and appetite disturbed; skin in good condition. Other systems functioning, apart from instability and limited mobility. Some self-neglect from emotional upset.

Psychosocial. Agitated, emotionally labile and depressed. Limited insight. Low motivation at present. Still communicating but tending to withdraw. Open to family and friends. No request for spiritual help.

(ii) *Inter-personal factors*
Loving family relationships. Some loss of contact with friends and acquaintances in clubs.
Normally outgoing — currently flattened responses.

(iii) *Extra-personal factors*
Others in housing complex able to visit and support.
Community is an inner city area; heavy demand on health and social services. Limited places in day centres/luncheon clubs/community nursing services and social services below establishment.

(iv) *Problem formulation — priority rated and proposed health visitor action*

(a) Maintain safety and comfort.
Immediate referral for medical investigation; liaise with hospital staff for full data; contact social services; arrange for home help if possible. Later luncheon club placement; Transport for attendance at resumed club activities.
(b) Raise and maintain morale.
Treat underlying depression. Encourage friends and family to visit. Improve mobility; continue intensive short-term support.
(c) Maintain nutrition and dietary stability of diabetic state.
Determine accurate dietary intake, liaise with diabetic clinic and ensure correct balance. Discuss shopping and cooking arrangements with daughter and Warden, ? home help. Later possible use of luncheon club.
(d) Maintain integrity of skin.
Encourage attention to personal hygiene and reduce risk of skin infection.
(e) Review socio-economic state.
Relieve source of immediate anxiety by discussing needs with client and encouraging contact with local officer from Department of Social Security.
With client permission, discuss position with Local Authority Social Worker. Advise on local voluntary services which may be able to meet needs for any pressing deficiency in requirements following removal from previous home.
(f) Once agitation has subsided assist client to gain insight into circumstances and re-establish independence in living.
Encourage client to talk out difficulties and consider problem-solving measures.
Encourage client to take interest in new environment and to participate in activities held within the housing complex.
Inform about local-based group activities which she may wish to join, as substitute for some previous activities.
Assist client to regain full equilibrium and maintain stable state as long as possible: gradual withdrawal of intensive support.

Summary
Normally resilient individual.
Flexible line of defence breached by stressor — loss of husband
Normal line of defence breached by stressor — loss of health
Inner line of defence breached by stressor — loss of old home.
Requires help to recover equilibrium.

REFERENCES

Akinsanya J A 1989 Introduction. In: Akinsanya J A (ed) Theories and models of nursing. Recent advances in nursing. Series No 24: Churchill Livingstone, Edinburgh, p 1–11

Allen M N, Hayes P 1989 Models of nursing: implications for research in nursing. In: Akinsanya J A (ed) Theories and models of nursing. Recent advances in nursing series, No 24. Churchill Livingstone, Edinburgh, p 77–93

Arygris S, Schon D A 1974 Theory in practice: increasing professional effectiveness. Jossey Bass, San Francisco

Becker M H (ed) 1974a The Health Belief Model and personal health behaviour. Health Education Monographs 2: 324–473

Benner P 1983 Uncovering the knowledge embedded in clinical practice. Image 15: 41

Benoliel J 1983 Grounded theory and qualitative data: the socialising influences of life-threatening disease, on identity development. In: Wooldridge P, Schmitt M H, Skipper J K Jnr, Leonard R C (eds) Behavioural science and nursing theory. Mosby, St Louis, p 141–187

Binnie A, Bond S, Law G, Lowe K, Pearson A, Roberts R, Tierney A, Vaughan B 1984 A systematic approach to nursing care. Open University Press, Milton Keynes

Bradshaw J 1972 A taxonomy of social needs. Oxford University Press for Nuffield Provincial Hospitals Trust, Oxford, p 69

Burgess W, Ragland F C 1983 Community health nursing: philosophy, process, practice. Appleton-Century-Crofts, Norwalk, Conn.

Caplan G 1964 Principles of preventive psychiatry. Basic Books, New York

Caplan G 1974 Support systems and community mental health. Basic Books, New York

CETHV (Council for the Education and Training of Health Visitors) 1967 The functions of the health visitor. CETHV, London

CETHV (Council for the Education and Training of Health Visitors) 1977 An investigation into the principles of health visiting. The Working Group, CETHV, London

CETHV (Council for the Education and Training of Health Visitors) 1979 Principles in practice. The Working Group, CETHV, London

Chalmers H A 1989 Theories and models of nursing and the nursing process. In: Akinsanya J A (ed) Theories and models of nursing. Recent advances in nursing series, No 24. Churchill Livingstone, Edinburgh, p 32–47

Chao Y 1989 Theoretical thinking in nursing: implications for primary health care. In: Akinsanya J A (ed) Theories and models of nursing. Recent advances in nursing series, No 24. Churchill Livingstone, Edinburgh

Clark J 1982a Development of models and theories on the concept of nursing. Journal of Advanced Nursing 7: 129–134

Clark J 1982b A way to get organised: trying out principles in practice. Nursing Times Community Outlook (11th Oct): 287–297

Clark J 1983 Integration and the future of health visiting. In: Owen G (ed) Health visiting. Bailliere Tindall, London, p 360–361

Clark J 1985 The process of health visiting. Unpublished Doctoral Thesis, CNNA and South Bank Polytechnic, London

Copp L 1987 The implications of epidemiological research. In: Cahoon M (ed) Research methodology. Recent advances in nursing series, No 17. Churchill Livingstone, Edinburgh

Dickoff J, James P 1968 A theory of theories. Nursing Research 17: 3, 197

Dobson S 1987 Transcultural nursing: the role of the health visitor in multi-cultural studies. Unpublished PhD Thesis, University of Edinburgh, Edinburgh

Dobson S 1988 Diagnosis and the health visitor. Senior Nurse 8 (4) (April): 15–17

Dobson S 1989 Conceptualising for transcultural health visiting: the concept of transcultural reciprocity. Journal of Adv. Nursing 14: 97–102

Dubos R 1959 Mirage of health: Utopias, progress and biological change. In: Ansen R N (ed) World perspectives. Harper and Row, New York

Dunn M 1959 High level wellness for man and society. American Journal of Public Health 49 (6): 786-792

Dunnell K, Cartwright A 1972 Medicine takers, prescribers and hoarders. Routledge and Kegan Paul, London

Ebersole P, Hess P 1985 Towards healthy aging; 2nd edn. Mosby, St Louis

Falco S M 1989 Major concepts in the development of nursing theory. In: Akinsanya J A (ed) Theories and models of nursing. Recent advances in nursing series, No 24. Churchill Livingstone, Edinburgh

Fawcett J, Downs F S 1986 The relationship of theory and research. Appleton-Century-Crofts, Norwalk

Goodwin S 1987 Stress in health visiting. In: Littlewood J (ed) Community nursing. Recent advances in nursing series, No 15. Churchill Livingstone, Edinburgh

Hobson W, Pemberton J 1956 The health of the elderly at home. British Medical Journal 1: 587–593

Hockey L 1979 A study of district nursing: the development and progression of a long-term research programme. Unpublished PhD Thesis, City University, London

Holter I M 1988 Critical theory: a foundation for the development of nursing theories. Scholarly Inquiry for Nursing Practice 2: 223–232

Houldin A D, Saltstein S W, Ganley K M 1987 Nursing diagnoses for wellness. Lippincott, Philadelphia

Hunt M, Montgomery-Robinson K 1987 Analysis of conversational interaction. In: Cahoon M (ed) Research methodology. Recent advances in nursing series, No 17. Churchill Livingstone, Edinburgh

Janz N K, Becker M H 1984 The health belief model: a decade later. Health Education Quarterly 11: 1–47

Jennings B M 1987 Nursing theory development: success and challenge. Journal of Advanced Nursing 12 (1): 63–69

Kim H S 1989 Theoretical thinking in nursing: problems and prospects. In: Akinsanya J A (ed) Theories and models of nursing. Recent advances in nursing series, No 24. Churchill Livingstone, Edinburgh

Lau R R, Williams S, Williams L C, Ware J E, and Brook R H 1982 Psycho-social problems in the chronically ill. Journal of Community Health 7: 250–261

Leininger M M 1987 Importance and use of Ethnomeds: ethnography and ethno-nursing research. In: Cahoon M (ed) Research methodology. Recent advances in nursing series, No 17. Churchill Livingstone, Edinburgh

Luker K 1982a Evaluating health visiting. Royal College of Nursing, London
Luker K 1982b Health visiting and the elderly: an attempt at process-outcome evaluation. British Journal of Geriatric Nursing(Sept–Oct): 5–8
Luker K, Orr J 1985 Health visiting. Blackwell Scientific Publications, Oxford.
McFarlane J 1977 Developing a theory of nursing: the relationship of theory to practice, education and research. Journal of Advanced Nursing 2: 261–270
Maslow A H 1954 Motivation and personality. Harper and row, New York
Maslow A H 1962 Towards a psychology of being. Harper and Row, New York
Maslow A H 1987 Motivation and personality. Revised by Frager R, Fadiman J, McReynolds C, Cox R. Harper and Row, New York
McClymont M E 1982 Where are they now and what are they doing? A follow-up study of 7 cohorts of health visitor students, 1967–1973. Unpublished MSc Thesis, University of Surrey, Guildford
Neugarten B L, Havighurst R J, Tobin B S 1961 The measurement of life satisfaction. Journal of Gerontology 16:134–143
Neuman B 1980 The Betty Neuman Health Care Systems Model: a total person approach to viewing patient problems. In: Riehl J, Roy C (eds) Conceptual models for nursing practice, 2nd edn. Appleton-Century-Crofts, New York
Neuman B, Young R J 1972 The Betty Neuman Model: a total person approach to patient's problems. In: Nursing Research 21 (3): 264–269
Parse R R 1987 Nursing science: major paradigms, theories and critiques. W B Saunders, Philadelphia
Passant H 1990 A holistic approach in the ward. Complementary therapies in the care of the elderly. Nursing Times/Nursing Mirror 86 (4) (24th Jan): 26–28
Price I 1981 The nursing process. In: Illing M and Donovan B (eds) District nursing. Bailliere Tindall, London
Raymond E 1983 Skills in health visiting. In: Owen G (ed) Health visiting. Bailliere Tindall, London
Riehl J, Roy C 1983 Conceptual models for nursing practice. Appleton-Century-Crofts, New York
Roper N, Logan W, Tierney A 1980 The elements of Nursing. Churchill Livingstone, Edinburgh
Roper N, Logan W, Tierney A 1983 Using a model for nursing. Churchill Livingstone, Edinburgh
Roper N, Logan W, Tierney A 1985 The elements of nursing, 2nd edn. Churchill Livingstone, Edinburgh
Roper N, Logan W, Tierney A 1990 The elements of nursing, 3rd edn. Churchill Livingstone, Edinburgh (in press)
Rosenstock I M, Strecher V J, Becker M H 1988 Social learning theory and the health belief model. Health Education Quarterly 15 (2) (Summer): 175–183
Roy C 1970 Adaptation: a conceptual framework for nursing. Nursing Outlook 18 (3): 42–43
Salmon P, Hodkinson H M 1989 Survey reveals surprising findings: happiness is worth measuring. Geriatric Medicine (August 1989): 11–12
Saxton D F, Hyland P A 1979 Planning and implementing nursing intervention. Stress and adaptation applied to patient care, 2nd edn. Mosby, St Louis
Selye H 1956 The stress of life. McGraw Hill, New York
Smith J A 1983 The idea of health: implications for the nursing professional. In: Smith D, Ranstrom M, 1983 (eds) Nursing education series. Teachers' College Press, Teachers' College, Columbia University, New York
Thorne S E, Robinson C A 1988a Reciprocal trust in health care relationships. Journal of Adv. Nursing 13: 782–789
Thorne S E, Robinson C A 1988b Health care relationships: the chronic illness perspective. Research in Nursing and Health 11: 293–300
van Maanen H M 1988 Being old does not always mean being sick. Perspectives on conditions of health as perceived by British and American elderly. Journal of Adv. Nursing 13: 701–709
Wahl P R 1980 Therapeutic relationships with the elderly. Journal of Gerontological Nursing 6 (5): 261–267
Walker J M, Campbell S M 1989 Pain assessment: nursing models and the nursing process. In: Akinsanya J A (ed) Theories and models of nursing. Recent advances in nursing series, No 24. Churchill Livingstone, Edinburgh
Williams I 1979 The care of the elderly in the community. Croom Helm, London

CHAPTER CONTENTS

6

Caring for elderly people within various community settings

As already indicated in Chapter 5, the effective health care of older people depends upon both carer competence (be they lay or professional carers) and organisational efficiency. In earlier chapters we have discussed what is involved in professional ability, responsibility and accountability, and their relationship to professional commitment. In this chapter we focus on some of the administrative settings within which health visitors may work and the different forms in which care may be organised for elderly people. We do so in the awareness that organisations are shaped and moulded by many influences, both national and international. These are mainly social, cultural, economic and political influences.

The main purpose of the chapter is to emphasise the preventive and educative thrust of the health visitor's work, irrespective of organisational structures, and to discuss the different methods which may be adopted to identify and contact vulnerable older clients. The importance of compiling community profiles is stressed, as these provide the basis for providing a locally oriented service, acting as a necessary prelude to discovering the prevalence of health and social problems within different age groups. 'Targeting' vulnerable groups is one selective response, which may involve the health visitor in intervention in earlier age groups, in order eventually to benefit older people, for example The Oxfordshire Heart and Stroke Project. Thus there may be some moves away from traditional patterns of health visiting, with complementary approaches being utilised.

Inevitably the administrative structures within which health visitors work will constrain, or facilitate, their activities. Moreover, growing world inter-dependence means that international health policies may affect national health goals. In turn this can have repercussions on aims and objectives at local level. For this reason we discuss both the WHO Targets, as part of the global strategy for 'Health for All' by the year 2000, and neighbourhood nursing services. Primary health care serves as the inter-linking factor.

Similarly, the need for multi-disciplinary and collaborative approaches to the care of elderly persons is considered; hence team work and the concept of co-operation are examined. Additionally, in outlining some of the issues concerning screening, case-finding, functional assessment and surveillance, we have sought to show the crucial role which health visitors can play.

THE GLOBAL STRATEGY — 'HEALTH FOR ALL' BY THE YEAR 2000

In the Alma Ata Declaration, the World Health Organization adopted the goal of 'The attainment by all citizens of the world, by the year 2000, of a level of well-being that will enable them to lead a socially and economically productive life' (WHO 1978).

The involvement of individuals in primary health care was seen as the way to achieve this goal. Primary health care was viewed as meeting the basic needs of each community '*through services provided as close as possible to where people live and work; easily accessible — acceptable to all — and at an affordable cost*'.

This goal was adopted because the health state of the world population was not commensurate with available knowledge or technology. Nor did it reflect the amount of time and money being spent on health services. There were, and are, wide discrepancies in health experience. For instance, there is a 20-year difference in life-expectancy between different European countries. Even in the United Kingdom, after four decades of a comprehensive national health service, the 'health divide' still exists, and is widening (Whitehead 1987).

In an attempt to redress the present position, the European member states of WHO set out their first common health policy. They selected 38 specific health targets to be achieved (hopefully) by 2000 AD. In so doing they accepted that certain prerequisites are necessary for health for all: namely, peace, social justice, enough food and safe water, adequate education and a useful role in society for everyone (WHO Nurse/Euro 1986).

Each of these prerequisites clearly impinges on the health of older persons, everywhere. Furthermore, six major themes underpinned this important policy declaration:

- Equity
- Health promotion
- Disease prevention
- Community participation
- Multi-sectoral co-operation
- The adding of life (quality) to years.

Although many of the 38 targets apply to older people, we have selected some which we consider particularly relevant. It should, of course, be appreciated that they also have general applicability across other age-groups. We have grouped them according to time-scale, and the square brackets contain our insertions.

By 1990 all member states should

- have a Primary Health Care System (Target 30)
- have legislative, administrative and economic mechanisms which resource and support healthy lifestyles and ensure the effective participation of [older] persons in policy making (Target 13).

By 1995

- there should be significant *increases* in positive health behaviour in [older] people, related to nutrition; non-smoking; appropriate physical exercise; stress management (Target 16)
- there should be significant *decreases* in health

damaging behaviour, in [older] people, related to the over-use of alcohol; pharmaceutical preparations; dangerous driving and violent social behaviour [this latter largely affecting older persons as victims] (Target 17).

By 2000

- inequalities in health status between/within countries should be reduced by at least 25% (Target 1)
- [older] disabled persons should have the opportunity to develop their health potential and live fulfilling lives (Target 3)
- there should be a *10%* improvement in the average number of years [older] persons live free from major disease/disability (Target 4).
- life expectancy at birth, within the countries of the European Region, should be at least an average of 75 years. This can only be achieved if every member-state reduces by *25%* the differentials currently existing between geographic areas, the sexes and socio-economic groups (Target 6).
- accident mortality in [older persons] should be reduced by at least *25%* (Target 11).
- current trends/rises in suicide and parasuicide rates [in older people] should be reversed (Target 12).
- research must be developed to support 'Health for All'. It is particularly required in the following areas:
  - descriptions of the health of the [older] population
  - ascertainment of the biological factors that determine health in [older] people
  - the effects of lifestyle on health [in old age]
  - the effects of the environment on health
  - the best ways to deliver appropriate care to [older] people
  - improvements needed in policy-making, planning and management (Target 32).

(WHO 1985)

The relevance and the immediacy of these targets will strike readers. Furthermore, as the United Kingdom was a signatory to this policy declaration, and assented to each of these targets, it is clear that our current and future national health policy and administration will be strongly influenced by them. Hence the development of the health visiting profession, and the organisation of health visiting services, must be viewed in this context.

CARE SECTORS

Primary

In the United Kingdom, Primary Health Care Services are usually generic and continuing. They represent the first point of contact individuals have with the health care system, and they are the services most often utilised.

They include community medical and nursing services; community midwifery and health visiting; general medical, dental, ophthalmic, pharmaceutical and chiropody services. Supporting services such as physiotherapy, occupational and speech therapy are also included, where these are provided as community services by District Health Authorities. Although located within hospitals, Accident and Emergency Services count as primary care services. Additionally, occupational health services, currently outside the NHS, are also primary. Of course not all these services are utilised by older people.

Secondary

Secondary care services are those hospital and specialist services to which persons may be referred for consultation and intermittent specialist help. They cover a wide range. However, the division is somewhat artificial, since, in an integrated service, staff from both sectors mingle and liaise. This contact is likely to increase in the future, particularly as gerontological teams promote interest in combined work with older people. Also, as the notion of 'shared care' develops, joint priorities will be set up between clients, health and social services.

CURRENT ADMINISTRATIVE STRUCTURES

Health visitors are almost always located within the primary sector, which means they form part of the community nursing services. They maintain their contact with clients and colleagues in secondary sectors through formal liaison schemes, informal visits, planned meetings and case conferences. Telephone communication, records and reports, joint study days and shared in-service courses also assist understanding.

In each of these activities it is necessary to recognise the part played by clients/patients and to respect and appreciate the roles of the various carers and workers involved in helping older people.

Within the community nursing services health visitors form part of the line-management structure, currently being answerable to Unit Managers. This hierarchical pattern is similar to that prevailing in social work, but is in direct contrast to the collegial organisation of general medical practice. Except where joint appointments occur, the present position requires health visitors to surrender their direct client-service skills, if they wish to enter full-time teaching, or management. Health Visitor Tutors then transfer to educational settings, while Health Visitor Managers assume responsibility for the service. Hence facilitating and supporting staff; the transmission and implementation of District Health Authority policies; the deployment of services; the monitoring of standards and quality control, all form part of the managerial role.

Although it can be argued that such a dichotomy enables effort to be concentrated on either education and training, or efficient organisation, some observers contend that it negates professional autonomy at field level. It may restrict interaction, affect innovation, and reduce both educators' and managers' appreciation of the intensity and type of problems met within fieldwork practice.

Another view is that this pattern of requiring senior staff to surrender fieldwork could be interpreted as devaluing direct client-services. Such a situation would be highly detrimental to older people, who require optimum level competence from those who care directly for them. In order to minimise these possible adverse effects, the following need to be provided and maintained:

- channels for regular intra-disciplinary communication and consultation
- scope for intra-disciplinary innovation and creative problem-solving
- encouragement and support for fieldworkers acting as agents of social change
- means whereby fieldworkers' views can be fully represented and considered.

Organisational patterns at field level

At field level, health visiting is usually organised on either a geographic basis or by attachment to general medical practice. The relative merits and demerits of each type are well documented. Each has its ardent supporters (see Luker & Orr 1985). In either case the staff establishment is usually based on the total population served; although little research has been conducted to determine viable health visitor–population ratios. Actual caseloads frequently consist of extrapolated vulnerable persons from different age-groups, rather than the total geographic or practice population.

Geographically-based health visiting

This is the traditional administrative pattern. Health visitors relate to a population which is geographically defined. Within such an area they may assume responsibility for the care of elderly clients, either within a generic or specialist caseload. Although not exclusively so, this pattern has tended to be more common in inner-city areas, where there are many single-doctor medical practices and often a multiplicity of health and socio-economic problems.

In more rural areas, where this geographically-based pattern prevails, the 'patch' covered by general practitioners, district nurses and health visitors may well coincide. This co-terminosity of catchment areas encourages teamwork and has very many advantages for co-operation.

THE INTRODUCTION OF NEIGHBOURHOOD NURSING

Since the introduction of general management at Unit level and the publication of the Community Nursing Review Committee Report (known popularly as The Cumberlege Report) (DHSS 1986), fundamental changes have taken place in many geographically-based community nursing services. In general, health visitors have welcomed the underlying principles of the Cumberlege Report, which envisages a far more autonomous community nursing workforce than exists at present. The health visiting profession has long advocated consumer involvement in planning and evaluation of care, urging greater availability and accessibility of services to clients. The concept of a neighbourhood nursing team, in which *nurses* look at *nursing needs* and so structure their practice to meet them, can but benefit consumers and enhance worker job satisfaction. A new focus has, therefore, been provided which offers great scope to transmogrify practice, particularly within geographic settings.

However, there have been mixed responses. Some anxieties have been expressed that common planning, joint caseloads, and greater role flexibility could lead to the introduction of an all-purpose worker. This could undermine professional identity and specific discipline expertise. It would also contradict the views of the UKCC in Project 2000, where a distinct role for the specialist in health promotion is envisaged (UKCC 1986).

Advocates of the 'Cumberlege approach' counter these views by stressing that, within these nursing teams, disciplines remain separate, while expertise and knowledge is pooled. Hence professional identity is retained. Another expressed fear is that generic management at neighbourhood level could leave health visitors without direct professional support if a manager, without health visitor preparation, were to be appointed, who did not understand their specific role and needs. Conversely it can be argued that professional support, advice and development are so important that they require distinct provision, separate from the managerial function (King's Fund 1988a).

The management of change is a highly sensitive area, which requires in-service education for existing staff and 'common core preparation' for potential staff. Improved education and preparation of generic neighbourhood managers is also essential.

The implementation of the Cumberlege Report

The implementation of 'Cumberlege' has been on rather an ad hoc basis. Many District Health Authorities have decentralised their nursing services, although there are wide variations in the types of structures. Most commonly, Units have been divided into 'localities' or 'patches' rather than neighbourhoods, although it is not always clear which criteria have guided their formation. In some Authorities, Nursing teams have been established, mainly incorporating District Nurses, School Nurses and Health Visitors. Occasionally, Community Psychiatric Nurses have been included. Variation in the type of management has also occurred, the most common being generic management. For reports on the introduction of neighbourhood nursing services in two inner-city areas, see Dally (King's Fund 1988b) and Brown (King's Fund 1988c).

OLDER PEOPLE AND NEIGHBOURHOOD NURSING

The Cumberlege Report specifically addresses the health needs of older people, as part of an overall programme of neighbourhood nursing. It sees some team members as acquiring specialist skills with older adults, in order to enhance team services. It advocates that each District Health Authority should have a clear statement of its policy aims for older clients, about which all community nursing staff should be informed. They should be clearly aware of their part in policy implementation.

The Report

- recognises that older people need relevant health information and advice, so that good health can be encouraged and competence and confidence in self-care be increased.

It urges

- reduction of unnecessary hospital admissions for older people
- the specific visiting of those 'at risk'
- personalised, participative, planned nursing care for sick elderly people, available on a 24-hour basis
- improved resources
- adequate systems for determining priorities
- specialist advice and support to meet the needs of frail, mentally infirm older clients and their carers.

It emphasises

- continence promotion
- respite care
- support and help for all informal carers, especially those who are themselves elderly
- efficient systems for co-ordinated care.

It recommends

- written guidelines for the identification of elder abuse, and for the action to be taken
- greater professional support and a wider range of resources to deal with this problem
- a nursing key-worker for older clients receiving multi-agency care.

These details have been given in full because they represent a blueprint for effective team care, being offered to older people.

The concept of neighbourhood nursing thus appears to combine many of the advantages and to reduce a number of the disadvantages of traditional geographic work-patterns. It allows health visitors to identify more strongly with a particular population, making it easier for them to recognise prevailing culture patterns and to discover the indigenous and informal networks which sustain older people. Moreover, because they become more familiar neighbourhood figures, health visitors are likely to be approached more readily for ad hoc help and advice. This is of great significance when it is appreciated that over 85% of all health problems are dealt with directly on a self-care or lay-care basis.

A neighbourhood structure also allows health visitors to become more aware of, and co-operate with, local health initiatives (see Ch. 8, pp. 174–177). Examples of co-operative ventures with various community groups are reported by Drennan (1984), Cotton & Sharp (1989) and Jones (1989).

Opportunities for observation, liaison and participation

Working within a circumscribed locality also affords opportunity for the observation of older people as they go about their daily activities, such as shopping, visiting friends, attending luncheon or social clubs or community centres. Such information and unobtrusive observation may prove invaluable in detecting need, or determining coping ability. Health visitors identifying with a specific locality may also find it easier to locate and hence visit and liaise with staff in sheltered housing complexes, day centres, day hospitals, or residential accommodation for older persons. Such staff can provide valuable information which may subsequently affect health visitor interventions.

In return they may welcome guidance on the management of older persons with whom they are involved. This reduces the risk of fragmented or overlapping care. Differing workers provide alternative perspectives on the needs of older persons and ways of meeting these, so broadening overall understanding. Workers can thus encourage each other, spurring each other on to desirable action. Areas for research can also be highlighted.

However, without specific attempts to create teamwork, geographic health visiting can mean fragmented care. There may be difficulty maintaining contact with a number of different general practitioners and nursing colleagues. There is then a risk of conflicting advice. Health visitors may become professionally isolated from peers and colleagues, so that work may assume a particular idiosyncratic emphasis, without being challenged.

Nevertheless, many health visitors enjoy geographic placement, and maintain essential health promotion, educational and supportive roles. Since the advent of computerised information systems, their need for accurate, relevant local data has been more widely recognised. This should make it easier to obtain material for compiling and updating community profiles, which are essential tools for effective practice, especially with older people.

COMMUNITY PROFILES

The compilation of a community profile begins with a Community Assessment. (An outline guide for the latter is given in Appendix 1.) It involves the collection of comprehensive data, incorporating not only topographical, geographic and relevant historical features, which hold implication for modern life, but considerable social and demographic information as well.

Patterns of employment and unemployment impact strongly on health. In turn they affect well-being and socio-economic status at retirement. Hence details about the occupational life of the community are highly pertinent. Other factors affecting community functioning which need to be considered include:

- housing status — types, provision, waiting lists
- transport — amount, modes, suitability of provision for older people
- provision/utilisation of education, leisure, health and social services
- religious activities and community involvement
- environmental services — specific problems
- legislative and protective services — adequacy and acceptability for older people

The collection and analysis of mortality and morbidity data is also essential. Not only do they yield incidence and prevalence rates, indicating local health problems, but they should enable comparison to be made against national standards. It is of course necessary to use age-specific, as well as sex, ethnic group and socio-economic status rates, when making comparisons.

Mortality data are comparatively easy to obtain, although their limitations as a reflection of the health status of a community should be recognised. Doubts, too, exist about their accuracy, by cause of death, except where post-mortem has been undertaken.

Morbidity data are clearly more sensitive indicators of community health. Their paucity is currently hampering health visiting activity. Pressure to rectify this is an example of how health visitors can influence policies affecting health.

Such quantitative data are, however, insufficient. They do not reflect the values and priorities of a community, nor address the different beliefs, customs and traditions that affect individual and family health, or community reactions to health promotion measures. For such detailed socio-cultural information, qualitative data are required.

An ethno-methodological approach can be adopted. This involves obtaining the views of a range of individuals. It means talking with people who live and work in the particular community and use, or refuse, its various services. In the context of older people, it means finding out what they feel about the locality; and what they wish to see improved, preserved or altered. Linking qualitative data and quantitative data in this way, allows a more holistic view.

This integrated material can then be used to prepare a profile of both the entire community and specific sub-populations such as the elderly. Through systematic analysis the strengths of the community, and of specific aggregates within it, can be assessed. Resources, assets and requirements can be identified, both personal and material, as well as specific needs and problems. Thus priorities can be determined and participative plans made. In some cases such planning may involve 'targeting' specific groups. Health visitors will be aware that such selectivity is an expedience, and that the ability to survey the whole field at risk, and so provide a universal service, is their ultimate and continuing aim (Denny 1989).

Maintaining profiles, evaluating work

Obtaining and maintaining profiles requires time, skill and adequate resources. These latter include relevant, discipline-related software packages for use with computerised information systems. It is noteworthy that in the Oxfordshire 'Change for the Better' Project, described by Dauncey (1989), staff were given time and replacement help to enable them to prepare such profiles from data provided. These profiles can now be used as a basis for evaluation and review of activity, against set goals. Such an audit is necessary if work is to be effective. The significant point to note is that *attempts to measure outcomes can only be valid if appropriate inputs have been made.*

Using community profiles to advantage is a skilled technique, necessitating critical analysis and synthesis. Excerpts can be highlighted, in order to publicise local problems. Reasons for proposed changes in services can be demonstrated. This has been done in a number of localities — for example, Leighton Buzzard, where articles in the local press explained to residents how and why health visiting services were being broadened to take account of community needs. The rationale for a new, evening 'drop in' Clinic, for clients of all ages, was given by the Neighbourhood Care Manager, who pointed out endeavours to offer available and acceptable services (Stone & Wallace 1988). Thus an ability to work with the media is an additional requirement in planning and promoting change.

Community data were also utilised by Jarman (1984, 1985, 1988), in his research, to establish scores for the detection of underprivileged areas. His material is now servicing health visitors in several localities. This focus on community appraisal and associated risk analyses is discussed by Hamilton (1983), McCarthy & Dally (1984) and Fawcett-Henessy (1987).

GROUP AND INDIVIDUAL RISK APPRAISAL

From such community data, especially morbidity/mortality material, average risk estimates for particular conditions, for specific groups, can be obtained. Examples include 'the young elderly'; 'the older elderly' and 'the very old'. This enables special measures to be adopted to reduce group risk.

Individualised 'at risk' scores can then be gleaned from the standardised group data, and

Table 6.1 Some prognostic categories for certain major causes of death amongst older people

Cause of death	*Some prognostic categories — identified risk factors*
Accidents	
Home	Alcohol habits — increased intakes Drugs and medications Mobility problems Reduced sensory acuity Stress
Motor vehicle	Alcohol habits Drugs and medications Reduced reaction time Mileage driven each year Seat belt use (failure to use)
Arteriosclerotic heart disease	Raised blood pressure Raised cholesterol levels Cigarette smoking Diabetes mellitus Family history of heart disease Obesity Insufficient exercise
Cancer	
Breast	Family history Personal history benign breast disease Non-use of self-examination Pregnancy history (nulliparity)
Colon/rectum	Family history Prior polyp Undiagnosed rectal bleeding
Lung	Smoking habits
Uterus	Undiagnosed vaginal bleeding — post menopausal
Cerebrovascular accidents	Raised blood pressure High cholesterol levels Diabetes mellitus Smoking habits Reduced exercise
Respiratory disease	
Bronchitis/emphysema	Smoking history/habits Occupational history
Pneumonia	Personal history of bacterial pneumonia Alcohol habits Smoking habits

Based on data derived from:
Geller-Gesner Tables. In: Hall J H, Zwemer J D (eds) 1979 Prospective medicine. Department of Medical Education, Methodist Hospital of Indiana, USA
Donaldson R J, Donaldson L J 1983 Essential community medicine. MTP Press, Lancaster, p 61–164
Central Statistical Office 1989 Social Trends No 19. HMSO, London

adjusted to take account of personal and family health history and lifestyles. Individuals can then be shown how they may possibly reduce *their* risks and increase the probability of *their* survival and well-being.

Many prognostic categories are now well recognised, which have been derived from research studies, actuarial findings and professional reports. They can be used with all ages, once adequate data are confirmed (La Dou et al 1975, Hall & Zwemer 1979, Alderson 1986).

Table 6.1 sets out some prognostic categories for major causes of mortality in older persons. Nevertheless, it should be appreciated that there is, as yet, insufficient evidence linking risk reduction and an increase in survival. Risk appraisal can serve as a basis for specific health promotion/education activities with older people, provided that excessive client anxiety is avoided, as this may create negative response.

There are those who argue that it may be easier to develop individualised preventive strategies of this nature within the ambit of general medical practice. Here more than one team member may be involved with the older client. Even so, it is clear that there are a range of methods available to geographic-based health visitors, which enable them to discover and then provide a needs-based service (Golding et al 1986, Horrocks 1986, Hunt et al 1986, McEwen 1989). Integrating these various notions will go some way towards enabling the WHO Targets for older persons, to be met.

HEALTH VISITING BASED WITHIN GENERAL MEDICAL PRACTICE

Under this system health visitors relate to a population who have registered with a general medical practitioner, or a group practice. Such schemes have been in existence since the 1950s. Those who introduced them were enthusiastic about their potential. Since 1974 this pattern has been preferred government policy, being reiterated in the White Paper 'Promoting Better Health' (DHSS 1987).

Primary Health Care Teams have been defined in the Harding Report (DHSS 1981). The beliefs underlying this pattern of work include the following.

1. Augmented care is potentially more comprehensive and continuing than that given by individuals.
2. Resources within teams are likely to be used more economically and rare skills utilised more appropriately.
3. Standards of care are likely to be raised through discussion, informal learning and peer group influence.
4. Working together is likely to improve communication, raise morale, foster inter-dependence and encourage co-ordinated care.
5. Diversifying talents and skills is likely to increase job satisfaction.
6. Working together enables team members to deepen their awareness of their own roles, and to respect and acknowledge the roles of others. These beliefs can equally apply to neighbourhood nursing teams.

However, in spite of sound ideals and logical arguments, not all primary health care teams function at this level. Health visitors and other team members have at time expressed disquiet and disenchantment. There are several reasons why this is so.

Teams have sometimes been constituted without adequate preparation, or prior consultation, so that not all members have necessarily been committed to the concept. The differing values and assumptions underlying specific forms of professional work have not always been explored and acknowledged. Environments have not always been conducive to collaborative work, and essential tools such as age–sex registers, have not always been available.

Merely placing people together in an administrative structure does not constitute 'a team'. Many so-grouped have discovered that dynamic forces within groups can have positive or negative effects. *'Pulling together'* is an art to be learned — sometimes through disequilibrium and conflict (Dingwall 1982, McClure 1984, Westrin 1986). These problems may equally apply to neighbourhood nursing teams.

Improving the chances of team success

Some common barriers, which stand in the way of teamwork, have been identified by Hunt (1983). They include:

- inadequate educational preparation of team members
- role ambiguity and incongruent expectations
- status differentials
- authority and power structures
- leadership styles.

Accepting such barriers as 'inevitable', and concluding that primary health care teams 'do not work', would clearly be inappropriate. Effective teamwork is essential for certain health and social services goals to be achieved, particularly with older people (MacLean 1989). Hence, those concerned to develop high-level collaborative care will doubtless wish to consider those factors consistently identified as contributing to effective team functioning. These are as follows.

1. The quality and partnership of all team members should be recognised. At different times any member can serve as the point of first contact, or be the most appropriate person for consultation or referral.
2. Roles should be clarified, so that they can be mutually acknowledged, recognised and respected. To avoid ambiguity, role-conflict, or role-overload, role-expectations should be clearly defined and communicated.
3. Team goals should be mutually determined. They should be clear, relevant and feasible. Each member should understand and assent to their adoption, and should recognise their part in achieving them.
4. Time must be found for formal and informal communication. This is helped if members are housed under one roof, if meetings are scheduled, if feedback and interaction are encouraged, if leadership is apparent but not dominant, and if everyone appreciates that renegotiation is a continuing process.
5. Team members should be flexible within roles, sometimes allowing working practices to overlap. However, this does not mean that roles are interchangeable.
6. Team members should have a firm commitment to, and agree with, the team concept. These factors have an equal application to neighbourhood nursing teams.

The value of shared learning

The value of shared learning, as a concept, has long been recognised by those engaged in community health and social worker education. However, practical implementation of the idea has proved somewhat difficult, on account of the variation in length and format of courses. The recommendations contained in the Cumberlege Report, for similar-length courses and common core preparation for all community nurses, would go some way to solving this difficulty. However, trainee general practitioners, to date, are less often involved in such College courses. There is, therefore, scope for greater in-service multidisciplinary education, especially during supervised practice and in the first year after qualification.

In their study of the health assessment of elderly people at home, Buckley & Runciman (1985) made a plea for for all such education to be 'reality-based'.

They considered educational resources should be made available to primary health care teams, to allow them to examine their practice for effectiveness. The crucial role of Field and Practical Work Teachers, in promoting multi-disciplinary learning and working, was also identified.

Promoting inter-professional co-operation

It is, however, not only during preparation for qualification that shared learning and co-operation needs to be encouraged. It is an essential part of every professional's ongoing education. The recent founding of The Centre for the Advancement of Inter-professional Education in Primary Health Care (CAIPE) is therefore to be welcomed (Fawcett-Henessy 1989).

NEIGHBOURHOOD NURSING SERVICES AND PRIMARY HEALTH CARE TEAMS

The Cumberlege Report regarded neighbourhood nursing services as 'comprehensive reinforcement for primary health care teams'. It saw nurses as enhancing general practice, through their knowledge of the neighbourhood population. The Report recommended

- formal agreements
- the formation of multi-disciplinary teaching practices
- the extension of the nursing role within practice settings.

More controversial points, which would have implications for the care of older people, include the possibility of limited nurse-prescribing and the development of the nurse-practitioner role.

The Community Nursing Review Team in Wales similarly recommended direct access and self-referral to nurses in primary health care settings. They advocated (Welsh Office 1987)

- formal identification of shared objectives and priorities
- frequent, regular review meetings between team members
- the development of effective performance indicators.

THE ROLE OF DOCTOR IN GENERAL PRACTICE

There are some 30 000 general medical practitioners currently operating within the United Kingdom. Average list size is 2000 (Central Statistical Office 1989).

However, this may change, if the proposals for the reform of the NHS are implemented, since these contain distinct incentives to doctors to increase their list sizes (Dept of Health 1989).

Approximately 60% of general practitioners work in group practices, of between 2 and 10 members. Some 30% are housed in health centres.

Since 1981 all doctors entering general practice have had to undergo 3 years post-registration vocational preparation. During this period there is an emphasis on socio-medical care and the roles of other team members. Not all general practitioners prepared before 1981, necessarily recognise the difference between medical and primary health activity. Nevertheless, since 1983, there has been a move away from the perception of the general practitioner as a reactive worker, and a greater emphasis on prevention and anticipatory care (Royal College of General Practitioners 1983, Pereira Gray 1987, Taylor & Buckley 1988). This has significance for the care of older people.

The impact of NHS reform proposals on general medical practice

Under the new NHS proposals, far-reaching changes are envisaged, both for general practitioners and family practitioner committees. Practices with more than 11 000 registered patients could become budget holders (NHS Review Working Papers 3 1989). Budgets could then be used to cover the costs of in-patient care, day care procedures, and most outpatient services for the practice population. No decision has yet been made about the cost of investigations associated with prevention and screening. Since, under the proposals, certain hospitals could achieve self-governing status, general practitioners could obtain services for their patients from NHS Hospital Trusts, any appropriate District Health Authority, or from the private sector (NHS Review Working Papers 1 1989). This could complicate liaison work and might mean some older persons being treated some distance from their homes. Conversely, it is possible that a broader range of options could improve choice, and might speed up the time spent waiting for treatment.

Other proposals (NHS Review, Working Papers 4, 6 and 8 1989) which could radically affect the role of general practitioners, and hence the care of older people, include

- indicative prescribing budgets
- medical audit and peer review

- changes in the structure, membership and function of family practitioner committees.

Although at present much medical opinion is opposed to these changes, their implementation could have serious repercussions for community nursing services. There is considerable disquiet that older people may suffer as a result of the changes, since they are heavier utilisers of services. The proposals are being closely monitored by the various professional organisations (RCN 1989 Lampada Supplement, Poulton 1989).

Patterns of work and consultation in general medical practice

Doctors bring a wealth of clinical knowledge to the PHC team. A significant point to note is that in any one year they are likely to see *over* 75% of all older persons registered with them. In an average practice of 2000–2500 population, there are likely to be approximately 350 persons aged 65 years and upwards; 120 of these are likely to be 75 years or more (DHSS 1987). However, in 'preferred retirement areas' the proportion of older persons in a practice could rise from around 17% to over 40%. This is a factor to be borne in mind, when realising that the 'very old' are likely to require more home visits, so increasing time spent travelling. Furthermore, the non-specific nature of illness in old age may entail that more time is required for diagnosis.

Some idea of the amount and distribution of work in general practice can be seen from Table 6.2(a). This shows that some 17% of older people aged 65–74, and 22% of those aged 75 years or more, consulted their GP in the fortnight prior to interview for the General Household Survey 1986 (OPCS 1989). This represents a slight increase over previous years. The average number of consultations were 5.5 and 7.5, respectively (Table 6.2(b)).

Although older people are higher utilisers of the health services than most other groups, except young children, two main points should be noted:

1. The sizeable minority of older people who do not consult and appear well
2. The differences in the pattern of illness:
   a. much self-reported sickness, among older people, seems due to chronic illness (Fig. 6.1(a))
   b. in approx 25% of those older persons reporting long-standing illness, their condition also causes restricted activity (Fig. 6.1(b))
   c. acute illness affects comparatively fewer persons, generally, but is more common in the older age-groups (Fig. 6.1(c)).

Recognising and promptly treating acute illness in older people is very important, requiring expert diagnostic skills. However, caring for those with chronic or long-term illness or disability can be

Table 6.2(a) Percentage contacting general practitioner in the 14 days prior to interview, shown by sex and age, 1986

Age group	Males (%)	Females (%)	Total (%)
0–4	21	21	21
5–15	10	10	10
16–44	7	17	12
45–64	13	15	14
65–74	17	17	17
75+	22	22	22
Average over all age groups (rounded)	14	17	15

Based on data from General Household Survey 1986, Series GHS No 16. Office of Population Censuses and Surveys, Social Survey Division 1989, HMSO, London

Table 6.2(b) Average patterns of consultation with general practitioner by sex and age, 1986

Age groups (years)	*Number of consultations per person per year*		
	Males	*Females*	*Total*
0–4	6	7	6.5
5–15	3	3	3
16–44	2	6	4
45–64	4	5	4.5
65–74	5	6	5.5
75+	8	7	7.5
Average over all age groups	4.6	5.6	5.0

Based on data from General Household Survey 1986, Series GHS No 16. Office of Population Censuses and Surveys, Social Survey Division, 1989. HMSO, London

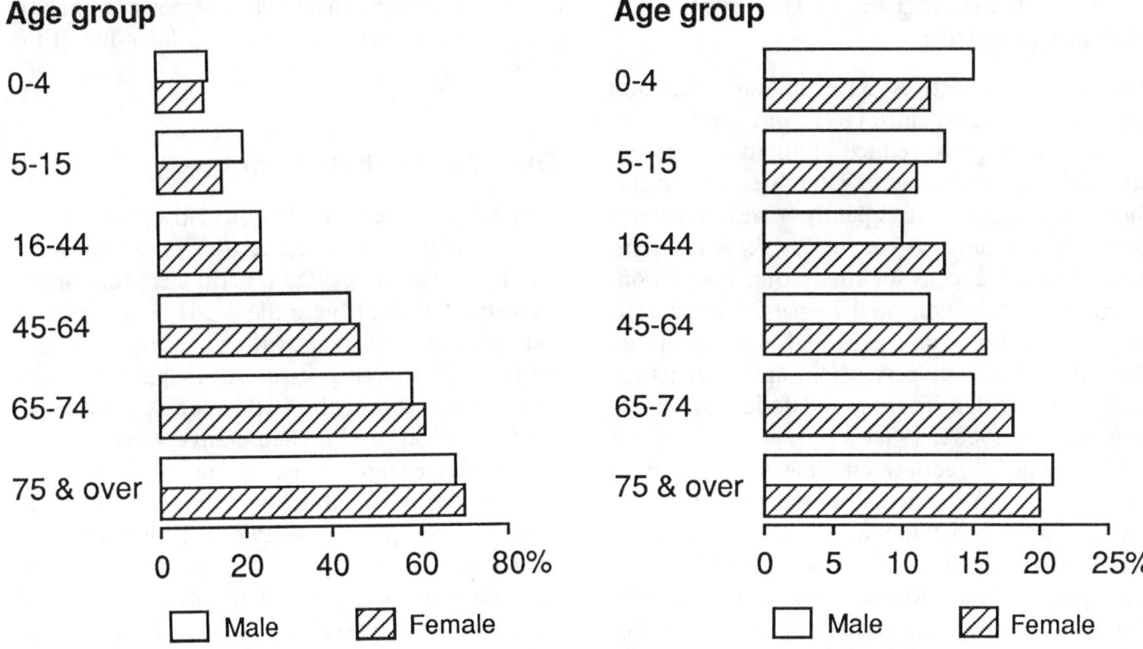

Fig. 6.1(a) Comparative picture of persons reporting long-standing/chronic illness, within a 2-week period prior to interview for the General Household Survey 1986 (OPCS 1989; reproduced by kind permission; Crown Copyright).

Fig. 6.1(b) Comparative picture of the percentage of persons reporting restricted activity arising from long-standing/chronic illness, within a 2-week period prior to interview for the General Household Survey 1986 (OPCS 1988; Crown Copyright).

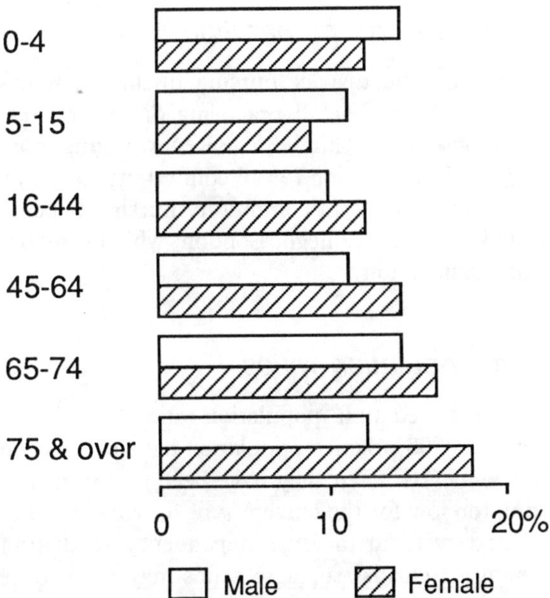

even more challenging than dealing with acute, specific and frequently self-limiting disorders (Graydon 1985, McClymont 1985, Roberts 1985, Rowatt 1985). It may carry less job satisfaction, reminding doctors of their limitations and frustrating their efforts to cure.

Familiarity with persons who have complaints of long-standing may sometimes blunt one's perceptions of what can be done to help them. It is important for all team members to recognise these difficulties which their colleagues may face, especially when caring for older people. In this way it is possible to offer more support and encouragement to try new ideas.

Fig. 6.1(c) Comparative picture of the percentage of people reporting acute illness within a 2-week period prior to interview for the General Household Survey 1986 (OPCS 1988; reproduced by permission; Crown Copyright.

Preventive strategies in general medical practice

Some medical practices have initiated schemes based on The Oxfordshire Heart and Stroke Project, in an attempt to reduce premature mortality and disabling conditions in later life. Under this scheme a Facilitator (frequently a health visitor) assists PHC teams to set up systematic, standardised health checks for their adult population. Information is disseminated to participating staff and patients. Protocols are devised, e.g. for the accurate detection of hypertension, and systems are set up for the identification and follow-up of patients (Astrop 1988a, 1988b).

Opportunistic recruitment takes place from those aged 35–64 years who are attending the practice for a consultation. Once agreement to participate has been given, personal health histories, smoking and alcohol consumption habits, blood pressure readings, and weight/height ratios are obtained.

- Those with blood pressure readings below 160/90 mm Hg are advised 5-yearly checks.
- Those with blood pressure readings of between 160/90 and 180/90 mm Hg are advised annual checks.
- Those with blood pressure readings above 180/90 mm Hg are considered for therapy.
- Those found to be overweight, on the basis of standardised tables, are given dietary advice and regular monitoring.
- Blood sugar estimations are taken in those who are 30% or more overweight, or who have a family history of diabetes.
- Blood lipid levels are measured in those with blood pressure readings 160/90 mm Hg or above, and/or in those with personal or family histories of coronary heart disease occurring before the age 55 years.

Audits taken so far, in these 'intervention practices', have shown improvements in recording, monitoring and recalling. The low-cost, low-technology method appears acceptable to patients, and, once running, can be continued by practice nurses (Fullard et al 1987). Although longer-term research is obviously needed to judge effectiveness, it is thought that such schemes are likely to effect improvements in health in later life (Fries 1988).

The role of district nurse

Over 60% of the workload of district nurses, and 75% of their time, is concerned with the care of elderly people. As skilled practitioners they are responsible for identifying the needs of sick persons and planning and providing appropriate programmes of nursing care. Although their main contribution within the PHC team is oriented towards clinical and rehabilitative care, district nurses increasingly assist in the promotion and maintenance of health, by education and preventive techniques (Ross 1987). With multi-disciplinary teams developing, opportunities exist for role expansion and role extension, especially with older people (Kratz 1980, McCabe 1984).

Increasingly, registered district nurses work in skill-mix teams, heading up the work of enrolled district nurses, or nursing auxiliaries. They carry out assessment, planning, implementing and evaluation, and delegation, supervision and control activities. They liaise with a wide range of voluntary and statutory personnel.

Education and preparation

Since 1982 the district nursing qualification has been mandatory for all practising district nurses. In response to the Cumberlege Report urging more integrated preparation for all community nurses, a new degree course in community nursing is being started at King's College, London, which provides dual qualification.

Staff–population ratios

Recommended staff–population ratios of 1 district nurse to 2500 practice population have never been fully achieved; even they have been questioned as being too low for the current type of work. Studies are underway to measure dependency in district nursing caseloads, so these ratios may have to be adjusted. Similarly the ratio of 1 district nurse to 1 GP has never been reached. Currently it stands at 1 to 1.8

Role relationships

Surveys show that over 70% of district nurses report 'good relationships' with general practitioners. Where disquiet is expressed it appears to relate to a lack of reciprocity (Dunnell & Dobbs 1982, Phillipson & Strang 1984). Similarly, over 80% of district nurses report 'good relationships' with health visitors. Although their roles may sometimes overlap, especially in the care of older persons, they remain distinct and complementary. 'Good relationships' may sometimes represent superficial contact, marked either by an avoidance of conflict, or attitudes of subservience or compliance. If this is so, it may not be to the advantage of the team, or to the benefit of clients. The true partnership of district nurses and health visitors can result in great strength for older people.

Sources of work and referral for district nurses

Within their work with older people district nurses receive open referrals in approximately one-third of cases (Ross 1987). Doctors, however, still shape their work, although their referrals are sometimes inappropriate and often too late (Cameron *et al* 1989). This is regrettable, particularly with very old people and in terminal illness. These researchers also found that ethnic minority elderly persons were under-represented in district nurses' caseloads, often because of the misconception that certain ethnic minority groups 'prefer to care for their own elderly'. Because of their role with the very old, the sick and the disabled, district nurses are in a prime position to discover informal carers, especially those who may themselves be elderly. They can then alert the team to their needs. Thus the district nursing contribution to preventive activities in screening, case-finding and research within general practice settings is likely to increase, complementing their clinical skills.

New developments affecting the role of district nurse

Although the traditional skills of district nurses remain and are being extended, the intensity of their workload has, and is, expected to increase. Demands are, and will be, generated from developments in neighbourhood nursing; from the proposed reforms in the NHS; from the increased throughput of hospital patients being discharged early into the community, for cost containment reasons, and the need to deal with waiting lists. In turn these changes impinge upon the health visiting service and the care of older people.

Some major issues likely to affect the role include

- the need for closer liaison with general practitioners in view of their changed contracts and increased responsibilities with older persons aged 75 years and more
- the potential risks versus safeguards, in terms of planned and continuing care, for older patients being treated under new contractual arrangements related to general practice budgetary control
- the increased use of more sophisticated technology in nursing patients within the community (such as in The Hospital at Home Scheme, in Peterborough) (Mowatt & Morgan 1982)
- the increasing use of home care-assistants: social services aides and future support workers.

It is noteworthy that Local Authority Social Services have now extended their home help services into more personal forms of care. In consequence district nurses have to consider their relationship with these workers, particularly regarding delegation, monitoring, supervision, responsibility and accountability. There is also the question of education, training and support for these workers, which similarly concerns health visitors.

Many of these issues are also relevant to a consideration of the interface between district nurses and practice nurses, within the PHC team. With the employment of a greater number of practice nurses and improved education and training available for them, district nurses and health visitors need to be aware of the many opportunities, and the potential difficulties which may arise (see Hockey 1984, Marsh 1985, Cater & Hawthorn 1988, MacLean 1989).

THE PRACTICE NURSE AND THE NURSE PRACTITIONER: ROLES AND RELATIONSHIPS

The practice nurse

The nature of the practice nurse's role has been a subject of controversy for several years. Some argue it is a responsibility of community nurses to provide a service for patients, within the Surgery or Health Centre. Others favour privately employed staff. The Community Nursing Review Team, in the Cumberlege Report, urged the phasing out of privately employed staff, by a withdrawal of their salary reimbursement to general practitioners. This was in line with professional organisation recommendations. In return it was envisaged there would be expansion of District Health Authority provision. Strong opposition by General Practitioners and many of the 4000, mostly part-time, practice nurses resulted in government continuance of the reimbursement system.

What is not in doubt is the need for a nursing input on medical practice premises. Practice nurses carry out a range of prescribed treatments; investigation and screening measures; monitoring and follow-up; prophylaxis such as vaccination and immunisation; health promotion and health education activities. Many of these duties benefit older people.

Research studies have shown that there are marked differences at present between the work of privately employed staff and that of community nurses acting within practice premises (Cater & Hawthorn 1988). Most of these differences relate to the amount of time which is allocated to practice nursing work. Community Nursing staff spend an average of 1.3 hours per week on practice duties, whereas directly employed staff spend an average of 9.7 hours weekly. Clearly this time differential affects the volume of work which can be undertaken.

Education for practice nurses has received considerable impetus over the past 5 years. This is in line with envisaged role expansion and role extension. Two recent developments are likely to accelerate these role changes:

1. The availability of Open Learning Packages (Newsline 1989)
2. The appointment of a Practice Nurse Adviser, with a remit to increase the range of work, provide guidance and support for those initiating new schemes, and to promote research (Hoddinott & Martin 1989).

Such developments could enhance work with older people, but some observers point out the risk of overlap, or fragmented care. The issues surrounding the practice nurse's role are of course far more complex than that of inter-professional rivalry. They involve such questions as

- medical delegation and responsibility
- nurse autonomy and accountability
- identifying education appropriate for an extended clinical role
- legal constraints on nurse-prescribing (although this is likely to be modified shortly)
- professional support for, and management of, role-holders.

For a review of such issues see Bowling (1988).

Meantime, developments in this sector hold implications for the work of health visitors with older people, especially in view of the changed nature of general practitioner contracts, due to be implemented in April 1990.

Nurse Practitioners

Nurse Practitioners made their debut in the 1960s. Their introduction was based on concern over the shortage of primary care physicians and the changing health needs of society. Not to be confused with Medical Assistants, Nurse Practitioners were regarded as

Registered Nurses who have successfully completed a formal programme of study designed to prepare them to deliver primary health care.

(American Nursing Association 1975)

Components of work included:

- assessing the health status of individuals, and families, through health histories; performing clinical examinations; ordering laboratory tests and X-rays; making initial diagnoses
- performing minor surgery, using local anaesthetics as required
- independently recommending non-prescription drugs
- writing prescriptions on blanks pre-signed by doctors
- initiating and modifying drug therapies using designated protocols
- prescribing medications
- dispensing from clinic stock
- carrying out physical and psychosocial assessments and screening procedures, and preventive measures
- carrying out health promotion. (Based on material from Leitch & Sullivan Mitchell 1977, Watson et al 1983 and Stillwell 1988a.)

However, the Nurse Practitioner role is seen as offering a different service to that of doctors, in that it includes responsibility for the planning, implementing and evaluation of nursing care needs as well.

The Alma Ata declaration (WHO 1978), gave considerable impetus to the development of Nurse Practitioners, world-wide. They are, however, a comparatively recent introduction in the UK (Stillwell 1988a). One health visitor considers that this is a preferred role for some health visitors to undertake, especially with older people (Betterton 1989).

The Cumberlege Report recommended that consideration be given to the deployment of this role within the context of neighbourhood nursing. Evidence of the acceptability of the service to consumers, and its effectiveness regarding care-outcomes, gave impetus to their recommendation (see Sox 1979, Fagin 1982, Sullivan 1982, Molde & Diers, 1985, Kenkre et al 1985). However, there are many implications and debatable points surrounding open access and autonomous functioning (Bowling 1988, Carr 1988, Stillwell et al 1988). Surveys of client/patient attitudes towards the availability of a Nurse Practitioner within general medical practice, in the UK, have shown positive responses (Kenkre et al 1985, Stillwell 1988b). These workers were regarded as: 'approachable', 'easy to talk to', 'did not appear rushed'. The latter comment should be studied in relation to the average length of consultation — 22 minutes — per person.

If the health status of the fast-increasing older population is to be improved, it may be that one way is through the development of this role, in line with WHO recommendations (WHO 1986).

THE ROLE OF HEALTH VISITOR WITHIN GENERAL MEDICAL PRACTICE

As the team's health promotion and disease prevention specialist, the health visitor can make a distinctive contribution to the care of older people, within the practice setting. The strength of this lies in the educational orientation, and in the continuing contact with families in health and disease. However, health visitors face a difficult task. The very versatility of their preparation places them at risk. Within general practice the secondary and tertiary preventive elements of their work can increase, to the detriment of steady primary prevention. Also, competing demands for their services make it difficult for them to demonstrate their role fully with any one age group.

There is evidence which suggests that the self-initiating and educative nature of health visiting work, and its social orientation, may be less readily understood than the overtly displayed clinical skills of doctors and nurses. The latter tend to share activities more often within the framework of the medical model. Hence role facets such as client-advocacy or project initiator may be less readily perceived or appreciated. Research shows that the different value-bases between doctors, nurses and health visitors may be an important contributory factor in explaining the varied perceptions and expectations of the team. Moreover, there is evidence to suggest that health visitors prefer scheduled team meetings, mutually determined team goals and regular evaluation, whereas doctors and nurses tend to rely more on ad hoc and informal contacts (Gilmore et al 1974, McClure 1984).

Another factor which may impinge upon relationships is the low ratio of health visitors to doctors: this is currently 1 health visitor to 2.4 doctors. This means that health visitors cannot always give sufficient time to deepening rapport and expanding their role. Sometimes this creates a sense of disenchantment amongst those general practitioners who perceive the potential of health visitors. This point is discussed by Barley (1987), when commenting on the ever-growing opportunities for work with older people. He envisages a need for a total health visiting work force of 19 000 if the recommendations contained in the joint policy statement of The British Geriatrics Society and the Health Visitor Association (1986) are to be realised. Nevertheless there is a great need for health visitors to adopt more flexible approaches in their work within the practice setting.

Identifying vulnerable client groups

Within a well-run practice there is great scope for identifying vulnerable persons and groups. Setting a practice profile against a community profile can enable analysis to take place and inferences to be drawn for care. Such utilisation of the search principle makes it possible for health visitors to then detect unmet needs in a subset of the practice population, who may not necessarily refer themselves. In spite of the fact that older people have generally higher levels of chronic disorder, their well-being can still be promoted, as can that of their carers. This particularly utilises the concept of health as adaptation (see Ch. 5).

While essential tools for the task, such as age–sex registers and vulnerability indexes are easier to obtain since the advent of computerised information systems, it must be appreciated that not everyone registers with a general practitioner. Hence some very vulnerable members of society can be 'lost', unless health visitors also retain a strong community dimension to their role.

Despite some health visiting consultations being held within 'surgery hours', allowing older people to receive counsel and health guidance during a visit to their doctor, the need for home visiting still remains. Full assessment depends on obtaining comprehensive data and on establishing relaxed and informal relationships with older persons (see Age Concern/Health Education Authority 1987, Martin 1989, McNaught 1987 and Appendix 4).

Like district nurses, health visitors have a large role-set. Increasingly they are receiving self-referrals from older clients and carers. In particular they need to liaise with community psychiatric nurses. Policies of discharging mentally disordered persons into the community, many of whom are older adults, have strengthened this need for liaison, especially as promoting the health of the mentally frail is an important element within health visiting (Colles 1989).

The work undertaken by health visitors with individuals, and their families, within the practice, is complemented by work with groups (see Ch. 8). Enabling older people to deal with their problems on a participative basis, is an increasing part of health visiting activity (Balter et al 1986, Drennan 1988). Demonstration of the effectiveness of health visiting for older people has been shown by Vetter et al (1984, 1986), Harrison et al (1985) and Kemp (1986). Tighter evaluation of outcome measures is, however, advocated by Clayden & Newman (1984).

PROMOTING HEALTH AND FACILITATING COLLEAGUES

As health promoters, health visitors not only have a direct interest in enhancing the well-being of their older clients (see Ch. 7, pp. 150–156), they are also concerned to enable and facilitate their colleagues. In the context of care of older persons within general practice organisation, this entails

- being conversant with the volume of work colleagues carry and the types of problems they face when caring for older people

- appreciating colleagues' aspirations and expectations
- recognising their disappointments and frustrations and providing support at such times
- respecting their goals of care and enabling them to achieve these as far as possible.

This need to facilitate colleagues also applies in the field of health visitor/social worker co-operation.

The role of social worker

In some practices social workers form part of the nuclear PHC team. Their work frequently impacts with that of health visitors and may at times overlap. They provide a valuable source of help for older people. Services include support and counselling, the provision of social and recreational facilities, casework and services for the mentally infirm and older disabled persons.

Through social workers, respite care and/or recuperative holidays can be arranged, as well as Day Centre placement and residential accommodation as necessary. They can also offer help with the elderly abused. There are also other workers within Local Authority Social Services (LASS) who can offer valuable services for older people, ranging from home helps and care assistants through to occupational therapists and community transport officers.

Positive efforts need to be made by health visitors and social workers to see how best their complementary roles can benefit older people. Apart from joint learning, joint assessment may be another way of achieving greater understanding and co-operation (Stevenson 1989). Shared responsibility for carer support groups and or pre/post-retirement courses are other examples.

Some indication of current demands made by older persons on selected health and social services is shown in Table 6.3. It will be noted that the percentage of older persons increases with advancing age. Nevertheless the overall use remains quite small. Consumer evaluation research is needed to see if this results from lack of information concerning the availability of services; service accessibility; or resource constraints.

Table 6.3 Use of some health and social services by elderly persons, within a l-month period prior to interview, 1986, by sex and age

Services used	Sex of User	Age groups using services (%)				
		65–69	70–74	75–79	80–84	85+
Chiropodist	M	4	6	10	12	8
	F	8	12	16	20	23
Day-centre	M	2	4	3	3	5
	F	5	6	8	11	7
District nurse	M	3	2	4	7	12
	F	2	2	7	12	23
Health visitor	M	0	0	1	2	2
	F	0	1	2	2	4
Home help	M	2	3	7	17	25
	F	1	7	13	24	39
Luncheon club	M	1	2	2	2	8
or centre	F	3	4	4	8	8
Meals-on-	M	1	1	3	4	2
wheels	F	0	1	3	7	11

Source of data: Office of Population Censuses and Surveys 1989 General Household Survey No 16: 1986

A survey of consumer attitudes and levels of satisfaction, in relation to services received, was undertaken in Wales, by Salvage (1986). It showed from a sample of persons aged 75 years and over, receiving health and social services, that recipients had generally high levels of satisfaction. There were, however, some areas of disenchantment. For example the timing of meals-on-wheels services, and the types of food served, evoked some disappointment, as did the hours of work and limited range of domestic work undertaken by some home helps. Because of a lower awareness of some services, Salvage recommended greater dissemination of information for older clients, concerning luncheon clubs, day hospitals, incontinence laundry services, bath attendants and sheltered housing.

The wider team

In endeavouring to offer a comprehensive service to older people, PHC team members have widespread liaison responsibilities. Wider team members include geriatricians and other hospital staff, paramedical personnel, social, education and housing staff and a host of voluntary workers. There is much scope therefore for shared learning and communication, which health visitor educators and managers might well consider.

THE GERIATRIC LIAISON HEALTH VISITOR

Drawing the PHC team members and the wider team together is part of the role remit of the Geriatric Liaison Health Visitor. This role may be undertaken on a rota basis by a number of health visitors within general practice settings, although, of course, geographic-based health visitors may also fill this role. Duties include acting as

- a point of contact, channelling information between client and professionals working in the community and in hospital
- an adviser on health promotion / disease prevention activities for older clients and carers
- a health counsellor offering education, support and rehabilitative guidance for clients and families
- a mobiliser of services
- an educational resource person.

Geriatric Liaison Health Visitors also participate in screening and case-finding activities and undertake a range of tasks including initiating new schemes.

SCREENING AND CASE-FINDING

Reference has been made earlier to screening and case-finding as important secondary preventive strategies, frequently undertaken within general medical practice settings. It may therefore be timely to clarify the meaning of these terms, which are often used interchangeably, thus causing confusion.

'*Screening*' is defined as

> the seeking out of persons with no overt symptoms, and asking them to undergo examination, to see if any disease is present.
>
> (DHSS 1976)

'*Case-finding*' is considered to be

> the detection of overt but unacknowledged or disregarded symptoms.
>
> (Williamson 1981)

Another way of putting it is given by Freer (1988). He sees screening as 'searching for conditions hidden to the person' and case-finding as 'searching for conditions hidden to the doctor'.

It is important to appreciate the difference between these two forms of detection, even though at a practical level they may both seem equally useful. The difference lies in the underlying principles, in the theory base, and in the detailed criteria developed to determine the efficiency and effectiveness of screening procedures (see Kemp 1986).

The principles of screening

The principles of screening relate to the disease, the test to be applied and to the proposed treatment.

1. The disease or condition being searched for should be an important health problem, for both the individual and society.
2. The natural history of the disease, including its development from the latent to the manifest stage, should be fully known.
3. Precursors of the condition should be identifiable.
4. Factors determining responses to treatment should be evaluated.

Rigour must equally be applied to the screening tests to be used. These should be

- simple
- acceptable
- accurate and precise
- cost effective
- sensitive
- specific

(Donaldson & Donaldson 1983).

Tests which are non-invasive, or involve simple observation and little or no undressing, such as tests of sight or hearing, are more likely to evoke co-operation, whereas painful and time-consuming tests are less likely to be accepted.

In general the benefits derived from early detection and treatment of the disease should justify the costs of the screening programme.

Tests must be reliable, giving consistent results. For instance the problem of obtaining reliable blood pressure readings, on account of subject and observer factors, are well known (Fullard et al 1987, Astrop 1988b).

Screening tests must also be sensitive and specific.

Sensitivity means the ability of the test to give *positive results* when the disease being screened for *is present*.

Specificity, however, means the ability of the test to give *negative results* in healthy individuals *without the disease*.

Ideally both sensitivity and specificity will be 100% each. That is, the test will give all true positives and all true negatives. However, this is only achieved when the normal and the diseased populations are widely separated, according to the test used (Fig. 6.2).

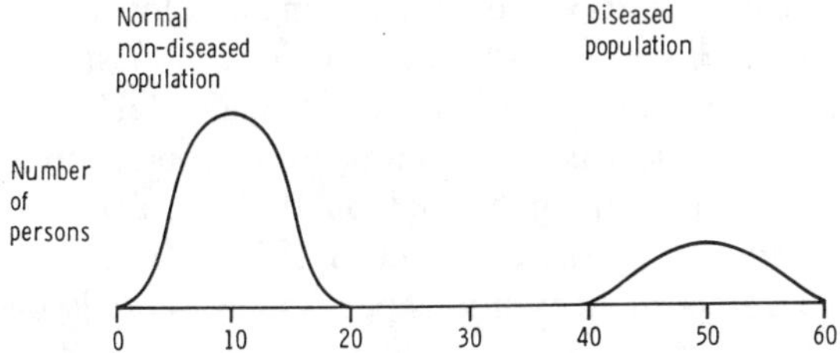

Fig. 6.2 An hypothetical screening test.

Unfortunately, in real life, the situation is seldom so clear cut. The normal and the diseased populations often overlap. Consider for example, the measurement of intra-ocular pressure, in order to screen for simple glaucoma, where there is an overlap between persons with non-glaucomatous eyes and those with glaucomatous eyes (Fig. 6.3).

Those with intra-ocular pressures below 22 mm Hg will all have non-glaucomatous (i.e. '*normal*') eyes. Those with values above 26 mm Hg will all have glaucomatous ('*diseased*') eyes.

However, for those with values of 22–26 mm Hg, it is not possible to say to which group a particular person belongs. The degree of sensitivity and specificity of the test will be varied, depending on which screening values are adopted. Thus, if the values of 26 mm Hg and over are chosen, the test is 100% specific. All persons with normal eyes will be excluded; therefore there are no false positives. Nevertheless this is at the expense of excluding some persons with values of 22 mg Hg or more, but below 26 mm Hg, who may have glaucomatous eyes. They therefore form a false negative group.

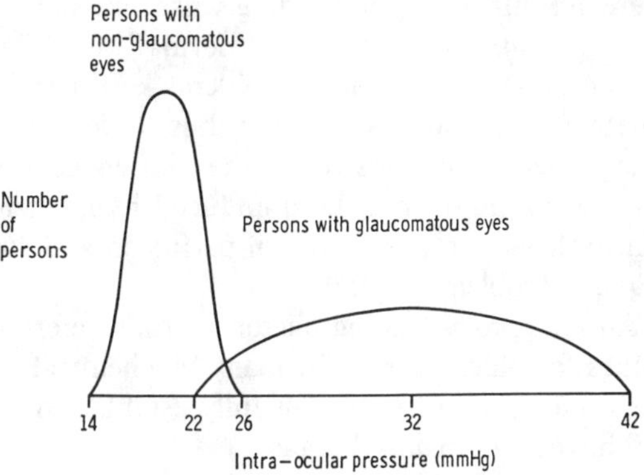

Fig. 6.3 Specificity and sensitivity of tests for persons screened for simple glaucoma (hypothetical values).

Conversely, if the value is set at 22 mm Hg and above, the test becomes 100% sensitive. All the persons with abnormal eyes have been covered, but this is at the expense of including a few people with normal eyes, who now form a 'false' positive group.

Clearly very careful judgement has to be exercised when determining the values which will be used for demarcation purposes, so that individuals are not 'missed cases' on the one hand, nor exposed to needless anxiety and the risk of hypochondria on the other.

This issue is sometimes compounded further, because of the difficulties which may arise in determining 'normality'. For instance, when screening for anaemia, the usual definition of 'a value less than 12 g Hb' is of limited use, since vascular and psychomotor symptoms do not appear until values of about 8 g Hb/100 ml are reached. Similarly, in screening for hypertension, there are difficulties in deciding what levels of systolic pressure to accept as 'normal' for older persons. There are also problems in deciding whether, and how best, to treat those older people who appear hypertensive by the chosen criteria, yet are symptom free. Drug-induced hypotension can itself lead to poor cerebral perfusion and subsequent problems.

Another complicating factor is that reference values for older people, for many biochemical and haemotological tests, are not fully established.

This occurs mainly because

1. the value of many 'norms' have been derived from population studies of younger persons; these may have no applicability to older people
2. there has hitherto been a difficulty finding sufficient disease-free older persons in order to establish 'older norms'.

However, this picture is changing. Research on 70-year-olds in The Gothenburg Longitudinal Study, is already yielding valuable data (Svanborg 1985, Ciba Foundation 1988). These findings are stimulating further focused research, which should provide guidelines in future.

Ethics apart, there is little point in screening persons for any condition unless the treatment for the condition is available, acceptable and effective. This is of paramount importance with older people. A high detection rate can swamp existing treatment facilities, causing frustration and distress to staff and patients alike. A necessary maxim is to always calculate beforehand the effect, on others, of instituting any change in programme.

TO SCREEN . . . OR NOT TO SCREEN?

One should not necessarily infer, from this discussion, that screening for older people is *undesirable*, but rather that it should be undertaken with caution, in the understanding that it is more problematic. Some attempt to identify pre-symptomatic disease *is* carried out for older people, e.g. biochemical assays of thyroid function, or blood glucose estimations. Multiphasic screening, which produces biochemical profiles of elderly people, may show unsuspected disease, but there seems little correlation between these results and subsequent death (Murray & Young 1977).

A trial of multiphasic screening in South-East London found there was no significant difference, 9 years after initial screening, between screened and control groups, in any outcome measures tested (South East London Screening Study Group 1977).

Curiously enough, some individuals who have been screened and been found to have the condition sought for, have refused treatment. A salutary reminder that decisions ultimately rest with the client/patient!

SEARCHING FOR UNREPORTED MORBIDITY: CASE-FINDING

In earlier life, the application of secondary prevention methods, in the form of screening, may lead to early detection and possible cure. In later maturity, however, there may be less scope for cure, so the emphasis must rest on the implications of detected conditions for functioning and for quality of life. Pioneering studies, undertaken post-war, but before the beneficial impact of the NHS had occurred, identified high levels of unreported morbidity in older people (Sheldon 1948, Anderson & Cowan 1955, Williamson et al 1964). An average of 3 unreported conditions per person were discovered.

Such unreported illness thus came to be known as 'the iceberg of morbidity'. The submerged portion of the iceberg showed a characteristic pattern, with the bulk of 'unknown' conditions being locomotor problems, foot conditions, visual and hearing defects, urinary tract disorders, depression and dementia.

A decade or so later, further studies confirmed a similar level of hidden morbidity (Barber & Wallis 1976, Abrams 1978, 1980). However, since then it has been suggested that an important secular change may be occurring in the attitudes, behaviour and health status of *some* older people (Tulloch & Moore 1979, Ebrahim et al 1984). Improved utilisation of health services, and rising standards of well-being in some groups of older people, who therefore rarely need to use the services, may account for this change.

This phenomenon is matched by a paradox, mentioned by Svanborg (Ciba 1988). He and his colleagues found that while studies generally show *under-diagnosis* to be common in older people, *over-diagnosis* also occurs. Particularly, this seems to happen in such cases as congestive cardiac failure, dementia and hypertension. Over-medication can then result.

Bearing these complexities in mind, it is not surprising that the major focus of prevention in later life has shifted from the detection of asymptomatic disease, to discovering those poorly-reported conditions which have implications for function and quality of life. Hence multifunctional assessment has become a preferred activity (Fillenbaum 1984).

Economic constraints and demographic changes provide the impetus to identify valid, rational bases for health care policy. This issue was addressed in The Harrogate Symposium on Preventive Care for Older People, reported by Taylor & Buckley (1988):

> Health care planners and practitioners are both looking for efficient and effective ways, which will distinguish between those older people, who *do* require comprehensive assessment and those who *do not*.

Health visitor assessment and case-finding: alternative methods

Examples of attempts by health visitors to identify, assess and then survey all older people in a given sub-population are reported by MacLeod & Mein (1988) Killingbeck & Sanderson (1988), Steel (1989) and Martin (1989).

A further study is reported by Phillips (1987). In this research study 215 older persons, aged 65–75 years, attending 'Well Pensioners' Clinics' in Lewisham, were assessed, using an health visiting tool based on Orem's model of self-care (see Appendix 3 and Appendix 4). Personalised health promotion was undertaken with all participants, on the basis of this assessment. In addition 31% of participants were referred to their GPs for further consideration. 60% of these subsequently required medical treatment.

There are distinct advantages to the use of this method of case-finding, by contrast to some others, e.g. a differentiating questionnaire or letter (Barber & Wallis 1982) (see also Table 6.5):

1. Assessment is perceived as an integral part of a well-persons' clinic activity.
2. It provides a benefit for all participants, in terms of subsequent personalised health promotion, apart from any required medical intervention, as a result of the detection of unreported conditions.
3. Referral of a proportion of persons with hitherto undiscovered morbidity allows surveillance to be subsequently undertaken.

Phillips estimated that it would be possible to provide a District-wide service, which would allow every local person aged 65–75 to receive one such assessment, on a 3-yearly basis, if every Clinic/Health Centre in the District mounted one weekly session. This was calculated to require 1 health visitor and 1 clinic nurse, per session, per week. This contrasts with Killingbeck & Sanderson (1988) who estimated that it would require 7–8 health visits per week in order to provide a home-visiting surveillance programme, on a 5-yearly basis, for all 70–80-year-old clients, in their Health Centre.

Clearly, local factors and manpower resources have to be taken into account, as well as other differences between home-based and clinic-based health appraisal and assessment.

It should be noted that in each of these examples, considerable pre-planning was necessary; criteria were determined after consultation with colleagues; consumer evaluation was undertaken and all the rigour associated with research method was applied.

Sometimes other workers can assist in such projects, allowing health visitors to conserve their skills, particularly for primary preventive activities. In two programmes, volunteers were trained to act as initial data collectors, under supervision (Beales 1988, Carpenter & Demopoulos 1988). In each instance the projects were considered practical, low-cost and effective ways of reaching large numbers of older people.

Other methods

In a study in Stirling (McIntosh et al 1988, McIntosh 1989), an enrolled nurse, working in liaison with health visitors, proved to be highly effective and economic as a case-finder. Patients aged 75 years and over were identified from the age–sex register, and a process of opportunistic and domiciliary organised assessment was carried out. Tools used included standardised, numerically scored, serial medical, social and functional assessments. Those at 'high risk' (35%) were identified by a series of scores in several dimensions; they received quarterly surveillance visits thereafter. The 41% found to be moderately impaired received 6-monthly visits, and the 24% deemed healthy were seen annually. Surveillance input increased by 9%, but on-demand crisis intervention *decreased considerably*. High input services and aids, offered on a pre-determined support plan, improved standards of care and helped older people remain at home longer.

Selection of 'at risk' groups

As the examples of Phillips & McIntosh et al have shown, one way of identifying 'high risk' groups is to carry out 'universal' assessment first, and then concentrate on surveillance of those found to have problems. Another way is to endeavour to determine vulnerability on the basis of some disadvantage, or life-upheaval experience. The problem with this latter method lies in being sure one has identified correctly! Several predetermined 'at risk' groups have been used in different research studies (Williamson 1981). Table 6.4 sets out some research-identified 'at risk' categories. However, it should be noted that the researchers have subsequently concluded that such a 'priority risk group' approach is less efficient than an individual method using a differentiating letter (Taylor & Ford 1988).

One such letter, devised as an initial 'screening out' device, was developed by Barber & Wallis (1982). It was used at Woodside Health Centre, Glasgow, and is shown in Table 6.5. Tests show it to be highly sensitive and specific, but rather 'costly', as it requires 80% of the particular popu-

Table 6.4 Potential high risks groups among elderly persons, ranked in priority order

Category 1 Elderly potentially at highest risk
Divorced/separated
Recently discharged from hospital
Recently moved/relocated
The very old (80+)

Category 2 Elderly potentially at medium risk
Recently widowed
Living alone
Poor
Social class V category

Category 3 Elderly potentially at lowest risk
Isolated persons
Single persons
Childless

Based upon data given by Taylor R, Ford G, Barber H 1983 The elderly at risk. Research Perspectives on Ageing, 6. Age Concern Research Unit, Mitcham

Table 6.5 Postal questionnaire as sent out to selected high-risk groups of elderly from Woodside Health Centre, Glasgow (accompanying letter not shown)

Name
Address

e.g. Do you live on your own?	Please circle the answer applicable to you	
Do you live on your own?	Yes	No
Are you in the position of having *no* relatives on whom you can rely for help?	Yes	No
Do you need regular help with housework or shopping?	Yes	No
Are there days when you are unable to prepare a hot meal for yourself?	Yes	No
Are you confined to your home through ill health?	Yes	No
Is there any difficulty or concern over your health you still have to see about?	Yes	No
Do you have any problem with your eyes or eyesight	Yes	No
Do you have any difficulty with your hearing?	Yes	No
Have you been in hospital during the past year?	Yes	No

Thank you for answering these questions. Would you please return this form to me at the surgery? A stamped addressed envelope is enclosed.

Reproduced by kind permission of Dr J H Barber and Miss J Wallis H V

lation to be contacted initially, in order to yield full results. Efforts are now in hand to refine the instrument, and to obtain a more 'economical' but equally sensitive and specific tool.

Health visitors will appreciate that the use of any differentiating mechanism can only be justified, in terms of resource-costs, if it reveals a substantial proportion of persons with 'unknown' problems. At the same time, 'knowing' about a problem does not guarantee it will be dealt with, or ameliorated. If quality of life for clients and carers is considered important, then the use of a differentiating device, be it an assessment form, or a letter or questionnaire, may enable health visitors to offer more targeted surveillance, while retaining health promotion activities for all.

In this connection, the imaginative Edinburgh Birthday Scheme has much to commend it (Porter 1988). Here a variant of the Woodside questionnaire is sent, with a short, friendly letter, offering health visiting services. This is enclosed in a simple but attractive birthday card. A pre-paid envelope is enclosed for a reply. The card is sent to older persons aged 65, 70, 75 and 78, on the anniversary of their birth-date. From 80 years, cards are sent at 2-yearly intervals, changing to yearly intervals after 90 years. Home visits are paid if the reply indicates need, or if there has been no reply after 3 weeks.

Over a 2-year period (April 1985 to March 1987), 565 cards were sent out, 94% of questionnaires were returned, and 814 clients were subsequently identified (Stanton 1987, 1988). An audit sheet is completed, which enables continuing evaluation of the service. The scheme appears highly acceptable to clients, inexpensive and feasible to organise. One feature has been that 16% of clients have subsequently utilised the health visitor service, but *when they have chosen to do so*. This is the essence of any empowering activity.

Other selective groupings

Other selective groups have been used by health visitors, in their attempts at case-finding and surveillance. In her study, Phillips (1987), showed that five pre-determined groups of potentially 'at risk' elderly yielded high levels of health need and required more health visitor intervention than did a matched comparison group. These pre-determined groups were:

- those recently attending Accident and Emergency Departments
- those recently discharged from hospital
- those recently moved address
- those referred by general practitioner
- those referred by self.

However, Phillips findings could not confirm that these specific groups are the ones which would be *most* likely to benefit from health visitor assessment and intervention. Other similar examples are provided by Coupland (1986) and Tierney (1989).

There are thus a number of preventive strategies which can be used in health visiting older people, under different organizational patterns. However, two points must be noted. The first is that whichever method is used, it must be carefully planned and implemented and fully evaluated. A flow chart, showing some of the content of these stages, is given in Figure 6.4. The second point

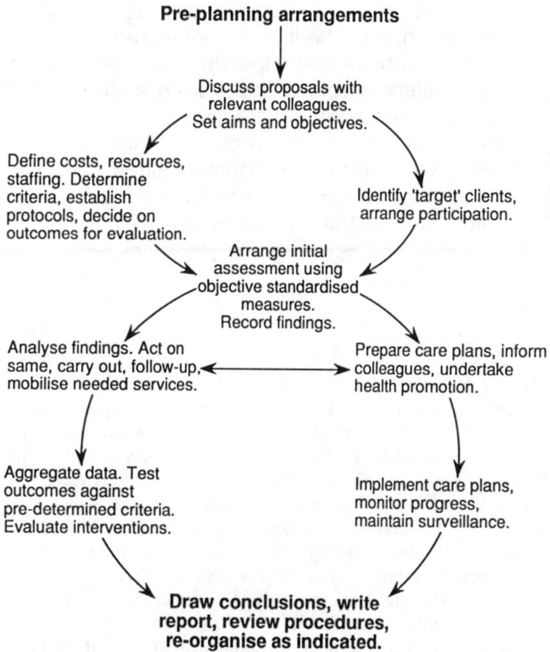

Fig. 6.4 Steps in a screening or a case-finding project programme.

is that, in spite of the evident enthusiasm with which some health visitors have undertaken work with older people, the overall involvement of the profession has not significantly increased in the last decade (see Table 1.4, Ch. 1).

It is clear that whatever organisational structure is operative, all health visitors must acknowledge that they have a responsibility towards the health needs of those in later maturity (Lowe 1988). To facilitate the practical health visiting care of older persons, a check list is given at the end of this chapter

SUMMARY

This chapter has focused on three specific areas.

1. The broad international perspective of health care delivery, with particular reference to WHO Targets for 'Health for all' for older people, has been described. This also showed how international goals impact on national and local health policies and hence administrative structures.

2. Geographic and practice-based health visiting, neighbourhood nursing services, and primary health care teams have been discussed. Roles of specific members have been given, with the intention of increasing respect for these and improving co-operation. Issues affecting role-changes were stated.

3. The meanings of screening and case-finding, in relation to older clients, have been given and their respective values discussed. The need for quality care and evaluative research has been stressed.

REFERENCE

Abrams M 1978 Beyond three score years and ten: a first report on a survey of the elderly. Age Concern, Mitcham

Abrams M 1980 Beyond three score years and ten: a second report on a survey of the elderly. Age Concern, Mitcham

Age Concern/Health Education Authority 1987 Chatteris Age Well Club and screening programme. Age well ideas sheet No 5. Health Education Authority, London

Alderson M 1986 An ageing population: some demographic and health trends. Public Health 100: 263–277

American Nursing Association 1975 Guidelines for the Nurse Training Act. In: Bliss A A, Cohen E D (eds) (1977) The new health professionals: nurse practitioners and physicians' assistants. Rockville, Maryland

Anderson W F, Cowan N R 1955 A consultative health centre for older people. Lancet 2: 239–240

Astrop P 1988a Facilitator: the birth of a new profession. Health Visitor October 61: 311–312

Astrop P 1988b What the facilitator can do for the practice nurse. Practice Nurse (May): 13–17

Balter D, Daniels H, Finch J, Perkins E R 1986 Training health visitors to work with the community groups. In: Perkins E R (ed) Nottingham Practical Papers in Health Education, No 14. Education Department, University of Nottingham, Nottingham

Barber J H, Wallis J B 1976 Assessment of the elderly in general practice. Journal of the Royal College of General Practitioners 26: 106–114

Barber J H, Wallis J B 1982 The effects of a system of geriatric assessment and screening, on a general practice work-load. Health Bulletin 40 (3): 125–132

Barley S 1987 An uncompromising report. British Medical Journal 294: 595–6

Beales D L 1988 The use of trained volunteers in a screening programme: an evaluative study. In: Taylor R C, Buckley E G (eds) Preventive care of the elderly. Occasional Papers No 35: The Royal College of General Practitioners, London

Betterton S 1989 The Nurse-Practitioner role at Buntingford Health Centre. Personal communication.

Bowling A 1988 The changing role of the practice nurse in the UK, from doctor's assistant to collaborative practitioner. In: Bowling A, Stilwell B (eds) The nurse in family practice. Scutari Press, London, p 13–29

British Geriatrics Society/Health Visitor Association 1986 Health visiting for the health of the aged. A joint policy statement. BGS/HVA, London

Buckley E G, Runciman P J 1985 Health assessment of the elderly at home. University of Edinburgh, Edinburgh

Burke V, MacCartney J, Pearson A 1986 The needs of retired people. Health Visitor, 59 (October): 302–303

Cameron E, Badger F, Evers H 1989 District Nurses and General Practitioners. In: Primary Health Care (7) (July): 14–15

Carpenter G I, Demopoulos G P 1988 The use of a disability rating questionnaire, in a case-controlled screening surveillance programme. In: Taylor T G, Buckley E G (eds) Preventive care of the elderly. Occasional Papers No 35. The Royal College of General Practitioners, London, p 11–12

Carr A J 1988 The implications of the Cumberlege Report for the development of a Nurse-Practitioner's role. In: Bowling A, Stilwell B (eds) The nurse in family practice. Scutari Press, London

Cater L, Hawthorn P 1988 Survey of Practice Nurses in the UK, their extended roles. In: Bowling A, Stilwell B (eds) The Nurse in Family Practice. Scutari Press, London

Central Statistical Office OPCS 1989 Social Trends No 19. HMSO, London

Ciba Foundation 1988 Research and the ageing population. Symposium No 134. Wiley, Chichester

Clayden A D, Newman C P S 1984 Effect of health visitors working with elderly patients in general practice. Randomised controlled trials. British Medical Journal 288: 1309

Colles S 1989 Account of role as Specialist Health Visitor (Psycho-Geriatrics), Balfour Day Hospital Edinburgh Personal communication

Cotton E, Sharp G 1989 Community health promotion and education: empowering groups. Account of activities in

Rochdale DHA. Personal communication
Coupland R 1986 Effective health visiting for elderly people — a specialist health visitor's perspective. Health Visitor 59 October: 299–300
Dauncey J 1989 Change for the better. Oxford District Health Authority, Oxford
Denny E 1989 The future of health visiting. Health Visitor 62 (August): 250–251
Department of Health 1989 Working for patients. HMSO, London
DHSS (Department of Health and Social Security) 1976 Prevention and health: everybody's business HMSO London
DHSS (Department of Health and Social Security) 1981 The Primary Health Care Team: report of a joint working group of the Standing Medical Advisory Committee and the Standing Nursing and Midwifery Advisory Committee (Harding Report). HMSO, London
DHSS (Department of Health and Social Security) 1986 Neighbourhood nursing — a focus for care. Report of the Community Nursing Review Committee, Chairperson: J Cumberlege. HMSO, London
DHSS (Department of Health and Social Security) 1987 Promoting better health. The Government's programme for improving primary health care. HMSO, London
Dingwall R 1982 Problems of teamwork in primary care. In: Clare A W, Corney R H (eds) Social work and primary health care. Academic Press, London
Donaldson R J, Donaldson L J 1983 Essential community medicine. MTP Press, Lancaster
Drennan V 1984 A new approach. Nursing Mirror 159 (14) 17th October: Health Visiting Supplement px
Drennan V 1988 (ed) Health Visitors and groups. Heinemann, London
Dunnell K, Dobbs J 1982 Nurses working in the community. OPCS, HMSO, London
Ebrahim S, Hedley R, Sheldon M 1984 Low levels of ill-health among elderly non-consulters in general practice. British Medical Journal 289: 1273–1275
Fagin C M 1982 Nursing as an alternative to high cost patient care. American Journal of Nursing 82: 56–60
Fawcett-Henessy A 1987 The future. In: Littlewood J (ed) Community nursing. Recent advances in nursing series, No 15. Churchill Livingstone, Edinburgh
Fawcett-Henessy A 1989 Co-operation in the community. A new commitment in inter-professional working. Primary Health Care (5) 7th May: 1
Fillenbaum G 1984 The well-being of the elderly: approaches to multi-disciplinary assessment. WHO, Geneva
Freer C B 1988 Detecting hidden needs in the elderly: screening or case-finding? Part 2 Review Papers. In: Taylor R C, Buckley E G (eds) Preventive care of the elderly. Occasional Papers No 35. Royal College of General Practitioners, London
Fries J H 1988 Aging, illness and health policy: implications of the compression of morbidity. In: Perspectives in Biology and Medicine 31 (3): 407–429
Fullard E, Fowler G, Gray M 1987 Promoting prevention in primary care: controlled trial of low technology, low cost approach. British Medical Journal 294 (25th April): 1080–1087
Gilmore M, Bruce N, Hunt S M 1974 The nursing team in general practice. CETHV, London
Golding A W B, Hunt S M, McEwen J 1986 Health needs in a London District. Health Policy 6: 175–84
Gooding H, Williamson G H, Honeyman F D 1986 The value of a preventive care service for the elderly. Health Visitor 59 (October): 305–306
Graydon J E 1985 Coping with cancer: a chronic illness. In: King K (ed) Long term care. Recent advances in nursing series, No 13. Churchill Livingstone, Edinburgh, p 120–131
Hall J H, Zwemer J D 1979 Prospective medicine. Department of Medical Education, Methodist Hospital of Indiana, Indianapolis
Hamilton P 1983 Community nursing diagnoses. Advances in Nursing Science (April): 21–35
Harrison S, Rous S, Martin E, Wilson S 1985 Assessing the needs of the elderly: using unsolicited visits by health visitors. Journal of The Royal Society of Medicine 78 (July): 557–561
Hockey L 1984 Is the practice nurse a good idea? Journal of The Royal College of General Practitioners 3: 102–103
Hoddinott D, Martin C 1989 Practice Nurse Adviser — a new role. Primary Health Care 7 (5) (May): 16–17
Horrocks P 1986 The components of a comprehensive district health service for elderly people: a personal view. Age and Aging 15: 321–342
Hunt M 1983 Possibilities and problems of inter-disciplinary teamwork. In: Clark J, Henderson J (eds) Community health. Churchill Livingstone, Edinburgh, p 233–241
Hunt S M, McEwen J, McKenna S 1986 Measuring health status. Croom Helm, London
Jarman B 1984 Under-privileged areas; validation and distribution of scores. British Medical Journal 289: 1587–1592
Jarman B 1985 Under-privileged areas. In: Medical Annual. Wright, Bristol, 224–243
Jarman B 1988 Primary Care. Heinemann, London
Jones C 1989 Community health promotion initiatives with informal carers (Report of work in Christchurch, Dorset). Personal communication
Kemp L M 1986 Screening the elderly. Health Visitor 59 (October): 303–305
Kenkre J, Drury V W M, Lancashire R J 1985 Nurse management of hypertension clinics in general practice, assisted by a computer. Family Practice 2: 17–22
Killingbeck P, Sanderson C 1988 Use of a postal questionnaire in screening for common problems. In: Taylor R C, Buckley E G (eds) Preventive care of the elderly. Occasional Papers No 35. The Royal College of General Practitioners, London, p 16–18
King's Fund 1988a Introducing neighbourhood nursing: the management of change. Dally G, Brown P (eds), King's Fund Centre for Health Services Development, Primary Health Care Group, London
Kings Fund 1988b Can Cumberlege work in the Inner City? The Wandsworth view. Dally G, King's Fund Centre for Health Services Development, Primary Health Care Group, London
King's Fund 1988c Preparing for Cumberledge. Brown P. King's Fund Centre for Health Services Development, Primary Health Care Group, London
Kratz C 1980 The district nurse. In: Barber J H, Kratz C R (eds) Towards team care. Churchill Livingstone, Edinburgh
La Dou J, Sherwood J N, Hughes L, Health hazard appraisal in patient counselling. Preventive Medicine.

Western Journal of Medicine 122 February: 177–80
Leitch C, Sullivan Mitchell M A 1977 State by state report: the legal accommodation of nurses practising in extended roles. Nurse Practitioner 2: p 19–30
Lowe R 1988 Reform — or die. Nursing Times 84 (42): 74
Luker K, Orr J (eds) 1985 Health visiting. Blackwell Scientific Publications, Oxford
MacLean U 1989 Dependent territories: the frail elderly and community care. Nuffield Provincial Hospital Trust, London
MacLeod E, Mein P 1988 The nursing care team: a task force approach. In: Taylor RC, Buckley E G (eds) Preventive care of the elderly. Occasional Papers No 35. Royal College of General Practitioners, London, p 19–21
McCabe F 1984 The community nurse — lynchpin in liaison, in the care of the older housebound person. Coventry Health District, unpublished paper
McCarthy N G, Daly E A 1984 Community assessment a risk factor analysis. Journal of Nursing Education 23 (9): 398–401
McClure L M 1984 Team work — myth or reality: Community Nurses' experience with general practice attachment. Journal of epidemiology and Community Health. 38 (1): 68–74
McClymont M E 1985 Intervention and care in long-term nursing of the adult. In: King K (ed) Long term care. Recent advances in nursing series, No 13. Churchill Livingstone, Edinburgh
McEwen J 1989 Planning health care: the community approach. In: Warnes A (ed) Human ageing and later life. Edward Arnold, London
McIntosh I 1989 Comprehensive screening of the over-75s — a worthwhile objective. Geriatric Medicine 19(8): 18–20
McIntosh I B, Young M, Stewart T 1988 General practice surveillance scheme. Scottish Medical Journal 33(5): 332–333
McNaught A 1987 Health action and ethnic minorities. National Community Health Initiatives Resource Unit, Bedford Square Press, London
Marsh G N 1985 More nurses needed. Nursing Times, Community Outlook 81: 10–11
Martin A 1989 The Age Well Club, Chatteris, Cambs: a comprehensive and structured health visiting service for elderly people. Unpublished Paper. Church Lane Surgery, Chatteris, Cambs
Molde S, Diers D 1985 Nurse Practitioner research: a selected literature review. Nursing Research 34: 362–367
Mowatt L G, Morgan R T 1982 Peterborough's Hospital at Home Scheme. British Medical Journal 284: 641–643.
Murray T S, Young R E 1977 A laboratory survey in a geriatric population. Update 14: 191–196
Newsline 1989 Practice nurse training package. Primary Health Care 7 (5): 2
NHS (National Health Service) Review: Working Papers 1989
No 1: Self-governing hospitals. Department of Health, London
No 3: Practice budgets for general medical practitioners. Department of Health, London
No 4: Indicative prescribing budgets for general practitioners. Department of Health, London
No 6: Medical audit. Department of Health, London
No 8: Implications for Family Practitioner Committees. Department of Health, London
OPCS (Office of Population, Censuses and Surveys) 1989 General Household Survey 1986: No 16. HMSO, London
Pereira Gray 1987 Preventive care of the elderly. The Journal of The Royal College of General Practitioners 37 (296): 9
Phillips S 1987 Ageing well. A model for health visiting older people. Summary Report. Lewisham and North Southwark Health Authority, London
Phillipson C, Strang P 1984 Health education and older people: the role of paid carers. Health Education Council, in association with the Department of Adult Education, University of Keele
Porter A M D 1988 The Edinburgh Birthday Card Scheme. In: Taylor R C, Buckley E G (eds) Preventive care of the elderly. Occasional Papers No 35. The Royal College of General Practitioners, London, p 22–23
Poulton B C 1989 The White Paper: a continuing debate in the community. Primary Health Carere 17 (5) (May): 18
Roberts I 1985 The social and economic implications of chronic illness: a British perspective. In: King K (ed) Long-term care. Recent advances in nursing series, No 13 Churchill Livingstone, Edinburgh, p 71–96
Ross F 1987 District nursing. In: Littlewood J (ed) Community nursing. Recent advances nursing series, No 15. Churchill Livingstone, Edinburgh, p 132–159
Rowatt K M 1985 Chronic pain: a family affair. In: King K (ed) Long-term care. Recent advances in nursing series, No 13. Churchill Livingstone, Edinburgh, p 137–150
Royal College of General Practitioner 1983 Promoting prevention. Royal College of General Practitioners, London
RCN (Royal College of Nursing) 1989 Lampada supplement. The health challenge. (May): 1–4
Salvage A V 1986 Attitudes of the over 75s to health and social services. Final report (August), Research Team for the Elderly. University of Wales, Cardiff
Scottish Home and Health Department 1978 District nursing in Scotland (Hockey Report) HMSO Edinburgh
Sheldon J H 1948 The social medicine of old age. Oxford University Press, Oxford
South East London Screening Study Group 1977 A controlled trial of a multi-phasic screening programme in middle age: results of the South-east London Screening Study. International Journal of Epidemiology 6: 357–363
Sox H C 1979 Quality of patient care by nurse practitioners and physicians: a 10 year perspective. Annals of Internal Medicine 91: 459–468
Stanton A 1987 Screening/Case-finding in the elderly: The Edinburgh Birthday Card Scheme. Focus (6) (Spring): 18–19
Stanton A 1988 Case-finding in the elderly: The Edinburgh Birthday Card Scheme — An HV's perspective. Health Bulletin 46 (2). Scottish Home and Health Department, Edinburgh
Steel K 1989 Taking care to the over-80s: Case-finding in one practice. Geriatric Medicine (January) 43–46
Stevenson O 1989 Age and vulnerability: a guide to better care. Age Concern Handbook, Edward Arnold, London
Stilwell B 1988a Origins and development of the Nurse Practitioner role. In: Bowling A, Stilwell B (eds) The nurse in family practice. Scutari Press, London
Stilwell B 1988b Patients' attitudes to the availability of a Nurse Practitioner in general practice. In: Bowling A, Stilwell B (eds) The nurse in family practice. Scutari Press, London, p 111–120

Stilwell B, Restall D, Burke-Masters B 1988 Nurse Practitioners in British general practice. Scutari Press, London

Stone A, Wallace C 1988 Neighbourhood Health Care Services for the older client. Personal Communication 28th December, Bassett Road Health Centre, Leighton Buzzard

Sullivan J 1982 Research on Nurse Practitioners: process behind the outcome. American Journal of Public Health 72: 8–9

Svanborg A 1985 The Gothenborg Longitudinal Study of 70 year olds. In: Bergener M, Ermini M, Stahelin M B (eds) Thresholds in aging. Sandoz Lectures. Academic Press, London

Taylor R, Buckley E G 1988 Preventive care of the elderly: a review of current developments. Occasional Paper No 35. Royal College of General Practitioners, London.

Taylor R, Ford G, Barber J H 1983 The elderly at risk. Research perspectives on ageing. Age Concern Research Unit, Mitcham

Taylor R, Ford G, 1988 Functional geriatric screening: a critical review of current developments. In: Taylor R, Buckley E G (eds) Preventive care of the elderly. Occasional Papers No 35: Royal College of General Practitioners, London

Tierney B M T 1989 A feasibility study of health visitor intervention with older people, consequent upon their attending an accident and emergency department. Hounslow DHA, unpublished paper.

Tulloch A J, Moore V I 1979 A randomized controlled trial of geriatric screening and surveillance in general practice. Journal of The Royal College of General Practitioners 29: 733–742

UKCC (United Kingdom Central Council for Nurses, Midwives and Health Visitors) 1986 Project 2000. UKCC, London

Vetter N J, Jones D A, Victor C R 1984 Effect of health visitors working with elderly patients in general practice: a randomized controlled trial. British Medical Journal 288 (4th February): 369–372

Vetter N J, Jones D A, Victor C R 1986 A health visitor affects the problems others do not reach. The Lancet 5th July: 30–32

Watson A, Hawkins J B, Thibodeau J A 1983 The Nurse Practitioner: current practice issues. Tiresias Press, New York

Welsh Office 1987 Nursing in the community: a team approach for Wales. Report of the Community Nursing Review Committee for Wales. Welsh Office, Cardiff

Westrin C G 1986 Primary Health Care: cooperation between health and welfare personnel. Euro-Social Research Papers 8. European Centre for Social Welfare Training and Research, Vienna

Whitehead M 1987 The health divide: inequalities in health in the 1980s. Health Education Authority, London

WHO (World Health Organization) 1978 Alma Ata declaration. WHO, Geneva

WHO (World Health Organization) 1985 Targets for health for all. WHO, Geneva

WHO (World Health Organization) Nurse Euro 1986 Discussion Paper 8017. WHO, Copenhagen

Williamson J 1981 Screening, surveillance and case-finding. In: Arie T (ed) Health care of the elderly. Croom Helm, London

Williamson J, Stokoe J H, Gray S, Fisher M, Smith A, McGhee A, Stephenson E 1964 Old people at home: their unreported needs. Lancet 1 (23rd May): 1117–1120

CHECKLIST FOR HEALTH VISITORS WORKING WITH ELDERLY CLIENTS

Background data

Have I prepared/obtained a Community Profile? How aware am I of the number and distribution of older people within the community in which I work? Does my caseload reflect this distribution?

How familiar am I with pertinent epidemiological data affecting the elderly population in the community in which I work?

Do I know the major causes of mortality and morbidity amongst the elderly population and can I describe the trends? What steps, if any, have I taken to ensure that health visiting programmes relate to these needs. Do I participate in overall health care programmes designed to reduce these specific health problems? How effective are the measures taken?

Data related to specific settings

If I am undertaking geographic-based health visiting, what steps have I taken to effect liaison with others involved in the care of older persons? How far have we been able to agree joint goals and work towards meeting these?

If I am working in general-practice-based health visiting, am I aware of the distribution of elderly persons within the practice population? Have I a systematic and efficient method for identifying them and determining their level of vulnerability?

What steps, if any, have I taken to ensure that the general practice team, of which I am a member, studies the overall needs of the elderly within the practice population and sets joint goals in care?

How frequently do I attend meetings designed to evaluate action taken to meet such goals? How often do I participate in re-planning and re-organisation of joint-care programmes?

How ready am I to initiate and maintain contact with elderly clients when the onus is left to me?

How frequently do I liaise with other team members, particularly social workers and paramedical personnel such as chiropodists, dentists, occupational therapists, physiotherapists and speech therapists, opticians and pharmacists?

Do I have clear lines of communication with hospital personnel and am I familiar with the various policies for admission, discharge and follow-up of elderly patients? Do I have close contact with staff in accident, emergency and outpatient departments and with dieticians and other consultative personnel?

Do I clearly understand the policies of my employing authority concerning the care of the elderly?

Am I aware of the community facilities which exist for older people and do I attend co-ordinating meetings, case conferences and public meetings as necessary?

Preparation for visits

Before undertaking visits to the elderly, whether at their homes, in clinics, health centres, residential accommodation, day centres, clubs or other settings, how well do I prepare myself by scrutinising available data and checking out related material from colleagues and other agencies?

How do I ensure that advice and information I plan to give is based on sound scientific principles and is feasible for elderly client(s) or their carer(s) to implement?

How carefully do I structure the plan of my visit, in order to cover relevant problems of which I am aware? Do I use a clear model/framework? How ready am I to allow the agenda to be flexible, should the client wish to introduce new issues into the situation?

During visits

How carefully do I study the sociocultural background of my client(s) and their family(ies), in order to set them at ease? Work within their value system? Afford them dignity?

How thoughtful am I in ensuring that the language I use and the modes of approach I adopt are comprehensible and suitable for them? What steps do I take to gain and hold their confidence and respect? How ready am I to allow the client to take the initiative in identifying their needs, problems and goals? Am I an active listener and do I direct conversation into productive channels when necessary?

How ready am I to pay attention to both verbal and non-verbal communication from client(s) and carer(s)?

Do I give high priority to maintaining functional independence amongst my elderly clients?

How careful am I to ensure that I have collected data in all the realms of living, before making an assessment of situations?

Do I take advantage of the many opportunities I have for teaching, whether by example, demonstration or precept? Do I take time to study the learning style of individual clients, being aware of the emotional factors which influence learning, and taking time to evaluate if learning has occurred?

Do I elicit clients' coping abilities and build on and strengthen these, so that I utilise every resource the client has for his/her benefit?

Am I careful to place the client into the context of his/her family?

Do I study the family as a unit, recognising the needs of family members and perceiving the family in totality?

Do I recognise the contribution client makes to the family and the demands they place upon it?

Do I take into account the special needs that may be posed by the illness or disability of the elderly member?

Am I aware of family dynamics and of the environmental stresses they encounter? Is the advice and help I am able to give, adequate for the family's needs?

Do I perceive the relationship of client-family and community?

Am I able to interpret community policies and programmes for the benefit of client and family? Do I take full account of all the community influences that operate on the client and family?

At the close of the visit

Do I allow time for recapping on salient points?

Do I ensure that the client is fully aware of what has been discussed and decided between us? That the client and/or carer is quite clear about the responsibilities they have for putting any jointly prepared plans into operation? That client and/or carer know what action I have agreed to take and approve same? That client, carer and myself are clear about evaluation criteria? That I have written down all relevant material and left it in an accessible place for the benefit of client, carer and any professional personnel who may be involved?

Do I make sure that the client knows when to expect me again and knows how to contact me?

After the visit

Do I ensure a systematic format for recording significant data?

Do I check that the format is clear, concise, accurate and suitable for use within the health visiting organisation and amongst other colleagues?

Do my records make explicit the basis of my assessments and demonstrate my rationale in care?

Do I ensure that the documents are treated correctly, respecting confidentiality?

Within the team?

Do I seek to facilitate the work of other team members, especially in the care of the elderly? Do I try to understand their problems and support them as appropriate? Do I work constructively with them to improve our services, especially to the elderly population?

Do I respect the health visiting management and co-operate with them?

Research

Do I systematically read and evaluate relevant research reports, especially those relating to the care of older people?

Do I seek to apply relevant knowledge from research findings to my own field of work?

Do I participate readily in research projects, especially those affecting older people?

Do I keep abreast of current research issues, especially ethical issues in research with older people?

Do I indicate problems which require to be researched?

Do I undertake research activities, myself?

CHAPTER CONTENTS

7

Health promotion in later life — retirement

Retirement can be the passport to personal freedom — the gateway to renewed opportunity. However, the extent to which this possibility becomes a reality depends on a number of factors, not least of which is good health. This chapter, therefore, focuses on some of the many dimensions of retirement, within the context of health and health promotion. In adopting this approach, we have two main contentions: first, that health promotion is, and always has been, both a legitimate and desirable health visiting activity; second, that there are certain phases of the life-span when particular events occur which can cause individuals to reflect on their situation in relation to their health; they may then be more receptive to health-promoting ideas. Retirement may be one such time. Harnessing the potentially re-awakened motivations can be a major task, utilising all the identified health visiting principles.

Some may perhaps question whether health promotion is worthwhile in later maturity. Certainly, in order to derive the greatest benefit, it would appear best undertaken from the earliest years. Even so, it has particular impact in middle and later life. Evidence suggests that a number of older people appear to want to stay well (Maloney et al 1984). Older people do make lifestyle changes (Allen 1986a, Brown & McCreedy 1986). Furthermore, this motivation, the sense of personal involvement and these healthier lifestyles are often sustained (Schafer 1989).

Of course, health promotion means far more than raising personal consciousness about health and health-enhancing practices, important though this may be. It is concerned with complex action on economic, social, environmental, ecological and political fronts as well (Whitehead 1989). For these reasons it is necessary to review general concepts and principles, before considering specific topics and practical strategies applicable to health promotion activity in later life.

DEFINING HEALTH PROMOTION

Attempts to define health promotion are fraught with difficulty. In Chapter 5 we explored some of the ambiguities surrounding the concept of health. We saw how conceptual variation could lead to the devising of different frameworks and models of care. Similarly, the term 'promotion' holds different meanings. It is, for instance, an active 'go-getting' word, conveying the thought of movement, progression, advancement and elevation. To many, 'promotion' is associated with enterprise, enhancement and achievement. In the commercial sense the term carries a connotation of 'social marketing': the vigorous application of persuasive techniques, in relation to the presentation of products. This is done in the hope that potential customers will be convinced of the value of the products and hence will become purchasers. However, the promoters remain aware that consumer choice remains paramount. To yet others, 'promotion' may conjure up ideas of championing causes: conveying notions of commitment, advocacy, mediation and values.

With such a range of thoughts it is not surprising, therefore, that definitions of health promotion 'differ in scope and degree of attention to detail' (Tannahill 1985). Moreover, confusion often results because the term is frequently used synonymously with either 'health education' or 'disease prevention'. Such interchangeability is misleading. Each of these terms is conceptually distinct, although they are closely related and frequently overlap. Differentiation is therefore important.

According to Pender (1982, 1987), health promotion means

> all those activities directed towards sustaining or increasing the level of well-being, self-actualization or fulfilment.

This definition has much in common with wellness enhancement, as advocated by Ryan and Travis (1981) and Houldin et al (1987). These writings emphasise that health promotion involves

- *a choice:* decisions are deliberately taken to move towards optimal health;
- *a pattern:* lifestyles are deliberately adopted and life skills developed in order to achieve optimal well-being;
- *a process:* awareness is developed that higher levels of well-being can be achieved in the present but that there is no end point.

It is noteworthy that these ideas of health maintenance and enhancement of well-being apply equally to individuals, groups and communities, having both personal and environmental application.

DEFINING HEALTH EDUCATION

One means whereby the maintenance and enhancement components of health promotion can be achieved, is through the medium of health education. This is defined as

> consciously constructed opportunities for learning, which are designed to facilitate change in behaviour, towards pre-determined health goals.
>
> (Nutbeam 1986)

Thus there is a sense in which health education becomes a health promotion tool. It should be noted that health education also has an individual, a group and a community application.

Defining disease prevention

By contrast, disease prevention serves largely as dealing with health maintenance. It means

> the range of personal, medical, social, legal, fiscal and other policies, aimed at safeguarding health.
>
> (Tannahill 1985, Nutbeam 1986)

It includes the primary, secondary and tertiary levels of prevention, already mentioned in Chapters 1, 2 and 6.

An important stage in the clarification of the

meaning of these different terms occurred at the First International Conference on Health Promotion, held in Canada in 1986, when a charter was drafted. This set out what health promotion involves and pointed to various ways in which it could be implemented.

THE OTTAWA CHARTER

The Ottawa Charter declared health promotion to be '*the process of enabling people to increase control over and to improve their health, by empowering them . . . to identify and realise their aspirations . . . satisfy their needs . . . and change or cope with their environment*'. The Charter stressed health as a positive concept; a resource *for* living rather than an objective *of* living — and the enhancement of well-being as a continuing goal. It also placed health promotion firmly on the agenda of policy-makers in all sectors, requiring them to

- build healthy public policy
- create health-supportive environments
- strengthen community action
- develop personal skills in individuals
- re-orient health services.

Essential concepts underpinning health promotion strategies were seen to be *caring*, *holism* and *ecology* (The Ottawa Charter for Health Promotion 1986).

The significance of this Charter

Although being mindful of the dangers of rhetoric and conscious of the warnings of cynics that actions speak louder than words, one should not under-rate the importance of this declaration from this international source. It patently represents a major shift of emphasis, from professionally directed goals to people-directed ones. It implies that future health promotion activities should be client-centred and should focus more on group and community work — points reinforced by Duffy (1988) and by Green & Raeburn (1988). It also makes clear that inter- and multi-disciplinary co-operation will need to increase in future. Thus health visitors might expect to find that they are increasingly participating in joint health promotion programmes. A summary of these implied shifts of emphasis is given in Figure 7.1.

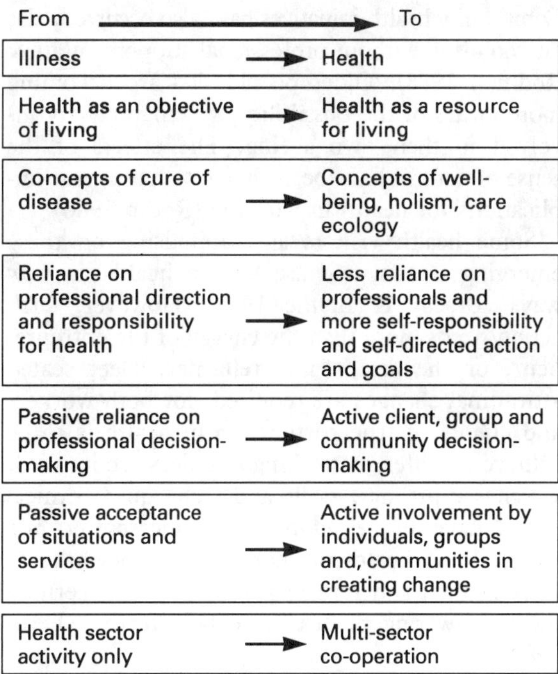

Fig. 7.1 Health promotion — shifting the emphasis. (Based on The Ottawa Charter 1986 and material from Cotton & Sharp 1989.)

Reasons for, and consequences of, change

These shifts of emphasis have not suddenly occurred; rather they represent gradual, cumulative client reactions to a prevailing sense of loss of control, world-wide. Negative attitudes towards medical dominance, and concern at the tendency to medicalise many problems, have been variously expressed. Some clients have demonstrated their sense of powerlessness by 'expecting a pill for every ill'. Others have shown their disillusionment with an over-emphasis on high technology by seeking alternative therapies, or ecological and environmental answers to health matters.

A plethora of self-help groups have arisen, offering information and support. They often initiate research and build up extensive specialised literature, as well as carrying out fund-raising.

Community health initiatives have also occurred, alas far too often without professional support (Watt & Rodmell 1988). Older people also are becoming more aware of the possibility of being actively involved in their own ageing. The effects of the sense of control have been shown to have great implications for health in later life (Rodin 1986).

Some health visitors are capitalising on these emerging trends, and are 'selling health' in new ways (Bracey & Blythe 1985). However, such action needs more than the energy of the entrepreneur, or the zeal of the reformer. Deep-seated attitudinal changes are required, for both workers and clients, if true partnership in health is to be achieved. Different working practices are implied, which require new skills and techniques. Ethical issues have to be addressed (Anderson & Fox 1987). Valid health promotion indicators have to be identified and refined if evaluation concerning the empowering process is to be effective (Dean 1988).

Empowerment

Empowering individuals, groups and/or communities, in health matters, represents an extension of the enabling process already familiar to health visitors. Some facets of the empowering process include:

- helping individuals and groups to recognise and present their aspirations as a valid activity
- facilitating the identification of health needs and providing information and help to assist clients and groups to meet these
- enabling individuals, groups and communities to create options, exercise choice, adopt healthy lifestyles and develop life-skills conducive to health, including changing their environment whenever necessary and/or possible
- offering interventions which reinforce such healthier lifestyles, enhance such life-skills, or effect environmental safeguards.

Each of these points applies to older adults.

While stressing the importance of personal responsibility for health, one should recognise the danger of over-emphasising this aspect (Syme 1986). To encourage older persons to exercise healthy choices, implies that alternatives are available to them. When this is not the case, despondency can be increased. Furthermore, one should recognise that improved health levels do not always result from individual health maintenance practices, however sound (Brown & McCredy 1986). There is then a risk of 'victim blaming' if desired outcomes are not achieved (Becker 1986).

It should also be remembered that individuals, faced with choices, may opt for less healthy options. Those faced with empowerment may choose to relinquish control in favour of greater dependency! When such is the case, these individuals must be allowed to exercise their rights without fear of recrimination (Kaplan 1988). These issues are further reflected in the next chapter, when we discuss group health promotion, specific strategies and topics.

PROMOTING HEALTHY RETIREMENT

Retirement can be classified from three dimensions (Streib & Schneider 1971, Murray et al 1980):

1. as a significant event
2. as a social status
3. as a developmental process.

Retirement as a significant event

The connotations of the term 'retirement' are many and varied. For some it means 'a moving on', for others 'standing down'. A few may react negatively, perceiving the event as one of retreat, 'carrying inuendos of passivity and seclusion', (Ebersole & Hess 1985). Conversely, those more positively inclined see it as 'a chance to do one's own thing'. Thus some look forward eagerly to the event, while others dread it, perceiving it as bringing only loss and social distress. Hemingway is reputed to have thought 'retirement' to be the vilest word in the English language! Indeed the event can sometimes propel persons from familiar roles and comfortable routines, into states of role-confusion and disequilbrium, thus posing threats to physical and mental health.

Successful negotiation of this transition is therefore crucial. It depends on many factors, including the following:

- personality attributes
- personal perceptions about work and worth, and the strength of the work ethic
- the extent of pressure upon the person to retire
- the level of information about retirement, which the person possesses
- the attitudes of self and significant others towards the event of retirement and its potential aftermath
- socio-economic circumstances
- physical and mental well-being pre-retirement.

Furthermore, it depends considerably on whether retirement implies complete cessation from employment; partial cessation; or leaving one post to assume another, albeit very different. It also rests on whether retirement is/was a personal preference; mandatory, but willingly accepted; compulsory but unwillingly accepted; forced on medical grounds; or retirement superimposed on a lengthy period of unemployment. Hence reactions are likely to be as diverse as the various categories. Most importantly, successful coping with the event of retirement appears to be related to adequate preparation (Beck 1983, Wan 1985). It also depends on the absence of concomitant disruptive life-events, such as other marked role-transitions, loss and/or bereavement (Wan 1985).

Preparation and planning

Since retirement heralds the onset of a further developmental phase, which can last 40 or more years, one might expect that it would be anticipated and prepared for, over a long period. Paradoxically, however, although we spend some 15–20 years preparing for adulthood and the world of work, few people give more than scant attention to how they will spend their latter days, until they are within immediate sight of pensionable age. Nevertheless, it is during the active phase of later middle life, when family and work roles have mostly been carved out, that thoughts can best be directed to planning for the years of change and increased leisure.

Furthermore, the period 45–64 years represents a time when mortality and morbidity risks increase steeply — indicating that health visiting contact might profitably be directed to this middle-aged group. However, apart from the pressures of high workloads and time limitations, which sometimes render it difficult for health visitors to engage with this vital group, some practitioners have expressed concern about how best to make contact. One approach has already been discussed in Chapter 6. Health visitors working in primary health care teams may use their age–sex registers to identify potential clients. These persons are then invited for screening checks, or health surveillance sessions, which afford scope for health promotion and/or health counselling.

Others prefer to use different methods, such as 'drop-in centres'; adult health clinics; Age Well Groups; health circles, or health clubs (Drennan 1988, Martin 1988). Some practitioners focus on the many self-help groups in their locality and liaise with them, using this to foster contact with middle-aged persons and those facing impending retirement.

Whichever method is adopted, the relevant issue appears to be *the presentation of positive concepts of health,* so that people do not become preoccupied with morbidity, but rather have their attention focused *on their health potential* (Ryan & Travis 1981, Houldin et al 1987).

Co-operation with occupational health nurses

Some health visitor practitioners work closely with their colleagues in occupational health settings, realising that by such co-operation both workers become better informed. Consequently, both are able to give more personalised help to individuals and their families and can set joint goals in care, which stimulates effort.

Because significant numbers of older adults work regularly, employing organisations offer great scope for health promotion activities in the pre-retirement period. They are also well placed to undertake evaluative research, which aids effectiveness. Moreover, employers (often acting out of enlightened self-interest) are likely to support many health promotion measures. Symbolic actions by senior staff at the worksite (e.g. senior managers giving up smoking), may help to change organisational norms and hence health values. These then may modify the values of older individuals in favourable directions (Allen 1986a, 1986b). Other advantages of co-operation in the workplace, between occupational health nurses and health visitors concerning older persons at work, include (Terborg 1988):

- greater convenience for group attendance on a formal/informal basis
- opportunities for environmental and social modifications in favour of health
- peer group support.

Such health promotion programmes offered to older adults, on a collaborative basis, can incorporate health counselling about age-related health risks; exercise and sports facilities; modified conditions of service to ease transition into retirement; and social facilities for older workers and retirees.

Pre-retirement courses

Another avenue of contact with the late middle-aged group is provided when health visitors participate in formal pre-retirement courses. These may be offered by progressive employers; Colleges of Further and Higher Education; or such organisations as The Workers' Educational Association, Age Concern, or The Pre-retirement Association.

However, such courses, while useful, are often provided quite late in the pre-retirement phase, which proves a limiting factor in relation to anticipatory guidance, education and change.

Such pre-retirement preparation usually encourages persons to think ahead and identify their expectations and potential problems. Guidance may be given on planning finances and on legal aspects. Housing and living arrangements may be discussed, persons usually being recommended to appraise and renew household furnishings where possible and necessary. Entering retirement in as well-equipped a manner as one can, may reduce subsequent anxiety regarding expenditure. Hobbies and creative leisure pursuits also form part of such educational content. Intending retirees are often encouraged to obtain needful tools and materials, while still working, as these may prove expensive on limited retirement income.

The sense of excitement and anticipation associated with preparing and planning for this important phase of life was aptly captured by Comfort (1977). He described retirement as

> entering a second trajectory, for which older people need to plan and get on a launching pad.

He clearly saw that older people had to shape society to expect every retiree to have an active and fulfilling retirement career. Already there are signs that some pensioners' groups are eagerly seeking such active involvement. Health visitors are well placed to help generate and sustain such self-help and enthusiasm.

Preparing significant others

Another facet of health promotion in the pre-retirement period, which may currently be underdeveloped, is the preparation of significant others. Retirement as an event can have a great impact on spouses, family members, relatives or friends. Furthermore the attitudes and reactions of significant others can profoundly affect the way impending retirees perceive themselves and their future. For instance, for some women who have not been actively engaged in the labour market, the concept of retirement may have little personal meaning. Because they continue to have active and multiple roles, interests and responsibilities in and outside the home, they do not undergo marked status change, or alter their lives profoundly when they grow older. Consequently they may not understand how a retiree may feel. They may thus find the retirement of a spouse, relative or friend a disruptive event. This can cause mutual distress. Such reactions may be particularly marked where couples have had widely segregated conjugal roles and different daily living patterns. As one woman pithily remarked:

I married my husband for better or worse, but not to get lunch for him every day!

Anticipatory guidance, a familiar health visiting technique, may have much to offer in such circumstances, since it has both educative and facilitating elements. Focused discussion may make it possible to enable others to appreciate how those contemplating change and loss of long-standing employment may feel and act. Hence they themselves may adapt accordingly and so enable mutual adjustments to take place. Of course, many significant others look forward eagerly to the retirement of their spouses, relatives or friends, finding the post-retirement years ones of enrichment and enjoyment.

The time of retirement

Some employers, mindful of the effect of '*retirement shock*', have introduced flexible policies, whereby older employees can have a 'phased winding down'. This may take the form of gradually decreasing hours of work, a move to a part-time appointment, job-sharing, or planned early leaving. Gradual tapering off can help to promote positive adapation, thus encouraging employees to see the event of retirement as the culmination of one progressive, sequential career and the entrance to another. This perception is much helped if the financial accompaniments of the change are high, and alternative interests are available.

However, for those in whom the work ethic is deeply ingrained, or who regard retirement as the loss of valued social contact, there may be difficulties. Similarly, for those for whom the future seems but a dreary prospect of dependence upon limited financial resources, the outlook may appear bleak. Then the moment of severance from valued employment can be very traumatic.

Even the time-honoured rituals associated with leaving can heighten pleasure or increase despair, depending on the way they are perceived. The traditional gift of a timepiece, may be unintentionally cruel for some retirees dreading an unstructured day. Others may be given mementoes which recall past achievements, or presents which encourage them to look forward to the future.

Health promotion interventions can, however, help to influence customs and conventions associated with the event of retirement. More positive attitudes can be created and demonstrated through appropriate symbols. For instance, one health visitor was left in no doubt about the expectation of her colleagues concerning an active retirement, when her leaving present turned out to be a tricycle!

There are, however, many other complex factors associated with the event of retirement. Social upheavals, resulting from mass unemployment and/or redundancy, have introduced new dimensions into the issue. To older people who have not been gainfully employed for several years before reaching pensionable age, the accepted notions of retirement will be irrelevant. Research studies have shown the profound effects loss of employment have upon physical and mental health. These affect not only the individuals involved, but their families as well (OPCS 1984, Nuffield Centre 1984).

Other factors

Other factors, too, may affect the timing of retirement: the type of occupation undertaken; the harshness of climate or weather; the working conditions; or the years of service given. For example, athletes, gymnasts, footballers and tennis players often 'retire' before they are 40. Some may subsequently take up careers in other fields. Most, however, will have to make some transitional adjustments. Conversely, judges are not usually obliged to retire until they are 75 years of age; while politicians, some business personalities, self-employed traders, directors in industry, or those in the arts may not retire at all.

RETIREMENT AS A SOCIAL STATUS

Retirement denotes a new social position — a changed status. This may be officially marked by entitlements to age-related concessions, or specific

Table 7.1 Normal retirement age for certain countries

Country	*Women*	*Men*
Belgium	60	65
Denmark	67	67
Eire	65	65
France	60	60
Greece	57	62
Italy	55	60
Netherlands	67	67
Norway	67	67
Spain	65	65
Sweden	65	65
UK	60	65
USA	70	70
USSR	55	60
West Germany	65	65

Based on material from The Observer 5.4.86; Victor C R 1987 Old age in Modern Society. Croom Helm, London, p 164; Ebersole P, Hess P 1985 Towards healthy aging. Mosby, New York; and Central Statistical Office: Social Trends No 19, 1989.

contributory benefits. Although many countries use retirement as an administrative device to mark out this social status, the age they select for official retirement varies (Table 7.1).

Change of social status from an employed person to a retired person may profoundly affect some individuals, causing loss of self-esteem. Health promotion interventions can help to counter such adverse effects.

Promoting self-esteem

The maintenance of a positive self-concept is essential for morale and hence well-being in body, mind and spirit.

Continuity is strengthened by encouraging the recounting of past achievements. A sense of identity is fostered when interest is shown in any displayed symbols of success, or in retirement gifts and cards. Nevertheless research suggests it is important to stress an identity apart from the work role, and to emphasise the many opportunities there are to contribute to society, which exist in the present (Atchley 1979, Ebersole & Hess 1985, McGoldrick & Cooper 1989). Facilitating the recognition of coping abilities, and encouraging older people to assess their strengths and clarify their expectations, can lead to an appraisal of skills and interests. This can serve as a prelude to channelling future activities.

Cicero knew the value of wide-ranging interests in later life, as a means of catering for physical, mental, emotional, social and spiritual health needs. He engaged in horse-riding; kept busy in farming, gardening and tending his vineyards; met frequently with friends to converse over meals and participated freely in debates and civic affairs. He said:

> I study Greek literature. . . . I am examining the secular and pontifical law, and daily I practice the habit of the Pythagoreans, running over in my mind all I have said and done. In my old age these are my mental gymnastics: these the race-courses of my mind!
> (Falconer 1923)

Self-regard is also enhanced by appropriate attention to personal appearance, and by the maintenance of wide social relationships. Other vital elements appear to be:

- maintaining hope
- the perception of being needed
- feeling cared for/having a sense of belonging
- being able to communicate freely with others
- having a sense of control over one's personal affairs.

CASE STUDY

Mr John S, a recently retired bachelor, had become downcast and somewhat slipshod in personal habits, when a health visitor, who knew of his interest in, and talent for, photography, put him in touch with a local, mixed age and sex group. The members were keen to learn about this hobby.

John's outlook brightened considerably once his knowledge and skills were utilised. His personal appearance and social relationships improved. By the end of the year he was eagerly planning to help the group mount an exhibition of their work.

Changing relationships and status transitions

As part of the status transition of retirement, there can sometimes be an increased emphasis on parent–child relationships, with subtle changes in the giving and receiving of help. This may be very evident when the newly retired find themselves carrying responsibility for the care of their aged parents or other old relatives. With increasing numbers of people achieving longevity, this situation is likely to increase.

Sometimes considerable curbs may be placed on the activities of the newly retired because of demands from the 'older old'. Where such circumstances cause hurt or resentment, the health visitor's health promoting activity for both parties may lie in therapeutic listening, in health counselling, in imparting relevant information to empower the particular individuals, and in facilitating positive ways of resolving the situation. The tyranny of over-dependent old people can sometimes constitute a very real risk to well-being for some in later maturity.

Grandparenting and great-grandparenting

For some older people, the social status of retirement may offer greater scope for exercising a role as grandparents, or even as great-grandparents. Understandably, geographic or social mobility can affect the frequency, and possibly the quality, of contact between the generations. One researcher found that diversity in grandparenting function was largely social-class related (Clavan 1978). Other cross-cultural studies have shown similarities in role functions, obligations and family and social expectations, between American and Russian grandparents (Mills 1982, Coonrod & Lesnoff-Caravaglia 1982).

There seems much scope for research studies on grandparents and great-grandparents in the United Kingdom. Health visitors might wish to consider their specific health promotion needs. Alternatively they may wish to document the contribution which older people who are grandparents make to the well-being of families.

At different times, grandparents or great-grandparents can act as confidants, as representatives of family history and identity, as reservoirs of family wisdom, or as surrogate parents. They are frequently sources of additional fun or treats, and often act as complementary bankers! Encouraging positive interaction between great-grandparents, grandparents and their grandchildren can thus enhance the well-being of both groups.

A source of distress to some older grandparents may arise when divorce or family breakdown occurs. Access to their grandchildren may then be rendered difficult and the emotional strain of dealing with the divorcee-parents may prove traumatic. Such grandparents may welcome the therapeutic listening and practical information which health visitors can provide. (Information on the rights of grandparents is given by Atherton & Manthorpe 1989.)

Foster grandparenting

The notion of 'foster grand-parenting' is, as yet, little developed. However, some older people may have much to offer in this role. They must, of course, be carefully selected and briefed. Befriending children in long-stay hospitals, residential schools or homes is often welcomed. This may particularly apply when distance separates the children from their own families. Younger busy parents also often appreciate friendly contact and practical support, from an older, experienced individual, especially when they are without their own family support. This may be highly pertinent if there is a large young family, a sick mother, or a handicapped child. Health visitors may sometimes be involved in preparing suitable older individuals to undertake this task, usually in collaboration with their social work colleagues.

Selecting other roles in retirement

Once work roles have been relinquished, many people find it helpful to forge new roles quickly. Some do this by finding avenues of community service. This may involve acting as sources of local or social history, such as working as guides in museums, stately homes or similar places of historic or artistic interest. Some help local school children to discover their heritage. Others assist in hospitals, canteens, residential establishments for the elderly or handicapped, act as volunteers in Day Centres, or work in shops for charitable organisations. A number like to help out in Mother and

Toddler Groups, play groups or creches, youth clubs, or community centres. They may be utilised as general helpers, story-tellers, games partners, toy repairers, or craft teachers. Others become involved in Adult Literacy Schemes, or assist in libraries, transport schemes or other voluntary activities. It is important that such work is congenial, and *that it is undertaken by choice* and not from a sense of unavoidable obligation or coercion. Such latter attitudes detract from dignity and may fuel ageism.

Self-help groups and mutual-aid schemes

Apart from these community activities, or the many self-help groups in which older individuals can play a valuable part, there is also great scope for mutual aid and the bartering and marketing of skills. In some localities informal exchange schemes exist, with those offering skills such as gardening, carpentry, or home decorating, exchanging services with those offering help with washing, cooking, sewing, or shopping. Such activities frequently require someone to act as a catalyst, before others realise what they can do to create mutual support systems. Health visitors may sometimes find their skills are required in this way.

Alerting communities

Another facet of the health visitor's health promoting role, is that of alerting communities to recognise the needs of the newly retired, and to value their contribution. The provision of appropriate leisure facilities, sports amenities, educational courses, special interest sessions, or social centres, can all facilitate well-being. Health visitors may find themselves, therefore, developing greater links with district authority staff, various voluntary agencies, education personnel, or community groups.

Many commercial enterprises are also now recognising the social status of the retired. They may see these older citizens as a potential market for special holiday ventures, house purchasing, or mortgage schemes. Care has to be exercised, when any group is accorded a specific status, that they are not thereby exploited, nor a 'ghetto mentality' created.

INCOME MAINTENANCE IN RETIREMENT

Fundamental to successful retirement, and affecting health, social status and well-being, is the possession of an adequate income. Social policy advisers often recommend that a retirement income of 60–80% of previous earnings is required if lifestyle is not to be too severely disrupted. In spite of the growth of both private and occupational pension schemes, and the State retirement system, many retirees fail to attain these recommended income levels. Many fall far below this, although a minority are affluent. Research into poverty shows a relationship between this and old age (Townsend 1979, Victor 1987). There are marked regional variations, with Northern Ireland, Wales, Scotland and Northern England having higher levels of poverty than the South-West, East, and South-East of England.

Approximately 60% of retired persons' incomes are now derived from State Retirement Benefit, 22% comes from occupational pensions and the remainder from savings, investments and earnings (Fiegehen 1986). Approximately one-third of all retired persons now receive an occupational pension, although in many instances amounts are small. 'Young-elderly', and those from former professional occupations, predominate.

Income means far more than the wherewithal to adequately maintain oneself. It represents a measure of independence, the ability to give to others, and perhaps the chance to fulfil some long-cherished dreams. It also creates a sense of security, in old age, against a future which may sometimes appear threatening or unsure. Hence health promoters have to take cognisance of the financial aspects of retirement.

Although health visitors are not expected to know all the intricate details of a complex social security system, they have a responsibility to inform clients about their entitlements. At times they may also be required to act as advocates. An appreciation of the general principles underlying policy, and the major eligibility criteria, is therefore necessary. Most importantly it is essential to be aware of sources of further information and help. In discussing these points, specific details of monetary allowances are not generally given. This is because detailed amounts change frequently, as do some eligibility criteria. Health visitors therefore have a responsibility for regularly updating themselves in this as in other aspects of their knowledge.

Retirement pensions

As indicated above, State Retirement Pension forms one of the main sources of income for older people. Four schemes exist: two contributory and two non-contributory. The latter two are either for certain persons over 80 years, or the few who were already pensioners when National Insurance was introduced in 1946.

Contributory pensions

Contributory pensions are based either on a personal record, or that of a spouse. Contributions are paid as a percentage of gross earnings during working life and are collected as part of The National Insurance system. Credits are available in certain circumstances.

Entitlement to benefit depends on three factors:

1. National Insurance Contribution record
2. Number of qualifying years
3. Anticipated working life. (This currently equals 90% of expected working life, which is presently 40 years for women and 45 years for men.)

Hence, married women who have not paid full contributions, even if they have worked, may not receive a full pension.

At present, basic retirement pension equals 33% of the average national manual wage. However, it is possible to achieve additions, through state earnings-related contributions, or by deferring retirement date.

State Earnings-Related Pension Scheme (SERPS)

Some persons who retired after 1979 may have paid additional contributions related to their pay, and hence will receive extra benefit. The Social Security Act 1986 and The Finance Act 1987 (No 2) introduced radical changes to SERPS, as well as to occupational and personal pension schemes, mostly in favour of the two latter. The changes affecting SERPS will affect those reaching pensionable age by 1998. The significant point for health visitors to note is that since 1988 membership of certain occupational or personal pension schemes may allow contributors to opt out of SERPS. However, because there are complicated reasons concerning the advantages or disadvantages of opting out, for different individuals, those considering such a decision are advised to seek independent financial advice before making irrevocable choices.

Additional deferred payments

Where older individuals defer their retirement benefit they may receive extra pension, for each 7 weeks worked after pensionable age, up to a maximum of 5 years.

Amounts are small, and, since the abolition of the earnings rule for those pensioners working in the five years following reaching pensionable age, it may be advantageous to some individuals to receive their pension immediately. Pensions are taxable.

Review of rates for Retirement Pension

Rates for pensions are subject to regular review and updating, usually in line with inflation. Appropriate leaflets are available from the Offices of The Department of Social Security, from Citizens' Advice Bureaux, Post Offices and Welfare Rights Organisations.

Early retirement

Some older people who retire before reaching pensionable age may suffer financial disadvantage.

Under certain circumstances they may be eligible for Unemployment Benefit. However, from October 1989 there are disqualifying periods. Where such early retirement occurs on medical grounds, the individual may be eligible for Sickness or Invalidity Benefit. Those in receipt of the latter benefit may opt to continue it for the first 5 years of retirement, as an alternative to Retirement Pension. There are certain tax advantages, and receipt of Invalidity Benefit may enable an otherwise eligible individual to claim Housing Benefit or Income Support.

Severe Disablement Allowance

Severe Disablement Benefit (SDA), may be paid to persons with an 80% disability or more. Those of retirement age, who are already in receipt of the Benefit, are advised to remain on it, rather than transfer to Retirement Pension. It confers small tax advantages and may allow an older person to receive a Disablement Premium or Higher Pensioner Premium if they claim Income Support (see p. X159). (For further details about SDA see Chapter 10, p. 246.)

Attendance Allowance

Some retired persons may be eligible for this Benefit (see Ch. 10, p. 246). The allowance is tax-free and non-means-tested, hence it can be paid in addition to Retirement Pension and/or Income Support.

INCOME SUPPORT

Income Support (IS) is a non-contributory, means-tested Benefit, intended for those whose income falls below a designated level. It was introduced in 1988 to replace Supplementary Benefit.

Retired persons, working less than 24 hours per week, may be eligible either to IS as a full replacement income, or as a supplement to other, non-means-tested Benefits.

Currently some 2.5 million retired persons receive IS — that is, 24% of the retired population. The proportion rises with increasing age, recipients being concentrated mainly among those from former manual occupations. There is a marked sex disparity, with elderly widows predominating.

IS differs from non-means-tested Benefits, since the onus is on the claimant to initiate procedures. This means that less than 70% of those older people who are eligible to claim, actually do so (Victor 1987). Lack of information about its availability is a major reason for such under-claiming, but other disincentives include:

- bureaucratic complexity
- misconceptions about entitlement or eligibility criteria
- stigma
- passive acceptance of old age as a period of low income, or a pervading poverty culture.

Empowering older people as part of an overall health promotion strategy therefore involves:

- increasing their knowledge about the availability of IS
- providing information about application procedures and relevant eligibility criteria
- proffering assistance with form completion, where appropriate
- giving guidance on follow-up actions, with local DSS personnel
- offering advocacy if claim decisions are contested.

Eligibility criteria and benefit procedures

At the time of going to press, IS is available to those whose capital is £6000 or under, and whose weekly income is below a prescribed level. Capital between £3000 and £6000 is, however, deemed to produce a tariff income of £1 per week for every £250.

Benefit is paid weekly to the level of 'an applicable amount'. Such an amount is determined by

1. a specified personal allowance
2. any specific client premium.

This latter is a flat-rate amount, paid to certain client groups. The specified premiums for retired persons are currently:

- Pensioner Premiums for those 60/65–74 years
- Enhanced Pensioner Premiums for those aged 75–79 years
- Higher Pensioner Premiums for those aged 80 years and upwards.

In addition, Housing Benefit may be paid, up to 100% of rent and 80% of rates or community charges.

Income Support also serves as a passport to free ophthalmic and dental services, under the NHS.

Other benefits to which those pensioners already in receipt of IS may be entitled, include:

- cold weather payments
- funeral expenses
- payments from the Social Fund.

Cold weather payments

A person aged 60/65 years or more, with a qualifying capital of *£500* or less, can apply for cold weather payments if

1. They live in an area where, for a period of seven consecutive days, the mean daily temperature has been at, or below, 0° Celsius; this temperature must be confirmed by the local weather station
2. they had been in receipt of IS for at least one day during this period
3. the claim is submitted within 3 months from the last day of cold weather.

Where there are several periods of cold weather in any one year, claims can be submitted together, up to the 30th April of the relevant year.

Health visitors, concerned to reduce the risk of hypothermia or other cold-related disorders, will doubtless wish to note these regulations.

Funeral expenses payment

Any retired person, receiving IS and with a qualifying capital of *£500* or less, who is deemed responsible for funeral arrangements, can claim for certain specified expenses. Any insurance monies, or assets derived from a deceased person's estate, are set against the prescribed benefits. This payment replaces the non-means-tested Death Grant, previously available under National Insurance.

THE SOCIAL FUND

The Social Fund (SF) differs from other non-means-tested Benefit in that, at present:

- it is cash limited
- it is discretionary
- there is no right of independent appeal, although there is provision for independent review
- loan payments are recoverable from any future benefits.

The SF covers three discretionary payments:

1. Community Care Grants
2. Budget Loans
3. Crisis Loans.

Community Care Grants

A Community Care Grant, to which a pensioner-recipient of IS may be entitled, is paid to those 'who have special difficulties in special circumstances'. Understandably, this law is capable of wide interpretation. However, guidance notes are very specific, and many circumstances are proscribed. Notwithstanding, it is always advisable for older clients with a capital of *£500* or less, to claim, since discretion may be exercised in their favour.

Budget Loans

These are interest-free loans made to help a pensioner-recipient of IS 'meet the cost of a special event'. This term 'special event' usually refers to the obtaining of an item of high priority, such as essential bedding, furniture, non-mains fuel, or essential repairs for a home owner who cannot get a bank loan or mortgage. There are very precise guidelines about eligibility and many proscribed events. Maximum payment is set at £1000, repayable within 2 years. Critics have been most concerned that this Fund is cash-limited, since if a particular Benefit office (DSS) has exceeded its limits, no one, however deserving, can obtain a Budget Loan, or a Community Care Grant.

Crisis loans

These are interest-free loans intended to meet emergency payments arising from a disaster such as fire or severe burglary. The pensioner-claimant does not have to have been in previous receipt of IS, but must be without any funds, or any alternative source of help. The CL must represent *'the only way to prevent serious risk to health or safety'*. There is a ceiling of £1000, repayable within 18 months.

Housing costs and Housing Benefit

Housing costs can swallow up a large proportion of income, so that some older people experience difficulty in meeting these expenses. Housing Benefit (HB) is designed to assist those on low income to meet these costs. It is operated by Housing Authorities (usually District Councils), under The Social Security Act 1986, The Housing Benefit (General) Regulations 1987 and subsequent amending legislation.

As stated previously those in receipt of IS may also qualify for HB, although non-recipients may also claim. However, a formal claim has always to be made, *separately from any claim for IS*. Claims must be renewed at regular intervals, or when any change in circumstances occurs. Some older people may find this procedure confusing and may therefore welcome guidance to assist them to claim. Disseminating information about this Benefit and the associated claim procedures is therefore essential.

Claim procedures for those not receiving Income Support

Retired persons, not in receipt of IS, may be eligible to receive HB if they are required to pay rent, general rates, or community charges, for a dwelling occupied in Great Britain. Qualifying criteria include capital of £8000 or less, and a weekly income at, or below, an 'applicable amount'. As with IS claims, capital between £3000 and £8000 is deemed to produce a tariff income. HB works on a sliding scale, whereby eligible expenses are deducted from available income, and the results are compared with the pre-determined scale of 'applicable amounts'. There are certain proscribed costs. Because of the complexity of regulations, older persons should always be advised to claim. Readers requiring more detailed information on all forms of benefit are referred to the DSS, to Local Authority Housing Departments, or to Welfare Rights Organisations or Citizens' Advice Bureaux. Useful publications, apart from DSS specific leaflets, include the annual publications of The Child Poverty Action Group (Rowland et al 1989, Lakhani et al 1989) and The Disability Alliance (Disability Alliance 1989).

Other budgeting ideas

Although often reticent about their finances, older persons may welcome information about the monthly budgeting schemes operated by the Electricity, Gas and Telephone services. Certain fuel tariffs may also be financially advantageous, so older clients may find it helpful to enquire about these. For some older people, annuities may be appropriate. These are mostly paid for the remainder of a life, subject to a lump sum investment, or pledged collateral. Independent financial advice is usually to be recommended.

A number of Building Societies are now offering schemes for older homeowners, whereby a loan can be raised for a defined percentage value of their homes. The money raised can either be paid as a lump sum, or taken in a monthly income. Repayment is made when the home is eventually sold. Those contemplating such a move are recommended to seek independent legal and financial advice.

Earnings

Earnings represent one of the most obvious ways of complementing retirement income. There are several agencies who specialise in the placement of older persons in work, often of a part-time nature. This course of action may appeal to some retirees now that the earnings rule is abolished. Older people may, however, require information about income tax position, and may wish to know how age allowances may be affected if earnings reach a certain level. Employment opportunities for older persons are likely to be more favourable in the immediate future, because of the changing demographic structure.

RETIREMENT AS A PROCESS

As a process, retirement can be a period of development, moving on from the impact of the actual event, through changed status, to daily, dynamic adaptation. Major developmental tasks include learning to cope with changing personal and environmental demands; maintaining adequate nutrition; solving issues such as personal transport, household cleaning and management; laundry and shopping. Most importantly it means using increased leisure wisely; learning to obtain maximum benefit and enjoyment from each day; dealing with health problems as they arise; and making the necessary preparations for an eventually good death.

Facilitation of such adjustments can be made easier if there has been health visiting involvement from earlier years; if predictive judgment has been exercised and anticipatory guidance proferred. Crisis work in old age can often be reduced by unobtrusive surveillance and the use of efficient early-warning systems.

Retirement and health

There is a limited amount of research on retirement as a process, and the findings about the effects of retirement on health are equivocal (Parker 1982, Ekerdt et al 1983, Ebersole & Hess 1985, Wan 1985, McGoldrick & Cooper 1989). Some of the variations found in different research studies are probably related to methodological issues.

Available evidence suggests that retirement cannot be directly related to early mortality, although minor morbidity does seem to rise. In particular, problems of sleeplessness affect some retirees (McGoldrick 1989). General consensus seems to support the following pragmatic views.

- The process of retirement needs continual readjustment.
- Encouraging preventive health measures in the pre-retirement years enhances health in retirement.
- Prior health status is a strong determinant of health after retirement, hence the importance of sound health maintenance.
- Informal social networks are important in strengthening coping mechanisms. Pre-retirees should be alerted to maintain these in later life.
- The major life events which appear to have a deleterious effect on health in later life include declining economic status, changes in living arrangements, and bereavement, especially widowhood (Wan 1985, Vernon & Jackson 1989).

HOUSING

Housing is a significant dimension of living for older people. It not only serves as a means of shelter, but can facilitate or hamper physical or psychosocial facets of ageing. The domestic environment grows in importance when it is appreciated that many of those aged 80 and over spend long hours in the home, without outside excursions (Abrams 1980, Grundy 1989a). Furthermore, since the Second World War, there has been an increase in the number of old people living alone (see Ch. 1, p. 7). This clearly influences the degree of help and support available within the household.

Choosing where to live, and perhaps with whom, is one of the most important tasks in later maturity. Decisions may be made in the early post-retirement period, which have to be altered later should frailty intervene.

Housing standards

Table 7.2 shows that the proportion of older people who are owner-occupiers has grown over

Table 7.2 Tenure of 'retired' households in Great Britain, by age of head, for 1971 and 1986, shown by percentages

Age of head of household	Owner occupied		Rented local authority		Unfurnished private		Furnished private	
	1971	1986	1971	1986	1971	1986	1971	1986
60–69	48	56	32	35	19	9	1	–
70–79	46	51	31	36	22	12	1	–
80+	43	45	31	39	24	16	1	–

Source: Central Statistical Office Social Trends No 19: 1989. HMSO, London

the past 15 years to 50%. However, while conferring security, home ownership may carry anxieties associated with the physical and/or financial ability to sustain maintenance. While the principle of heterogeneity applies in this sector as with many others, older home owners and those living in the privately rented sector tend to be relatively disadvantaged regarding housing (Victor et al 1984, Victor & Evandrou 1986, Grundy 1989b). An average of 4% lack basic amenities, such as a fixed bath or shower, or an indoor WC. Access may also constitute a problem. Steep steps or stairs, especially when exposed to weather conditions, may render mobility difficult, thus keeping some older people unnecessarily housebound.

Heating

Heating constitutes a particular problem for older people. The risk of hypothermia and other cold-related conditions grows with advancing age, creating a topic of much current concern. The types and adequacy of heating in many old persons' dwellings compare unfavourably with other population groups, in spite of older people's spending, on average, a higher proportion of their income on heating (Victor 1987). Reasons for this situation include:

- fewer older households having central heating (see Fig. 1.6, Ch. 1).
- poor insulation in older dwellings
- housing constructed to lower than current standards
- deliberate restriction of heating costs, in order to conserve money, and fear of debt
- the reliance of a sizeable minority on coal fires, which require preparation and maintenance, which proves exhausting to frail elderly people.

Even so, 'staying put' in a home of long standing is often a preferred choice for older people. Home-owners may therefore welcome information on Local Authority Housing Grants, for prescribed renovations or essential repairs. Environmental Health Officers and Housing Officers are often valuable sources of information and practical help. Nevertheless, supplementary costs may sometimes constitute a barrier to claiming grants. Then voluntary agencies can sometimes help. Special schemes may be available through organisations such as The Anchor Housing Trust, Age Concern, or Shelter. Advice can also be obtained from Local Housing Aid Centres, Welfare Rights Organisations, or Citizens' Advice Bureaux.

Some owner-occupiers remortage their property, in order to upgrade their homes, and/or provide them with an income. Others, who feel that they can no longer sustain responsibility for maintenance, may sell their property to a Housing Association in return for lifetime accommodation and a cash adjustment. Some effect a 'gifted housing' arrangement, such as that operated by Help the Aged Housing Trust, whereby needful repairs are undertaken and individuals remain in life-tenancy, without further financial costs. Because all these schemes involve some element of risk, older clients should be urged to seek independent legal and financial advice before making decisions.

The right to buy

Council tenants, and some others, now have the right to buy their homes, at a discount price. The advantages of this for older peersons may be less obvious, especially if the property is in disrepair. As tenants, repairs and improvements may be dealt with more quickly. Transfers to more suitable property may be more easily effected. Conversely, rents may rise more steeply than mortgage costs, which may attract some income tax concessions. Such rent rises could wreck the budgeting plans of those who fall just outside the Housing Benefit regulations.

Private tenants

Where older tenants are living in private property they may face problems related to security of tenure, rent controls and obtaining repairs. They may at times need guidance on handling 'harassment', or pressures to quit the housing. Special difficulties may beset those older adults living in tied accommodation, or those rendered homeless.

Homeless elderly people

Approximately 1000 households containing an old person were dealt with in 1987 by Local Authorities under relevant legislation for certain categories of homeless persons (CSO 1989). This figure disregards the plight of older vagrants, or those who do not seek official help regarding their homelessness.

Housing policy

One advocated answer to the problem of homelessness is a definite housing policy for the older population, as mooted by the then Government (DHSS 1978). Since the publication of the White Paper on Community Care (DSS 1989), it may be that further encouragement will be given to Local Authorities and Housing Agencies to effect more urban renewal schemes, making it possible for older persons to remain in their own homes if they so wish. Alternatively, special housing provision for older people may be increased.

A concerted effort to re-appraise housing stock might lead to a more rational allocation of housing, especially where some older people are living in homes far larger than they require or can manage. However, great tact and sensitivity is required when making changes of this nature, particularly as enforced relocation can prove stressful and hence detrimental to health (Holmes & Rahe 1967, Lawton 1980, Ferraro 1982, Baglioni 1989, Thomas 1990).

Conversely, voluntary relocation can result in high levels of satisfaction, in spite of the major adaptations required (Kahana & Kahana 1983). Of course prior health status is strongly related to post-relocation well-being.

Residential relocation

Some elderly people decide to move to new homes in the country, at the seaside, to a 'preferred retirement area', or to be nearer relatives and/or friends who can provide valuable social support. This choice is sometimes exercised because of the perceived attractiveness of a particular area, ideas about the likely degree of family involvement (which may be misconceived), or the apparently favourable level of amenities available. Such migration can, however, have a marked effect on the recipient area, as well as the elderly people who move (Karn 1977). This latter study showed that a majority of elderly migrants who moved to the seaside tended to be childless, with fewer younger relatives to help them. In consequence health and social services in 'the reception areas' were severely stretched.

For these and other reasons, those contemplating a move to a 'retirement dream area' should be encouraged to spend time checking on local services, in relation to expected demand, and identifying specific difficulties. Desirably, they should spend some weeks in the locality, at least one month of which might be in the winter, before making their decision. Suggested checks might include the topography, climate, levels of air pollution and noise, transport facilities, accessibility to shops, churches, health and social services, availability of recreational and leisure amenities, and the convenience of the location for visiting relatives and friends. A couple contemplating such a move need to think well about how each would manage should they lose their partner. It is all too easy to become enamoured of a new area, without working through possible eventualities.

Sheltered housing

Sheltered housing consists of independent units, situated close together, sharing some common facilities and supervised by a warden or housekeeper.
(Bradley 1989)

These modern counterparts of older almshouses were mostly provided by Local authorities or some Housing Trusts during the post-war period. However, Housing Associations have considerably increased their provision in the past two decades, and the most recent phenomenon has been the spectacular increase in private units for sale.

There are marked differences in the social class distribution of residents and considerable variation in the geographic distribution of public and private sheltered housing. Not surprisingly, the latter is more commonly found in the more affluent South-East of England. Sheltered housing was envisaged as a means of enabling frailer older people to remain in the community rather than enter institutions. On entry, residents have to demonstrate independence in living, but often require Warden supervision if frailty increases.

Evidence quoted by Victor (1987) shows that residents in public sector sheltered housing receive comparatively high levels of community services, although they are not significantly more disabled than other elderly. This may be because they represent a more visible concentration of older people, or perhaps demonstrates the activity of Wardens and Housing Officers on their behalf.

Wardens in public-sector sheltered housing tend to experience considerable role ambiguity. Housing authorities often regard them as facilitators of care, while social services perceive them more as caregivers. This latter function is more in line with the realities of their work. Surveys which have examined characteristics and duties of Wardens have found that they often have diffuse job descriptions; experience isolation and a poor sense of occupational identity; lack support from managers; and often have little formal preparation for their important work, or in-service training (Butler et al 1983, Phillipson & Strang 1984, Bradley 1989).

Nevertheless, some Wardens go far beyond their expected duties of social surveillance, or good neighbourliness. They often have considerable knowledge of the needs of their elderly residents, and more of them are now extending their role towards older people in the surrounding community. There appears to be considerable scope for health visitors to develop a range of health promoting activities within sheltered housing complexes and to liaise more with Wardens. Issues currently arising from sheltered housing include:

- a need for clarification about the aims and purposes of such dwellings
- need to clarify and recognise the scope and limitations of the Warden role and to determine the necessary education for this role
- requirements for improved liaison between health care staff and Wardens
- the need for a greater emphasis on encouraging independence and providing residents with more contact with the wider community
- for those in privately constructed sheltered housing, the need to address the problems arising from escalating costs on imposed service charges and the restrictions on the re-sale of property.
  (Fennell 1985, Fisk 1986, Victor 1987, Bradley 1989, Grundy 1989b).

Nevertheless, sheltered housing may be an answer for a number of older people. Information from the various quoted surveys shows that turnover in such accommodation, for reasons other than death, is low. Thus it does appear to assist some older people to maintain relative independence in their later years. However, it is not a universal panacea. There may be no balance between the ages of residents, nor their levels of health or dependence, so that Wardens may sometimes find themselves facing heavy care demands. There is also a risk of segregating older people from the rest of the community and hence contributing to their marginalisation (Askham 1989). Health visitors may do a great deal to represent the needs of those older people in sheltered housing, in providing and supporting integrating activities, and in offering general health promotion interventions.

PROMOTING HEALTH IN BEREAVEMENT

One of the most frequent happenings which health visitors may encounter, when facilitating older people, is bereavement. This is because multiple loss is a prevalent theme in the life of an aged person. In the United Kingdom, over 70% of all the deaths that occur, do so in those aged 60 years and upwards. Major causes are heart and circulatory disorders, malignancy, cerebrovascular accidents and respiratory disease. Hence the death of contemporaries can be a fairly common experience for most older people.

At the turn of the century, when present-day elderly people were born, large families were the norm. Therefore, many older people have several siblings, as well as ramifications of other relatives, rendering them susceptible to repeated bereavement. Furthermore, concomitant losses can arise following deaths, such as loss of a home, or cherished possessions, which can add to grief. There may be loss of transport, loss of income, or changes in social identity, with the subsequent loss of some friendships.

'Older old' people (those aged 85 years or more) and elderly widows are most at risk of sustaining '*bereavement overload*'. This phenomenon, first described by Kastenbaum (1969), occurs when overwhelming grief is precipitated by a sequence of multiple losses, with little space for grieving time. It can lead to confusion, disorientation, a pervasive sense of helplessness and loneliness, and sometimes increased risk of suicide (Garrett 1987). Bereavement overload thus constitutes part of stress in later life. (The prevention and management of stress is discussed in Ch. 8, p. 202–204.)

As with retirement, bereavement can be studied as *an event*, *a status* and *a process*. Each phase calls for particular knowledge and skill on the part of carers, in order that intervention may be effective. Furthermore, health promotion in bereavement has an individual, a group and a community dimension. Figure 7.2 summarises the health visiting care at an individual level, in response to the different stages of client behaviour.

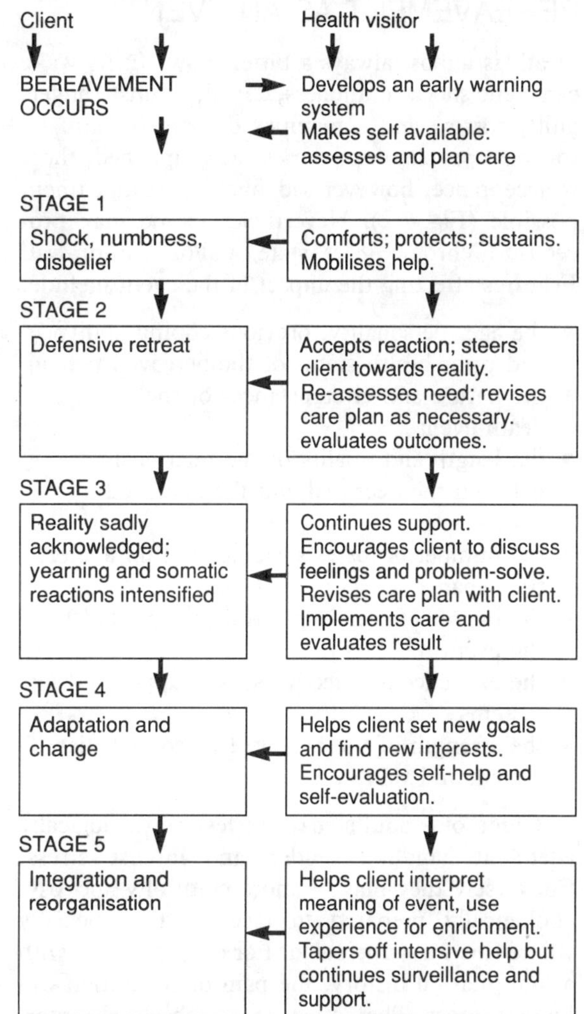

Fig. 7.2 Bereavement in later life and health visitor intervention. (Using a crisis intervention model, after Caplan 1964, 1974, to promote health and achieve adaptation — (see Appendix 3.)

Promoting healthy bereavement

It may seem strange to speak of promoting healthy bereavement, but that is exactly what health visitors seek to achieve. Recognising that death, grief and mourning are an inevitable part of the life-cycle, and moving healthily through the stages of bereavement to grief-resolution, can enhance emotional and spiritual well-being. However, the risk of unresolved grief and maladaptation is very strong.

BEREAVEMENT AS AN EVENT

Death is almost always a bitter blow. In its wake can come shock, numbness, denial, anguish, anger, guilt, sorrow and sometimes despair. Eventually for most people, grief-work is accomplished, there is acceptance, however sad, making readjustment possible (Fig. 7.2). Nevertheless some may proceed to chronic grief state and/or withdrawal. Features affecting the impact of the event include:

- the age, personality, previous coping ability and prior health status of the bereaved person
- the nature and circumstances of the death-event
- the length and quality of the relationship between the deceased and the bereaved person(s)
- the number of losses sustained within a short time-span
- the degree of social upheaval precipitated by the event
- the existence of effective social support systems
- the strength of the bereaved person's belief system and values.

'Older old' adults may be less physiologically adept at handling sudden and intense stress. Conversely they may be more culturally and psychologically prepared to face death, especially where this was anticipated. For conjugal pairs with a long marital history, the pain of separation can be very great. They often have such closely interwoven lives that the loss of the one may cut across the other's very existence (Raphael 1984).

Sudden death, especially under distressing circumstances, is often tragic. It may reactivate long-buried emotions and create psychological disturbance, especially guilt feelings. On the other hand, when illness has been prolonged, or suffering acute; where there has been care-giver strain, or there is a history of conflict, death may bring a sense of relief (Lopata 1973, Ferraro 1989). The deep sense of guilt or helplessness arising from undue dependency on the deceased person can also prove disruptive.

For these various reasons it is helpful if there has been effective health visitor contact prior to the event. This often means a relationship can be built upon. Client coping strategies can be understood and appropriate ones accordingly strengthened. The practitioner may have been familiar with the character of the deceased person and hence may provide more insightful support. It may also have been possible to have facilitated the dissipation of prior grief, or to have enabled potentially bereaved persons to brace themselves for the actual event.

Initial stages

Initial help in bereavement should be of a comforting and strengthening nature. Because numbness, shock and disbelief often predominate, immediate assistance may be welcomed in letting family and friends know of the sad event. Guidance concerning procedures, such as obtaining death certificates, registering the death and contacting a funeral director may also be required. In the event of an inquest, explanations may be needed and follow-up support required. Attention to basic needs, especially safety, are health-sustaining measures. In their grief elderly people may disregard these, especially eating, drinking and sleeping. Spiritual counsel may be valued. It should be mobilised only at client request, although the suggestion may need to be made. An awareness of cultural differences is also important. Recognising what death means to specific groups, and understanding ethnic and social rituals and ceremonies, are ways of offering health promoting support.

Grief reactions vary considerably. Some groups mourn overtly, others become silent and withdrawn, or 'aim to keep a stiff upper lip'. Each style requires different, but equally empathetic handling. Immediately following the loss of a significant other, behaviour may be somewhat bizarre. Examples include clinging to articles or garments belonging to the loved one, resistance to any change in the pattern of the old life, visits to the grave to 'talk things out', writing accounts of one's feelings to the dead person, and sometimes seeking an occasion 'to speak with the deceased'. As long as these activities are relatively short-lived, such 'strangeness' is not regarded as pathological (Garrett 1987).

BEREAVEMENT AS A SOCIAL STATUS

How people cope with bereavement may depend partly on their personal characteristics and partly on the social recognition afforded their bereaved status. For instance certain funeral rites are sometimes expected and these may prove comforting. Rituals such as specified mourning periods; wearing distinctive clothing; or permitted expressions of condolence such as wreaths, sympathy cards and letters may facilitate grieving.

There are marked gender differences in the social recognition of bereavement. For example, widowhood is normative for older women at present. It may therefore be easier for women, bereaved of a spouse, to obtain peer support than for men to do the same. Socially permitted expressions of grief also favour women. Whereas men, socialised not to express their feelings so readily, may be denied avenues of emotional release, or social support (Ferraro 1989).

Moreover, widowhood is a status, formally recognised by the State. Older widows may therefore welcome information on Widow's Benefit and other possible sources of financial or social help.

Organisations such as Cruse provide support for those suffering the loss of a spouse. However, the homogeneity of membership may again favour women. Furthermore, there is sometimes a tendency for other bereaved relatives or friends to feel 'left out'. They may, however, be grieving very deeply. Health visitors may find that more widely-based bereavement support groups meet health promotion needs in many localities.

It is perhaps at the community level where health promoting actions can make great impact. Enabling community members to understand and support bereaved persons is part of this aspect of the health visiting role. There is much evidence to suggest that close supportive relationships, and strong social networks, can buffer the adverse effects of life-crises, including bereavement (Stroebe & Stroebe 1983, Dimond et al 1987).

Research studies also show that those of high socio-economic status tend to fare better in bereavement. Higher education and income levels appear to confer benefits. Advantages secured include better health, larger social networks, greater coping resources. In a review of the literature, Ferraro (1989) concluded that 'in general, interventions should be geared to address those less fortunate on the socio-economic scale'.

BEREAVEMENT AS A PROCESS

Once shock has given way to denial, there is need to give older bereaved persons time to collect themselves (Fig. 7.2). This stage may be accompanied by mental mechanisms such as rationalisation or projection. Significant others may need an explanation of this, and about any resultant hostility, in order to avoid their feeling hurt or distressed.

As reality dawns on the bereaved person, sadness usually deepens. Somatic complaints may predominate and there is some evidence that these may be greater in 'older old' people (Garrett 1987). Medical aid may need to be invoked, but older people also respond well to empathetic listening, extra comfort measures, and kindly concern. They may find great solace in other family members, friends or pets. Reiterating the qualities of the dead person and cherishing their possessions may also prove consoling. Bereaved persons need help to realise that their reactions to loss are normal; that they can learn to accept them and to gain from them, hard as this may seem. They also need to discover that they can treasure memories without dwelling on them, and can develop new interests and activities. Thus, even in mourning, there is scope for health enhancement.

The adverse impact of bereavement on health

The symptomatology immediately accompanying bereavement is well documented. Cardinal signs include disturbances of sleep, appetite and weight; digestive and elimination upsets; headaches and liability to panic attacks. Depression is common (Parkes 1972, Fenwick & Barresi 1981, Ferraro et al 1984, Raphael 1984, Wan 1984). Underlying the older person's distress is a threat to the life of the survivor and a fear of, or anger at, being left alone. It is important for would-be helpers to appreciate the welter and depth of these feelings if support and health promoting interventions are to be effective, and emotional health maintained.

Epidemiological studies indicate that the impact of bereavement lasts for a considerable though variable period. An association between cardiovascular death and recent widowerhood was demonstrated by Parkes et al (1969), Ward (1976), and Helsing et al (1981). By contrast Maddison & Viola (1968), Jones & Goldblatt (1986) and Jones (1987) reported higher levels of both mortality and morbidity for widows during the first year after bereavement.

Another indicator of health status following bereavement is considered to be the use of health services, although clearly this is open to debate. In one study the utilisation of health services by the older bereaved appeared to increase between the 5th and 8th month after the event (Raphael 1984). However, in a subsequent study, Homans et al (1986) did not confirm this. Further details on the health effects of bereavement are given in Fuller & Larson (1980), Vachon et al (1982), Klerman & Clayton (1984), Lundin (1984), Rando (1986), Bowling (1987) and Ferraro (1989).

Implications and inferences

The significance of these various findings for health visitors would appear to lie in the direction of mobilising intensive initial support for all older bereaved persons, in providing continuing surveillance, health promotion and health education, and in ascertaining that acceptable continuing support is available, particularly between the 3rd and 9th months following bereavement. Since anniversaries of death, especially the first, are particularly poignant, unobtrusive visits to bereaved older persons at these times may prove valuable. Careful record keeping is therefore necessary, so as to readily identify such occasions, as part of efficient health visiting (Kubler-Ross 1969, 1975). Similarly, an awareness of male vulnerability, and the adverse effects of lower socio-economic status, may indicate some forms of 'targeting'.

SUMMARY

This chapter has focused on both retirement and bereavement, as an event, a status and a process, with the objective of promoting health, for those in later maturity. Through considering various definitions, the empowering, enabling and enhancing facets of health promotion were identified and seen to be clearly related to the health visiting role. Research studies have been cited as pointers for action. Although individual lifestyles, life-skills and behavioural practices have been seen to be important in enhancing well-being in retirement, it is at the community level where instigating, interpreting and influencing functions are most needed. The relationship between personal, environmental, socio-economic and political action and health promotion has been stressed, especially as they affect those in later maturity. This was because undue emphasis on personal responsibility for health can lead to 'victim blaming'. Detailed topics such as nutrition, safety and stress-control are important in relation to health promotion and are covered in the next chapter.

Health visiting involvement in the pre- and post-retirement periods has been seen to be ripe for development. Given that such development occurs, it may well be that in the future more preventive functions can be exercised, in preference to reactive care.

Given effective inter-sectoral co-operation in health promotion, it may be that future generations of old people may be able to say, with Cicero, 'nothing is more enjoyable than an active and leisured old age' (Falconer 1923).

REFERENCES

Abrams M 1980 Beyond three score years and ten: a second report on a survey of the elderly. Age Concern England, Mitcham

Allen J 1986a New lives for old: life-style change initiatives among older adults. Health Values: achieving high level wellness 10 (6): 8–18

Allen J 1986b Achieving health promotion objectives through cultural change systems. American Journal of Health Promotion 1 (Summer): 42–49

Anderson R C, Fox R 1987 Ethical issues in health promotion and health education. American Association of Occupational Health Nurses Journal 35 (5): (May) 220–223

Askham J 1989 The need for support. In: Warne A (ed) Human ageing and later life. Edward Arnold, London

Atchley R C 1979 Issues in retirement research. Gerontologist 19: 44

Atherton C, Manthorpe J 1989 The rights of grandparents. Age Concern England, Mitcham

Baglioni A J 1989 Residential relocation and the health of the elderly. In: Markides K S, Cooper C L (eds) Aging, stress and health. Wiley, Chichester

Beck S H 1983 Retirement preparation programmes: differentials in opportunity and use. Gerontologist 23: 294 (Special issue)

Becker M H 1986 The tyrany of health promotion. Public Health Review 14: 15–23

Bowling A 1987 Mortality after bereavement: a review of the literature on survival periods and factors affecting survival. Social Science and Medicine 24: 117–124

Bracey J, Blythe J 1985 Promoting positive health. Nursing Mirror 161 (6) (7th August): 17

Bradley L 1989 Sheltered accommodation: strengths and opportunities. Geriatric Medicine (August): 27–32

Brown J S, McCreedy M 1986 The hale elderly: health behaviour and its correlates. Research in Nursing and Health 9: 317–329

Butler A, Oldham C, Greve J 1983 Sheltered housing for the elderly. Allen and Unwin, London

Clavan S 1978 The impact of social class and social trends on the role of grand-parent. Family co-ordinator 17: 351

Comfort A 1977 A good age. Mitchell Beasley, London p 181–190

Coonrod C, Lesnoff-Caravaglia G 1982 The Soviet Babushka and the American Black 'Granny': coping models for older women. Paper presented at the meeting of the Gerontological Society of America, Boston, 22nd Nov (unpublished)

Cotton E, Sharp G 1989 Health promotion: shifting the emphasis. Personal communication, Rochdale District Health Authority, March 1989

CSO (Central Statistical Office) 1989 Social Trends No 19. HMSO, London

Dean K 1988 Issues in the development of health promotion indicators. Health promotion 3 (1): 13–21

DHSS (Department of Health and Social Security) 1978 A happier old age. HMSO, London

DSS (Department of Social Security) 1989 Caring for people: community care into the next decade and beyond. White Paper. HMSO, London

Dimond M, Lund D A, Caserta M S 1987 The role of social support in the first two years after bereavement, in an elderly sample. The Gerontologist 27: 599–604

Disability Alliance (ERA) 1989 Disability right handbook, 14th edn. Disability Alliance (ERA), London

Drennan V 1988 Celebrating age. Community Outlook (June): 4–6

Duffy M E 1988 Health promotion in the family: current findings and directives for nursing research. Journal of Advanced Nursing 13: 109–117

Ebersole P, Hess P 1985 Towards healthy aging. Mosby, St Louis

Ekerdt D J, Baden L, Bosse R, Dibbs E 1983 The effect of retirement on health. American Journal of Public Health 73 (7): 779–783

Falconer W H 1923 Translation of Cicero, De Sencute. Heinemann, London

Fennell G 1985 Sheltered housing: some unanswered questions. In: Butler A (ed) Ageing: recent advances and creative responses. Croom Helm, London

Fenwick R, Barresi C M 1981 Health consequences of marital status change among the elderly: a comparison of cross-sectional and longitudinal analyses. Journal of Health Social Behaviour 22: 106–116

Ferraro K F 1982 The health consequences of retirement. The Journal of Gerontology 37: 90–96

Ferraro K F 1984 Widowhood and social participation in later life: isolation or compensation. Research on Aging 6: 451–468

Ferraro K F 1989 Widowhood and health. In: Markides K S, Cooper C L (eds) Aging, stress and health. Wiley, Chichester, ch 4

Ferraro K F, Mutran E, Barresi C M 1984 Widowhood, health and friendship support in later life. Journal of Health and Social Behaviour 25 (3): 246–259

Fiegehen G C 1986 Income after retirement. Social Trends 13–15. HMSO, London

Fisk M J 1986 Independence and the elderly. Croom Helm, London

Fuller S S, Larson S B 1980 Life events, emotional support and the health of older people. Research in Nursing and Health 3: 81–90

Garrett J E 1987 Multiple losses in older adults. Journal of Gerontological Nursing 13 (8): 8–12

Green L W, Raeburn J M 1988 Health promotion: what is it and what will it become? Health Promotion 3 (2): 151–158

Grundy E 1989a Living arrangements and social support in later life. In: Warnes A (ed) Human ageing and later life: multi-disciplinary perspectives. Edward Arnold, London

Grundy E 1989b Longitudinal perspectives in the living arrangements of the elderly. In: Jefferys M (ed) Growing old in the 20th Century. Routledge, London

Helsing K J, Szklo M, Comstock G W 1981 Mortality after bereavement. American Journal of Epidemiology 114: 41–52

Holmes J, Rahe E 1967 The social readjustment scale. Journal of Psychosomatic Research 11 (Pt 8): 213–218

Homans S M, Haddock C C, Winner C A, Coe R M, Wolinsky F D 1986 Widowhood, sex, labor force participation and the use of physician services by elderly adults. Journal of Gerontology 41: 793–796

Houldin A D, Saltstein S W and Ganley K M 1987 Nursing diagnoses for wellness: supporting strengths. Lippincott, Philadelphia

Jones D R 1987 Heart disease mortality, following some results from the OPCS longitudinal study. Journal of Psychosomatic Research 31: 325–333

Jones D R, Goldblatt P O 1986 Cancer mortality following widowhood: some further results from the Office of Population, Censuses and Surveys longitudinal study. Stress Medicine 2: 129–140

Kahana E, Kahana B 1983 Environmental continuity, futurity and adaptation of the aged. In: Rowles G D and Ohta R J (eds) Aging and milieu: environmental perspectives on growing old. Academic Press, New York

Kaplan R M 1988 The value dimension in studies on health promotion. In: Spacapan S, Oskamp S (eds) The social psychology of health. The Claremont symposium on applied social psychology. Sage, New York

Karn V 1977 Retiring to the seaside. Routledge and Kegan Paul, London

Kastenbaum R 1969 Death and bereavement in later life. In: Kutscher A H (ed) Death and bereavement. Charles and Thomas, Springfield, Illinois

Klerman G L, Clayton P J 1984 Epidemiological perspectives on the health consequences of bereavement. In: Osterweis M, Solomon F, Green M (eds) Bereavement reactions, consequences and care. National Academy, Washington DC

Kubler-Ross E 1969 On death and dying. Collier MacMillan, London

Kubler-Ross E 1975 Death: the final stage of growth. Prentice Hall, Englewood Cliffs, New Jersey

Lakhani B, Read J, Wood P 1989 National welfare benefits handbook, 19th edn. Child Poverty Action Group, London

Lawton M P 1980 Environment and aging. Brooks/Cole, Monterey, California

Lopata H Z 1973 Widowhood in an American city. Schenkman, Cambridge, Massachusetts

Lundin T 1984 Morbidity following sudden and unexpected bereavement. British Journal of Psychiatry 144: 84–88

McGoldrick A E 1989 Stress, early retirement and health. In: Markides K S, Cooper C L (eds) Ageing, stress and health. Wiley, Chichester

McGoldrick A E, Cooper C L 1989 Early retirement. Gower Press, Aldershot

Maddison D C, Viola A 1968 The health of widows in the year following bereavement. Journal of Psychosomatic Research 12: 297–306

Maloney S K, Fallon B, Wittenberg C K 1984 A study of seniors, identifies attitudes, barriers to promoting their health. Promoting Health 5 (5): 6–8

Martin A 1988 Chatteris: Age-Well Club. Age well ideas sheet No 5. Age Concern/Health Education Authority, London

Mills L A 1982 Grandmother/child relationships: the grandmother perspective. Gerontologist 22: 105

Murray R, Huelskoetter M, O'Driscoll 1980 The nursing process in later maturity. Prentice Hall, Englewood Cliffs, New Jersey, p 137–156

Mutran E, Reitzes D C 1981 Retirement identity and well-being: realignment of role relationships. Journal of Gerontology 36 (6): 733–740

Nuffield Centre of Health Services Studies 1984. Unemployment, health and social policy. Nuffield Centre, 71–75 Clarendon Road, Leeds

Nutbeam D 1986 Health promotion glossary. Health promotion 1 (1): 113–127. Oxford University Press, Oxford

OPCS (Office of Population, Censuses and Surveys) 1984 Unemployment and mortality. Unpublished report, quoted in The Guardian, 17th September 1984

Ottawa Charter for Health Promotion 1986 Health Promotion 1 (4): iii–v. Oxford University Press, Oxford

Parker S 1982 Work and retirement. Allen and Unwin, London

Parkes C M 1972 Bereavement: studies of grief in adult life. Tavistock, London

Parkes C M, Benjamin B, Fitzgerald R G 1969 Broken hearts: a statistical study of increased mortality amongst widowers. British Medical Journal 28: 3–6

Pender N J 1982 Health promotion in nursing practice. Appleton-Lange, Norwalk, Conn.

Pender N J 1987 Health promotion in nursing practice, 2nd edn. Appleton-Lange, Norwalk, Conn.

Phillipson C, Strang P 1984 The role of paid carers. The Health Education Council in association with the Department of Adult Education, Keele University, p 93–110

Rando T A (ed) 1986 Loss and anticipatory grief. Lexington Press, Massachusetts

Raphael B 1984 The anatomy of bereavement: a handbook for the caring professions. Hutchinson, London

Rodin J 1986 Aging and health: effects of the sense of control. Science 233 (19th Sept) Articles 1271–1275

Rowland M, Kennedy C, McMullen J 1989 Rights guide for non-means tested benefits. Child Poverty Action Group, London

Ryan S, Travis J 1981 Wellness workbook. Ten Speed Press, Berkeley, California

Schafer S L 1989 An aggressive approach to health responsibility. Journal of Gerontological nursing 15 (4): 22–27

Streib G, Schneider C 1971 Retirement in American society: impact and process. Cornell University Press, Ithaca, New York

Stroebe M S, Stroebe W 1983 Who suffers more? Sex differences in the health risks of the widowed. Psychological Bulletin 93: 279–301

Syme S L 1986 Strategies for health promotion. Preventive medicine 15: 492–507

Tannahill A 1985 What is health promotion? Health Education Journal 44 (4): 165–168

Terborg J R 1988 The organisation as a context for health promotion. In: Spacapan S, Oskamp S (eds) The Social Psychology of Health. The Claremont symposium on applied social psychology. Sage, New York

Thomas S E 1990 Stress responses following relocation: a personal observation. Unpublished account

Thomson R 1989 Swimming upstream: a community nursing perspective. Primary Health Care 7 (10) (Nov/Dec): 6

Townsend P 1979 Poverty in the United Kingdom. Penguin, Harmondsworth

Vachon M L S, Sheldon A R, Lancee W J, Lyall W A, Rogers J, Freeman S J J 1982 Correlates of enduring distress patterns, following bereavement: social networks, life situations and personality. Psychological Medicine 12: 783–788

Vernon S W, Jackson G L 1989 Social support: prognosis and adjustment to breast cancer in later life. In: Markides K S, Cooper C L (eds) Aging, stress and health. Wiley, Chichester

Victor C R 1987 Old age in modern society: a textbook of social gerontology. Croom Helm, London

Victor C R, Evandrou M 1986 Social class and the elderly: an analysis of the 1980 General Household Survey. Paper presented at The British Sociological Association Annual Conference, University of Loughborough (unpublished)

Victor C R, Jones D A, Vetter N J 1984 The housing of the disabled and the non-disabled in Wales. Archives of Gerontology and Geriatrics 3: 109–113

Wan T T H 1982 Stressful life-events, social support networks and gerontological health. Lexington, Massachusetts

Wan T T H 1984 The health consequences of major role losses in later life: a panel study. Research on aging 6: 469–489

Wan T T H 1985 Well-being and the elderly. Lexington Books, Massachusetts

Ward A W M 1976 Mortality of bereavement. British Medical Journal 1: 700–702

Watt A S, Rodmell S 1985 Community involvement in health promotion: progress or panacea? Health promotion 2 (4): 359–368

Whitehead M 1989 Swimming upstream. King's Fund Institute, London

CHAPTER CONTENTS

8

Health promotion in later life — groups, strategies, topics

In the previous chapter emphasis was laid on the definition of health promotion and some of the implications it held for health visitors working with older people. Indication was given that future health visiting might focus more on work at group and community level, as a complement to that undertaken with individuals and families, where the weight is at present. Much of the existing work is undertaken in private homes, or clinic settings. Directing greater attention to aggregates is likely to both broaden the range of potential settings and increase the variety of contacts. However, this does not mean that home visiting and clinic work will not remain an important part of health visiting activity. Rather that this will be extended and hence reinforced.

Group and community work requires a re-orientation of thinking; it calls for a broader knowledge base and different methods of analysis and application. While core skills such as communication, organisational, perceptual and leadership skills remain important in any setting, facilitative, motivating, instigating and enabling skills may have to be further strengthened and adapted. Attitudes, particularly towards client participation and decision-making, may have to undergo change. A different set of assumptions may apply. Some practitioners may at first feel uneasy working in new ways, while others will welcome the opportunity to foster such developments.

In this chapter we briefly consider the principles underlying group and community work, and examine some of the potentialities and problems. In exploring possible strategies for use in health promotion with older people, some suggestions for practice are outlined. Priority topics are also presented and measures discussed as to how older people might be empowered to

- regard their aspirations in these various topic areas as valid and worthy of attention
- identify their particular needs and be enabled to discover how best to meet these
- increase their personal coping ability and personal sense of control
- develop more health-supportive environments.

Throughout, we are conscious of the need to be aware that health promotion is an inter-sectoral and collaborative adventure. The very nature of old age means that many needs cannot be directly met by clients themselves. Indeed, not all can be met by their informal carers, or the intervention of professional personnel. Changes may well have to be made in social, economic and environmental policies, at national and international level, in order to meet some needs. Hence the role of health visitors in influencing policies affecting health is regarded as highly pertinent (Orr 1985, Drennan 1988a).

COMMUNITY WORK

In Chapter 6 we stressed the importance of conducting community assessments and compiling community profiles. One of the several purposes underlying such an activity is that it enables health visitors to encounter and appreciate community networks.

Community networks

Much advantage for older people may be conferred through community networks. As secondary level relationships, they provide intermittent contact and hence may not always be immediately obvious to health visitors. This is why it is so important to take time 'Tuning In' to a community, before engaging fully in health promotion activities. The more formal social institutions of a secondary nature, such as church, educational, or voluntary organisations, will be more readily identified. Liaison is thus possible, and health promotion can form part of their programmes.

However, it is often the informal networks which, although diffuse, can serve to strengthen the coping abilities of older people. They help to maintain their sense of belonging, provide outlets for older clients to voice their concerns, act as channels for information and can offer practical help. Their representatives include hairdressers, post-office staff, pharmacists, milkmen, church workers, small shopkeepers and policemen. They can become valuable allies in health promotion activities, and can also serve as informal ways for health visitors to impart health information.

GROUPS

By contrast with the rather diffuse community networks, groups are often highly visible. They may be:

1. natural or informal
2. formal.

Natural or informal groups

Natural or informal groups, as their name implies, arise spontaneously, often out of shared concern or interaction. They have fewer goals, rarely expressed expectations, variable life-spans and operate with few restrictions. Examples include small clusters of older people, meeting within a luncheon club; or small groups of 'regulars' meeting in cafes, bars, parks, Day Centres or Community Centres. Some ad hoc leisure groups or church groups sometimes fall into this category.

Such groups should not be ignored. They often help old people to overcome loneliness, maintain self-esteem, release strong feelings, or deal with life-crises. They may also provide health visitors with valuable information about themes of common concern. However, it requires considerable skill and observation to identify and then utilise such opportunities. This calls for reflective practice.

Formal or formed groups

These are brought into being deliberately. In consequence they often have clearer goals, stated expectations and more structured membership. They may develop as a result of lay activity, as in the many self-help groups or health initiatives, or arise from professional sources. Among their many purposes such groups

> enable older people to exert control over their lives, through confronting and engaging some of the problems of living in either institutions or in the community.
>
> (Miller & Solomon 1979)

Examples might include patients' groups; reminiscent groups; groups for reality orientation; therapeutic groups; weight, smoking or stress control groups; exercise and fitness groups; or pressure groups designed to effect some specific social or health action.

Belonging to a group may be highly significant for some older people. Group procedures may enhance communication, develop personal skills, relay information, effect change, or prove therapeutic (Beaver 1983).

HEALTH VISITORS WORKING WITH GROUPS

Health visitors can work with a diversity of groups and in various ways. They may be invited to speak to group gatherings on a 'one-off' basis, or they may contact existing groups, build up relationships with them and then offer their services as resource persons. They may act as occasional or regular group leaders, especially in health-related discussions as Drennan (1988a) has shown. They may organise health courses, health forums, or co-operate in running Health Fairs or Festivals of Age (Drennan 1988b). They may conduct community outreach in response to local aspirations, as groups of older people declare their interest in health issues and demonstrate a desire to work together. Sometimes health visitors may join groups as 'grass-roots' members, working to secure social or environmental change, for their own as well as others' benefit. Some groups may not be exclusively for older people, but may have older persons among their members, pursuing general or specific health issues, for instance the Women's Health groups which have sprung up throughout the country. At other times health visitors may search for unmet needs and, if there is a confirmed response, may start new groups in an attempt to satisfy such needs.

Preparing and planning for new groups

It is necessary to undertake much preparatory work before launching new groups. Discussion is required to identify potential members, their level of interest, likely expectations and degree of commitment. Planning includes deciding on the optimum size of the groups, their number and membership structure. The frequency and length of sessions needs to be determined. When planning for older clients it should be remembered that they require time to assimilate new information or learn new skills (see Ch. 3, p. 59). They may, however, easily become fatigued if group sessions are prolonged. This then becomes counterproductive. Variety in the presentation of material, and in the deployment of time, helps prevent fatigue and create interest and enthusiasm among older members.

Venue and accommodation

Choosing a venue is important. However, options concerning location are often limited. Accessibility and safety are paramount considerations, especially where group members may have mobility problems.

Accommodation should be comfortable, kept at an even temperature (65–70°F), well lighted and ventilated and appropriately equipped for group purposes. Space is required for movement and fitness sessions; audio-visual material needs to be bright, bold, clear and varied.

To cater for relaxation sessions suitable chairs, mats and cushions will be required. Toilet facilities should be appropriate for older people, some of whom may have disabilities. Refreshment amenities are always welcomed. Other points include:

- security provisions
- insurance
- transport arrangements
- staffing and contingency cover
- finance
- publicity
- worker-support systems
- record systems
- evaluation measures
- procedures for dealing with group problems.

However, although resources need to be well organised beforehand and during sessions, these aspects are best undertaken unobtrusively. Group sessions need to be flexible and conducted in a relaxed manner, so that members feel at ease, discussion is facilitated and participation is encouraged.

Practitioners will appreciate that a collective approach is often desirable, so that continuity can be provided and activities shared. Many practical suggestions for those wishing to develop group work, especially with older people, are given by Burnside (1983), Ebersole & Hess (1985), Balter et al (1986) and Drennan (1988a).

Group dynamics and group development

There is a wide range of theories relating to group dynamics (for example, see Bion (1968), Cartwright & Zander (1968), Shaw (1971), Smith (1980) and Brown (1988)). Many of these ideas will be familiar to health visitors. The outline used later in the chapter represents one particular framework and serves to provide an illustration (Table 8.1). However, its use does not imply prior merit. Because of the great variety of health-promoting groups, the wide age range encountered among older people, together with their heterogeneity in health status, social skills and levels of organising ability, flexibility in approach is an essential requirement. Furthermore, practitioners may feel more comfortable using one theory than another.

Group membership

Group membership is best related to group purpose; hence there may be several different forms of group selection. Frequently, random self-selection is the format used, mainly for groups that are ad hoc, have broad general purposes, or are short-term. More structured or restricted membership may need to be used when specific issues or topics are to be addressed. For instance a smoking control group will likely only contain smokers, whereas a group for those who wish to consider 'how to cope with arthritis' will mostly likely be composed of sufferers and those more directly concerned with helping them, such as informal carers.

Group development

Early stages

Initially group members may exercise cautiousness, especially if they are unfamiliar with one another. Apprehension and anxiety may be shown, often dependent on the group purpose or topic. Time must be allowed for basic trust to be fostered — analogous with the early stages of human growth and development. As trust emerges, members are likely to relax and reach out to one another. Nevertheless group cohesion is not always easily achieved.

Middle stages

In the middle stage of group development, group leaders are required to be very active yet unobtrusive, skilfully handling group dynamics and steering the group towards closeness and effectiveness. Individual personality factors are likely to emerge more strongly during this stage, in drives towards greater autonomy and mastery. Some older members may become garrulous, over anecdotal, or monopolising of the group. Others may be excessively silent, sometimes because of depression. This can on occasions prove 'contagious'. It requires anticipatory planning, so that strategies for positive thinking can be quickly introduced when diffuse pessimism appears to be spreading.

There may be bids for leadership, or arguments, or 'subversive' behaviour, with some members operating on the fringe of the group. Learning may then be disrupted for all. Leadership style is all-important in handling such conflict. The democratic style allows for open discussion, release of strong feelings, or concerns, and subsequent resolution.

Later stages

As groups stabilise, communication usually becomes more effective. Energies can then be directed towards necessary tasks such as considering changing behaviour or lifestyles, problem-solving, or producing action to effect social or environmental change.

Other points may arise in group work with older people. Patterns of existing illness or disability may limit health promotion results. It is important that group leaders or members do not have unrealistic expectations. Cultural differences may affect responses, hence separate groups for older members of ethnic minorities may at times be necessary, especially when they have particular problems to face (Svedin & Gorach-Tomlinson 1984).

Cohort effects may need to be considered (see Ch. 3, p. 55–56). Illness and death may occur among members, creating an impact on the group. Some issues raised in discussion may confront health visitors with their own ageing. Attitudinal difficulties may then sometimes arise, which need resolution. All these eventualities are best thought out beforehand, so that possible responses can be carefully considered. Some form of counselling and worker support is also, therefore, required (Litwack et al 1980).

Nevertheless many groups of older people are lively, responsive and rewarding. Self-help and activist groups are often highly motivated and self recharging. Older members, especially from among the 'young elderly', who may have wide experience, frequently demonstrate great skill in leadership and organisation of such groups. They thus make a very positive contribution to the community.

STRIVING FOR EFFECTIVENESS IN GROUP HEALTH PROMOTION

One of the most imperative issues in health promotion concerns effectiveness. Health visitors engaging in this activity are aware of the competing demands for their time and the many constraints on resources. They know that health promotion activity is often long-term and frequently difficult. Understandably they wish their efforts with older people to be successful. For this reason they seek theoretical insights so that they can engage in research-based practice. As mentioned earlier, there are a number of theories which can be employed. We have selected one as an example: social learning theory (SLT), propounded by Bandura (1977a). We referred to SLT in Chapter 3, and we develop it here for three reasons, as follows.

1. The theory is gaining increasing social recognition.
2. Certain concepts, constructs and one model which derive from it relate strongly to health behaviour and change.
3. The theory appears to lend itself well to work with older clients.

Even so, other approaches may have much to offer.

Social Learning Theory

SLT is rooted in both stimulus-response theory and cognitive theory, with which health visitors will be familiar. It holds that behaviour is determined by expectancies and incentives (reinforcements) (Bandura 1986). Three types of expectancies are identified:

1. environmental expectancies
2. outcome expectancies
3. efficacy expectations.

Environmental expectancies

These are opinions and beliefs about environmental cues, about how events are connected and about the consequent results of specific actions.

Outcome expectancies

These are opinions and beliefs about how individual behaviour is likely to affect outcomes.

Efficacy expectancies

These are opinions and beliefs about one's personal competence to perform behaviours, deemed necessary to bring about particular outcomes.

Incentives

These are defined as 'the perceived value of a particular outcome'. The outcome may be a desired health status, physical appearance, social approval, economic gain or other consequence (Rosenstock et al 1988). For instance, under SLT, it is postulated that persons who value the perceived health benefits of a changed lifestyle (incentive), will attempt to model their behaviour in a similar direction, but only if the following apply.

- They believe their present lifestyle threatens a personally-valued outcome.
- This belief is reinforced by clues and cues in their environment.
- They perceive/believe that a specific behaviour change will both reduce the health threat and produce the desired outcome.
- They believe that they are personally capable of adopting and sustaining such behaviour.

Self-efficacy

Closely allied to SLT is the concept of self-efficacy, already mentioned in Chapter 3, p. 52–53. This is a *situation-specific concept*, propounded by Bandura (1977b) and elaborated by Schunk et al (1984), Strecher et al (1986) and Rosenstock et al (1988). It relates to an individual's or a group's belief about their level of ability and their competence to perform adequately in a particular way in a specific situation, e.g. ability to retain or regain mobility through following a specific exercise regime. Two conditions are necessary:

1. persons must have confidence in their personal competence (this = high self-efficacy)
2. persons must believe that particular behaviours will bring about desired (specified) outcomes/benefits.

This concept has relevance for health promoters because the hypothesis is that those with high levels of self-efficacy, who perceive related behavioural outcomes as beneficial, are more likely to attempt to produce the specific behaviour.

Conversely, those with low self-efficacy are likely to refrain from attempting the behaviour, even though they believe it could produce the desired outcome.

Proponents of this concept argue that it is possible to reduce the negative effects of low self-efficacy by

- demonstrating the particular behaviour in clear, related stages (modelling)
- verbally persuading the individual or group to attempt the behaviour
- providing spaced 'reinforcements' designed to encourage continuance of the behaviour
- offering feedback and 'rewards' for endeavour
- reducing anxiety through relaxation, reassurance and continuous encouragement.

Readers will recognise that these ideas underpin many group health promotion ventures, such as stress-control or assertiveness sessions. They also apply to rehabilitation.

The Health Locus of Control construct

A further construct which derives from SLT, and is pertinent for health promotion, is the Health Locus of Control (HLC) (Rotter 1966, Dabbs & Kirshott 1971, Best 1975, Best & Steffy 1975, Phares 1976, Wallston et al 1976a, 1976b, Wallston & Wallston 1978a).

This construct is not the same as the concept of self-efficacy, although it has much in common with it. A major difference is that it is a *generalised construct* about the self, in contrast to the *specific* nature of self-efficacy. As an individual difference construct HLC concerns *Internality* versus *Externality*.

The postulation is that 'Internals' are those persons who believe that the locus of control for health is vested within themselves. Hence they believe one becomes sick, or stays well, largely as a result of one's own efforts. Consequently 'Internals' display attitudes of high personal responsibility and autonomy. They are likely to be more successful in adopting and sustaining health-enhancing behaviours (Siegrist 1988). The factor within 'Internality' most highly correlated with the reduction of health-damaging behaviour, is thought to be 'Luck-denial' (Seeman & Seeman 1983).

Conversely '*externals*' are those persons who believe that the locus of control for health lies largely outside themselves. They therefore see health as mainly dependent on luck, chance, fate, or the actions of powerful others. Because of these perceptions 'externals' believe there is little they can do, themselves, to alter health status (Wallston & Wallston 1978a). For these reasons they are less likely to respond to health promotion initiatives which involve modifying health behaviour, unless they are exposed to specific methods.

A multi-dimensional scale to differentiate '*Internals*' and '*Externals*' was developed by Wallston et al (1978b). They postulated that different approaches would be required for each type. For a copy of this scale see Appendix 5.

Practitioners will doubtless appreciate that, through using such a tool, health promotion activities might be 'tailored' to suit each type. Some suggestions as to how these may be utilised are given later in this chapter.

The Health Belief Model

Arising also from SLT, and closely allied to both self-efficacy and the HLC, is the Health Belief Model (Rosenstock 1966, Becker 1974, Maiman & Becker 1974, Rosenstock 1974, Janz & Becker 1984, King 1984 and Rosenstock et al 1988). The Health Belief Model (HBM) is also discussed briefly in Chapters 3 and 5.

This model hypothesises that health-related action depends on the simultaneous occurrence of three factors, as follows:

1. Health motivations. (These are characterised by concern about health matters, readiness to seek health help, previous use of health services, and beliefs and behaviours commensurate with health.)
2. Perceived personal vulnerability to one or more health threats. (This is shown by an acceptance of being personally 'at risk' and by the perception of the potential severity of an illness or an accident, possibly related to previous experience.)
3. The perception that the benefits likely to be derived from specific health-behaviours

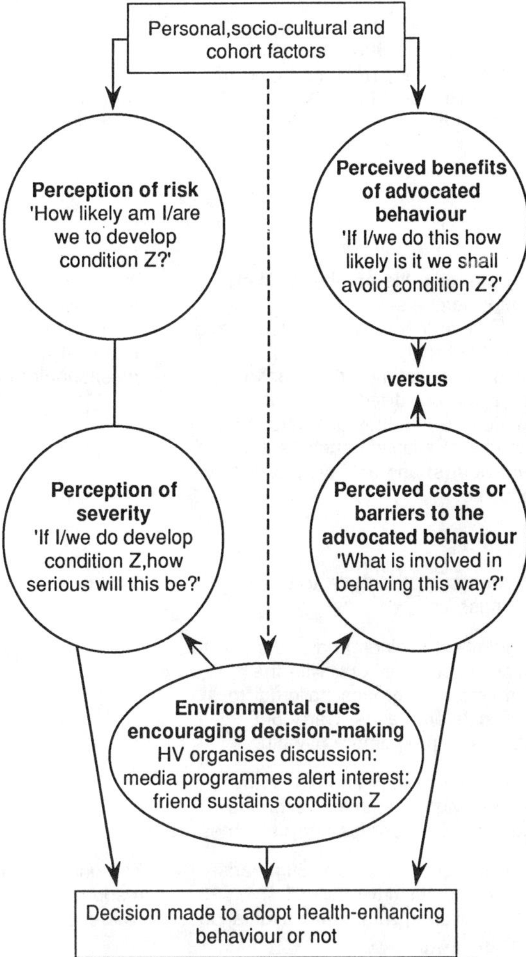

Fig. 8.1 The Health Belief Model. (Based on material from Rosenstock 1966, Janz & Becker 1984, King 1984, Rosenstock et al 1988.)

Table 8.1 A sample scheme for group health promotion, using Social Learning Theory, the concept of self-efficacy, the Health Locus of Control construct and the Health Belief Model

Activity	Methods of data collection	Theory — concepts, constructs and models used.
1. Ascertain health motivations among potential group members. Levels of general and specific health interest; current health themes. Relate to prevailing health policy. Reconcile where possible.	Brain-storming session; group discussion; health appraisal interviews; personal observation; scrutiny of quantitative data, e.g. local or national statistics; radio 'phone-in' programmes; health forums; questionnaires.	Incentives and health values.
2. Identify number of potential group members who personally believe they are at risk from a specific health threat, or who actually have a health problem.	Group discussion; health appraisal interviews; health forums; health polls; questionnaire responses. Relate to quantitative data such as incidence or prevalence rates, and to health service use.	SLT: — expectancies about environment. HBM: — perceived susceptibility; — perceived health threats.
3. Discover the proportion of likely group members who personally believe that the perceived threat to their health could be reduced by action on their part.	Group discussion; health appraisal interviews; multi-dimensional scale form to identify Health Locus of Control for each member, and determine Internality or Externality.	SLT: — outcome expectancies; Health Locus of Control construct. HBM: — perceived health threat — perceived severity — belief health action can reduce threat — perceived benefits of health actions vs. perceived costs of such actions.
4. Determine the number of likely group members who: (a) believe themselves susceptible to a health threat; (b) believe that their own health behaviour could reduce threat; (c) believe that they are personally capable of adopting such health behaviour(s) and achieving a desired outcome.	Group discussion; health appraisal interviews; results from the multi-dimensional scale re: 'Internality' or 'Externality'; questionnaire responses.	SLT: — environmental and outcome expectancies. Self-efficacy concept: — belief in personal competence and confidence. HBM: — belief in personal susceptibility; — belief action could reduce threat to health; — belief that benefits will outweigh costs or barriers.
5. Analyse data; relate to other findings.	Data from community assessment	
6. Interpret findings and use same to place group members, with their permission, in groups 'tailored' to their different needs. Carry out differential programme planning.		
7. Implement the various health promotion programmes, recording step-by-step progress and outcomes.		
8. Carry out evaluation. Summarise final outcomes; invite client participation in summative evaluation and review.	Personal interview; questionnaire responses; pre- and post-testing where appropriate.	
9. Reorganise as indicated.		

outweigh the costs involved in performing such behaviours. This is termed *Benefits versus Barriers*. (It is demonstrated by an account of personally perceived benefits, or valued outcomes; by the recognition of the likely cost involved in achieving such behaviours, but the expressed conviction that these outcomes would still be worth the effort/cost involved — this being accompanied by a belief in the efficacy of the health behaviour (see Fig. 8.1).

This model has been shown to be useful in explaining the take-up of preventive health measures, such as immunisation and vaccination, and/or cervical smear testing (Strecher et al 1986). It has been criticised as being less useful as a predictor of future health behaviour (Langlie 1977). It has been discussed by King (1984) in relation to nursing.

By now readers will likely have concluded that because there are strong similarities in each of these ideas, a combination might increase their explanatory power and hence their usefulness in practice. Indeed this is what is advocated by Rosenstock et al (1988).

PRACTICE IMPLICATIONS

Before applying these theoretical ideas to practice, considerable thought is necessary. The initial data collection may well prove time consuming, but might result in greater efficiency and effectiveness in the longer-term. This will of course require evaluation. A sample scheme, showing suggested stages for data collection and action, is given in Table 8.1. It is intended to stimulate thought rather than to be a blueprint, and health visitors will no doubt wish to modify it in line with their own further reading and thinking.

Having obtained data, as per the first five stages outlined in Figure 8.1, various approaches will have to be designed for the different types of group members. Some suggested approaches are given below. Health visitors will readily think of others. It will be apparent that some form of selective group membership will facilitate these various tailored approaches.

Those group members found to have high levels of health motivation

Potential group members found to have high levels of health motivation could be encouraged to get together and prioritise their health concerns, coming to a consensus about which health themes they wish to first address. Group programmes can then be formulated, to follow the priority list, harnessing the evident health motivations. Methods such as group discussion, which involve members in decision-making, are likely to be effective with this type of group.

Those group members found not to be highly interested in health matters

For those older group members found *not* to be highly interested in health matters, measures need to be adopted to increase motivation. Such individuals may respond to an exploration of their main aspirations and values. It may then be possible to relate these to health behaviour. For instance, where older persons show a low health motivation but a high value for independence, group members may be assisted, through discussion, to recognise that enhanced health levels may increase the chances of maintaining independence. Such older group members may also benefit from exposure to a general community campaign, designed to raise health-consciousness. Where appropriate, such a campaign could be linked to findings from community profiles.

Where a distinct health problem exists but is being ignored

If confronted by a situation where a distinct health problem exists, either within the entire community, or a specific subgroup, but is being apparently ignored, it is necessary to discover the reasons for this behaviour. Where apathy is shown, it may be dispelled by the dissemination of information and by encouragement to action. It is important to increase confidence of group members in the possibility of improving their situation. Where frank indifference is the cause, this may be challenged by 'confronting'. This may be done in a personal health consultation, or in small group discussions. Increased knowledge of relevant facts may then increase motivation and may lead to action. Where fear is the reason for ignoring a health problem, it may yield to reassurance and the clear presentation of facts. Older people who are fearful often have a low self-efficacy level and hence need considerable support and encouragement to action.

Those older group members who are currently unaware of the specific health risks posed for them by their present health behaviour

Where older group members are unaware of the specific risks they run because of their existing health behaviour, it is necessary to acquaint them of the facts. This can be done in a personalised risk-appraisal interview (as outlined in Ch. 6, pp. 122–123 and Fig. 6.1). Attempts to raise awareness of personal susceptibility must of course be accompanied by positive and repeated presentations of specific health-enhancing, threat-reducing health behaviours. Such behaviours should either be within the competence of the group members themselves to perform, or they should clearly understand how to obtain necessary help. It is important to avoid raising anxiety.

Those group members who are aware of personal health threats and who demonstrate high levels of personal responsibility, yet fear possible illness outcomes

Such older group members need quite different handling. They may respond to a clarification of the causes of such illness, and to the provision of information on the different levels of prevention which apply, as well as on particular therapies, should these be indicated. They should also be informed about services which can be mobilised to ameliorate any adverse outcomes. If such members are also '*externals*' (using the HLC construct), they may benefit from very specific instructions concerning the health actions to be adopted. Additionally, they may respond to role-modelling by powerful others, such as TV personalities demonstrating the preferred health behaviour.

Those currently aware that threats to their health may be reduced by appropriate self-action, and who display strong 'internality'

These older potential group members are probably the easiest ones with whom health promoters can work. They usually respond well to the presentation of factual, relevant information about health threats and health-enhancing behaviours. They often welcome details about alternative courses of action, and clear statements about necessary steps to be taken, and respond well to the recognition of their right to exercise informed choices. They require reinforcements designed to strengthen their sense of personal responsibility. They frequently benefit from 'contracting', whereby they agree to undertake certain health behaviour and to use health professionals as resources, to complement their own, informed, health actions.

Those currently aware of personal susceptibility and health threats, who recognise the behaviours needed to reduce such threats, but feel powerless to initiate such action

These older group members show low self-efficacy. If they are also '*externals*', they require approaches which strengthen their general expectancies, as well as education and training to develop greater '*internality*' (Green et al 1975, Tobias & MacDonald 1977, Wallston et al 1976b Wallston & Wallston 1978a, Seeman & Seeman 1983, Rosenstock et al 1988, Siegrist 1988). They are likely to benefit from being shown itemised steps to be taken; from selecting short-term/interim goals, the achievement of which provides reinforcement; and from encouragement and clear feedback.

'*Externals*' who demonstrate health awareness, but personal powerlessness, are also likely to be helped by social support systems, such as peer-group reinforcement, or from the interventions of powerful others. Contingency-contracting may also enhance self-efficacy and may modify 'externality'. The choice of goals, which will form the basis of the contracts, should be

- personally determined by the older client
- relevant to the older client's situation
- realistic and feasible of achievement within a given time-span and with the client's resources, or those available to the client from statutory or voluntary sources.

Successful accomplishment of small goals could lead to clients and groups accepting larger ones (Rosenstock et al 1988).

Whether these combined ideas *will* reflect increased effectiveness in group health promotion remains an empirical question at present. They offer one way of dealing with health promotion at group level. The answer concerning their effectiveness lies in the collection and analysis of comprehensive data, in the evaluation of both processes and outcomes, and in the generation and testing of subsequent hypotheses. This presents health visitors with considerable challenge.

PROMOTING THE HEALTH OF INFORMAL CARERS

Informal Carers represent one group whose health promotion needs are of particular concern to health visitors.

There is no widely accepted definition of 'informal care', but the DHSS defined Carers as

> persons who take primary responsibility, in the home, for the care of persons, who because of handicap or illness, need almost continuous care.
>
> (Social Work Development Group 1983)

Paid workers are regarded as 'formal Carers'.

Informal Carers are crucial to almost all major health and social policies. Their pivotal role has been recently re-emphasised in the Government White Paper on Community Care (DSS 1989). However, there is little evidence in the proposed legislation that the supportive services required to adequately meet carers needs will be forthcoming.

Demographic and social changes, and developments in medical treatments, have resulted in an increasing number of persons requiring informal care. In an attempt to ascertain the characteristics and needs of informal carers, the DHSS set up a research programme (DHSS 1984). This resulted in the publication of a Report, which health visitors will find useful (OPCS 1988).

Who cares?

There are currently estimated to be 6 million informal Carers in Great Britain ($3\frac{1}{2}$ million women and $2\frac{1}{2}$ million men). However, even this estimate may be an under-representation (OPCS 1988).

618 000 Carers (13%) are aged 65 years or more. Older men are more highly represented in this age group than in earlier ones, although male Carers are fewer in number than women because of sex disparity in longevity (see Ch. 1, p. 5–6).

Of those being cared for (termed 'dependants'), over 50% are aged 75 years of age or more. Thus elderly informal Carers, and Carers of the elderly, constitute a sizeable group for health promotion action.

Some idea of the strains imposed by 'caring', and the consequent threat to health, may be inferred from a scrutiny of some of the survey findings:

- 20% of all Carers look after more than one dependant.
- 59% of all Carers spend 50 or more hours per week caring for their dependant(s).
- 73% of all Carers look after physically disabled persons, two-thirds of whom are 65 years or more.
- 44% of all Carers report that they have suffered from '*long standing illness*' in the year prior to the Survey. This proportion rose to 50% for those aged 65 years or more.
- 21% of all Carers ($1\frac{1}{4}$ million persons), reported that their health '*had not been good*' in the year prior to the survey.
- 42% of all Carers with dependants living in the same household reported '*no one else available to look after dependant if I took a 2-day break*'. This proportion rose to 66% for Carers aged 65 years or more. Secondary support is available from within the

household for up to 50% of all cases, although less than 5% have paid help.

- Approximately 50% of all Carers (3 million persons) had been caring for at least 5 years prior to the Survey. 26% of them '*had not had any break since starting caring*', and 13% had '*not had a break from caring for 15 or more years.*'

Although it is difficult to grasp fully the import of such statistics, and while it is necessary to recognise the subjective nature of some of the comments, they do serve to highlight the constant nature of the caring activity.

The effects of caring on informal Carers

One theme arising from the literature on carers is the pervasiveness of the work, since it invades all realms, affecting physical, emotional, social and financial well-being (Groves & Finch 1983, Briggs & Oliver 1985, Wright 1986, Ungerson 1987, Hicks 1988). Because the work is at times heavy and unremitting, fatigue, back-ache, and ill-defined symptoms are common. Disturbed sleep reduces energy levels — particularly problematic where the carer has multiple household roles and may also be employed outside the home as well.

Role reversal between carer and dependant may be difficult to accept at first. Certain intimate personal tasks can prove repugnant to some informal Carers. Social life may be disrupted and there may be little personal time or privacy. Income frequently plummets, limiting possible diversions and possibly endangering future financial security. Career chances may be jeopardised. Where the dependant lives with the informal Carer there may be housing problems. Heating and telephone costs may soar, or furnishings may be damaged.

Relationships within the household may become strained, especially when other family members feel the dependant takes up a disproportionate amount of the Carer's time. Of course many informal Carers derive great emotional rewards from caring and feel privileged to undertake this task. There is little supporting evidence for the belief that the growth of welfare provisions has undermined the ability of families to care for their vulnerable members.

However, many informal Carers resent being '*expected' to care*, or having to do so for very long periods virtually unsupported (Ungerson 1987, Hicks 1988). Many contend that conventional statutory services fail to provide even basic levels of help. Indeed, for many such Carers, statutory services appear almost irrelevant (Jones et al 1983, Luker & Perkins 1987).

There is evidence to suggest that services are provided on other than rational grounds. 'Rationing' of services tends to occur according to unstated criteria. For instance, older persons, living alone, tend to receive rather more help than similar older persons living with others. Male carers tend to receive more help than females, in spite of such discrimination being illegal (Charlesworth et al 1984, Blythway 1987). However, Arber et al (1988) point out this discrimination may be less gender-related, but based rather on the Carer's marital status, age and household structure.

EMPOWERING CARERS

Empowering informal Carers begins with informing them about available services and how to contact them. Unfortunately, many Carers remain 'invisible' and often do not seek such information for themselves. They may, however, respond to overtures of support from health visitors and other professional workers. Some practitioners have found it helpful to mount a Carers' Day, or Carers' Forum, as a means of contacting people whom they cannot readily identify in other ways. One such venture in Rochdale resulted in 150 informal carers coming together and eventually forming a Carers' Support Group. This Group produced an information Handbook on available services and published a Carers' Charter (Weir 1987, Rochdale Carers' Group 1988, Cotton & Sharp 1989). A similar publication by The King's Fund (1989) offers many practical ideas for providing a new deal for informal Carers.

Among the various points advanced by these publications are the Carers' rights to

- be seen as individuals and included in discussions and care plans affecting their dependants
- ask questions about their dependant's health and medications, without having the answers side-stepped
- be given information and services that could ease the burden of caring at home
- be given support, respect and consideration by professionals
- have some time to themselves.
- receive respite care
- receive counselling during and after caring.

Additionally, induction processes for workers such as home helps and care assistants, and the curriculum for professional workers, should recognise the carer's contribution. Furthermore, all who come into contact with informal Carers should recognise their need to talk; hence the importance of listening is reinforced.

Health enhancement for informal Carers

Carers require information about how best to safeguard and improve their own health, as well as that of their dependant(s). Training needs, too, should be identified, so that Carers can work safely and efficiently. Courses for informal Carers might include:

- the management of common disorders and disabilities
- lifting techniques
- agency structures and functions
- services available and how to access them
- education on stress control and self-advocacy
- Welfare Benefits and rights.

(Based on information provided by Cotton & Sharp 1989 and Jones 1989.)

Anyone planning courses for informal Carers should take into account the need for a 'caring replacement service', for the period of the course, and possibly for the need for transport to allow Carers to attend easily. Quantitative and qualitative evaluation is also required.

Other functions which practitioners might fulfil as part of their health promotion activities include:

- supporting family groups while they recognise and resolve conflict related to caring
- drawing community attention in general, and service managers' attention in particular, to the shortage of provisions, such as Day Centres, respite schemes, voluntary visiting schemes and other home-based facilities.

Invalid Care Allowance

Invalid Care Allowance (ICA) is currently the only cash benefit specifically for informal Carers. Its limitations should be recognised. Intended as a 'replacement income', its eligibility is restricted to women aged 16–59 and men 16–64 who care for dependants for at least 35 hours per week. The dependant must be in receipt of either Attendance Allowance or Constant Attendance Allowance, and the claimant currently must not earn more than £20 per week. ICA is taxable and, because of the Overlapping Benefits Regulations, entitlement to Income Support is correspondingly reduced. Nevertheless there are some advantages to claiming, as follows.

1. ICA confers contribution credits for National Insurance purposes, which count for both retirement and sickness Benefit, although these cannot be claimed as well as ICA.
2. Recipients of ICA may receive the £10 Christmas Bonus.

Further details about this Allowance may be obtained from DSS Offices, from Welfare Rights Organisations, or from the Annual Publications of The Disability Alliance (Disability Alliance 1989).

The Disabled Persons Act 1986

One other piece of legislation holds out some hope for informal Carers, who, it is currently estimated, save the State some £6 billion per year on residential care and/or hospital services. This is the Disabled Persons Act 1986.

It does not provide for new services but when fully implemented will give Carers the right to have their needs, as well as their dependants, taken into account when care services are being planned. This may be particularly important in view of pending legislation on Community Care (DSS 1989).

Further information on the needs of Carers is available from The National Carers' Association (see useful addresses in Appendix 7).

PRIORITY TOPICS IN HEALTH PROMOTION

Exercise and fitness in later life

Independence within the community, and coping abilities in later life, depend on being able to perform a range of physical tasks and maintaining adequate levels of fitness. However, personal attitudes and cultural expectations, which have projected retirement as a time for 'taking things easy', result in a tendency for some older people to assume sedentary lifestyles. Consequently, the risk of 'disuse atrophy', a condition familiar even to Hippocrates, is ever present. It has been thought to account for up to *50%* of the physiological decline associated with ageing (Bortz 1982, Smith & Gilligan 1983, Speake 1987).

Health Visitors who wish to include exercise and fitness programmes within their health promotion initiatives for older people, will therefore need to

- review the physiological changes associated with ageing (see Ch. 2)
- appreciate the normal exercise responses which occur in older people
- take account of the benefits of exercise
- design appropriate activities for older clients.

Exercise-related physiological changes in later maturity

The major exercise-related physiological changes which occur with ageing can be summarised as follows:

- Decreases in
  - maximum oxygen consumption (VO_2)
  - vital capacity
  - maximum heart rate
  - exercise stroke volume
  - cardiac output
  - muscular strength and bone density
- Increases in
  - systolic pressure and peripheral resistance
  - airway resistance
  - vestibular hypersensitivity, affecting orthostatic tolerance and sense of balance
  - lipid levels, on account of decreased catabolism
  - muscle fatigue, because of fewer 'fast-twitch' fibres
  - calcium depletion.

(Based on material derived from Smith & Serfass 1981, Ciba Foundation Symposium No 134 1988, Marsiglio & Holm 1988, Webster 1988.)

These various changes, which are modified in different individuals according to the interplay of hereditary and environmental factors, are also liable to be affected by inter-current pathological conditions. Where disease does occur, it can sometimes lead to exercise being contraindicated. In such situations fitness is clearly compromised. Preventive action is thus the preferred choice (Gray 1987).

Exercise response in older individuals

Exercise can be classified as

1. Isometric or static type
2. Isotonic or dynamic type.

Isometric exercise uses few muscle groups. The normal response to static exercise includes an increase in heart rate, blood pressure, systemic vascular resistance and a slight rise in cardiac output. Stroke volume, however, remains unchanged.

Isotonic exercise uses large muscle groups, creates a volume-loading mechanism through rhythmic contractions, and increases heart rate, systolic pressure, cardiac output and coronary blood flow. It decreases blood flow to non-working muscles, and may reduce diastolic blood pressure (Marsiglio & Holm 1988, Webster 1988).

However, it is important to note that, while aerobic activities provide the most important cardiovascular benefits, they should always be preceded by isometric and isotonic stretching exercises, which gradually increase body temperature, improve circulation to muscles, decrease blood viscosity and render muscle contractions more efficient (Getchell & Anderson 1982, Marsiglio & Holm 1988, Webster 1988).

The benefits of exercise for older people

The probable physical and psychosocial benefits of exercise are well documented (they have been listed by Everard & Whelan (1985), Smith & Jacobson (1988) and Webster (1988). Results from research studies show that significant changes include: improved heart muscle tone, decreased blood pressure, reduced tension, increased high-density lipoproteins, decreased body fat, improved flexibility, increased ability to perform daily tasks with ease, and increased self-esteem (DeVries 1975, Sidney & Shepherd 1977, Sager 1984, Barr et al 1985, Larson & Bruce 1987, Smith & Jacobson 1988).

Women who exercise can help to reduce osteoporosis and orthopaedic problems (Riggs & Melton 1988). Additionally, older insulin-dependent diabetics who engage in regular exercise may find it easier to regulate their insulin requirements (Webster 1988).

Nevertheless, in spite of these clearly demonstrated benefits, and the changing concepts of fitness within the general population, some older people still under-estimate their own capacity to engage in physical activity. They justify their levels of inactivity on the grounds that 'vigorous exercise is dangerous in later life', and incorrectly assume that light sporadic exercise is more beneficial than sustained aerobic activity (Wells & Freer 1988).

Such attitudes are more likely to be displayed by those who have a high '*externality*' score on the Health Locus of Control Multi-dimensional scale (Wallston et al 1978b), or by those who incorrectly perceive their health status to be '*poor*' (Speake 1987).

Additionally MacHeath (1984) found that many professionals were even less likely than their older clients to rate exercise highly in later maturity. Consequently they tended not to encourage it in their clients/patients. All this lends considerable urgency to the need for health visitors to increase their health promotion input in this direction and to focus on creating a greater awareness of the importance of exercise and fitness in later maturity (Gray 1986).

Planning exercise programmes

The first step in planning exercise programmes for older adults is to obtain adequate data on organ function and physical status.

Ideally this should include a medical assessment of

- cardiovascular and respiratory status, including the results of an exercise stress test whenever possible
- resting heart rate, rhythm, body temperature and blood pressure
- haemoglobin levels and haemocrit rates, as low levels will increase the workload on the heart in its endeavour to maintain adequate oxygen supplies
- medication status, as certain drugs and medicines can lower exercise heart rates and hence complicate the assessment of target heart rates — e.g. beta-blocking agents.

Where there has been a history of disturbance of electrolyte balance, this and fluid balance should be assessed, as alterations may affect muscular irritability.

Absolute contraindications to exercise

It is important to remember the absolute contra-indications to exercise, which include the following:

- unstable hypertension and unstable angina
- atrial fibrillation, active cardiac myopathies and/or acute myocardial infarction

- recent pulmonary embolism or thrombo-phlebitis
- dissecting aneurysm
- anaemia and/or metabolic diseases.

Some other conditions may restrict mobility and hence modify exercise programmes. These include: arthritis, musculoskeletal disorders, intermittent claudication, emphysema and chronic bronchitis, and all conditions associated with pain (Marsiglio & Holm 1988).

Once clearance has been obtained for older persons to participate in regular exercise programmes, the following principles should be borne in mind

- Group activities must be safe, effective and sufficiently interesting to sustain motivation.
- Group members should establish mutually acceptable exercise goals.
- All programmes should commence at a low level of activity and should build up gradually to greater intensity. Surveillance of group members should be unobtrusively maintained.
- Every session should contain a 'warming up' and 'cooling down' session.
- Sessions should, whenever possible, contain the three primary types of exercise: namely, endurance, flexibility and strengthening exercises.
- Older people should not indulge in exercise immediately following a main meal and should intersperse activity with some periods of rest and relaxation.

Safety can mostly be achieved by ensuring that exercise takes place in the shaded outdoors whenever possible, or in rooms which are well lighted and uncluttered. Temperatures should be even (65°F whenever possible), and ventilation adequate. Clothing worn should be light, unrestricting but not flowing. Shoes should be supportive, supple, cushioned and have non-slip soles.

Effectiveness is best assured by choosing activities that have sufficient variation, intensity duration and frequency to derive optimum physical and psychosocial benefit. Those activities which are enjoyed are most likely to be sustained.

Suppleness and co-ordination may be achieved by flexibility and stretching exercises. They should be carried out 4 times a week to obtain maximum benefit.

For stamina and endurance, which enhances fitness, aerobic activities are needed. Types include brisk walking, cycling, swimming, dancing and some sports. Such activities should be taken 3–4 times weekly and continuously maintained for a minimum of 20 minutes. They should always be preceded by a 5–10 minute warm-up period and a similar-length 'cooling down'. *It is considered that $2\frac{1}{2}$–3 hours scheduled, sustained, exercise per week, should be well within the capacity of most well elderly.* Where specific fitness sessions are *not* available, brisk walking would appear to be the activity which health visitors can safely encourage, given that contraindications are observed.

Intensity of exercise

Some health visitors express concern about the intensity of exercise which they can safely recommend to their older clients. The intensity of exercise is measured in METS. 1 MET = a consumption of 3.5 cm^3 of O_2 per kilogram body weight per minute. Examples range from 1–2 METS expended when driving a car, watching TV or washing up, to 7–8 METS expended in hand-mowing a lawn, galloping on horseback, or chopping wood. Brisk walking, cycling at around 9 km/h, or ballroom dancing, utilises 3–5 METs, which is the level most health promotion practitioners recommend for desirable results (Cornett & Watson 1984).

Another approach to determining the appropriate intensity level of exercise for older people is *to aim to achieve a target heart rate.* This involves checking pulse rates beforehand, after 10 minutes of activity and then again after 20 minutes.

To determine a target heart rate in the absence of a graded exercise test following medical assessment, one *should add 20 beats to the normal resting heart rate.* Thus a healthy woman of 65 years, with a resting pulse rate of 72 beats per minute, can safely exercise up to 92 beats per minute. Clients can be taught to monitor their own pulse rate and how to modify exercise accordingly.

A more sophisticated formula exists where graded exercise tolerance tests are available (Webster 1988).

Very sedentary individuals may not achieve their target heart rate levels for several sessions. Group members should not be rushed, but encouraged to proceed at their own pace and to stop if they experience pain, discomfort or breathing difficulties.

Modifications of stretching and flexibility exercises can be undertaken sitting, for those with restricted mobility or impaired balance (Ebersole & Hess 1985, Graham 1988). Some activities can be done to music, which may increase enjoyment. Courses on suitable exercises for older people are offered by the organisation EXTEND (see Appendix 7).

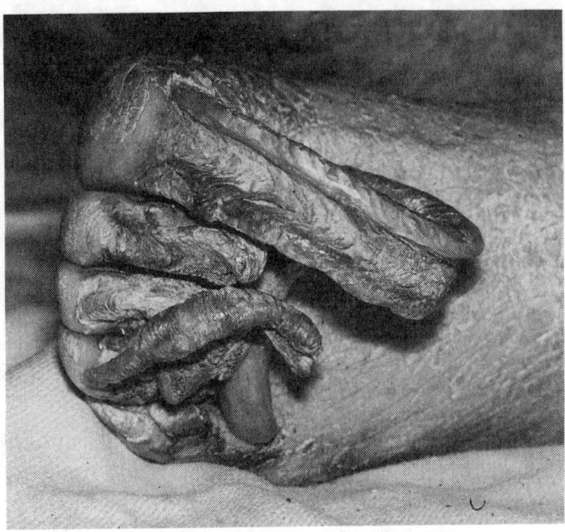

Fig. 8.2 Onychogryphosis in an elderly person.

PROMOTING FOOT HEALTH

The condition of the feet significantly influences the physical and psychosocial well-being of many elderly people, particularly affecting mobility and amiability. Health promotion goals for ageing feet should therefore be concerned with

- maintaining optimum function and mobility, through assessment, exercises and the prompt identification and treatment of conditions likely to threaten comfort and/or mobility.
- maintaining comfort via general foot hygiene and the prevention of infection
- preventing trauma by encouraging safe, appropriate footwear, that protects, stabilises and supports the foot and enhances mobility
- providing appropriate surveillance and guidance for those suffering from conditions such as diabetes mellitus, cardiac or renal disease, peripheral vascular or neurological disorders, the sequelae of cerebrovascular accident, or arthritis.

Older people often experience difficulty in caring adequately for their feet, because of poor vision, lack of flexibility, poor muscle strength, hand tremor, breathing difficulties or obesity. Nail care may be hindered because of thickening; nails then become extremely difficult to cut. In extreme cases onychogryphosis may occur (see Fig. 8.2). If nails cannot be softened easily with an application of warm oil, followed by 5–10 minutes soak in warm, soapy water, they need referral to a chiropodist, as do ingrowing toenails.

The nature of foot problems in later life

Podiatric difficulties most commonly encountered in later life include corns, callouses, ingrowing or involuted toenails, lesser toe deformities, hallux valgus, varicose veins, arthritis, pronated foot and foot oedema. In the most recent DHSS survey of foot problems in older people, over 86% of the sample reported some difficulty. 22% were found to have 'moderately severe problems', and 10%, 'very severe' problems (Cartwright & Henderson 1986). These researchers estimated that *the mobility of some 300 000 older persons in the UK is restricted because of foot problems. A further 700 000 could have their comfort and mobility improved by improved foot care.*

Clearly there is a need for some form of 'case-finding' service, since half of those affected in this survey were unaware of their need. However, in an earlier survey Chamberlain (1973) found Geriatric Health Visitors were not always effective in identifying foot problems among their clients. This was thought to be due to inadequate preparation, which may by now be remedied.

Empowering older people and their carers, in relation to foot health, may well involve health visitors in teaching and demonstrating effective foot hygiene, safe suitable foot massage, and in providing a surveillance service. Where practitioners are lacking preparation in this field, in-service education may be required. Additionally clients may have to be helped to obtain chiropody services. Liaison with both NHS and private sector personnel is therefore a necessary adjunct.

The NHS Chiropody service is currently understaffed in relation to the demands made upon it. Once clients have been referred to the service, long waiting lists can increase frustration. Moreover many older people suffer discomfort because of prolonged intervals between treatments. Drawing the attention of service managers to these unmet needs of older clients is thus one way of obtaining much needed improvements. Health visitors also need to liaise closely with their chiropody colleagues to assist them in determining priority needs.

One suggestion arising from the DHSS study (Cartwright & Henderson 1986) is that the work of foot-care assistants be extended, in order to provide a limited service within health centres and medical practice settings. So far no pronouncement has been made about this. Other much-needed improvements include an extension to the domiciliary chiropody service, or alternatively better transport schemes to enable disabled or housebound elderly people to attend chiropody clinics. Some older clients have benefited greatly from the use of complementary therapies concerned with foot health, and health visitors may wish to know about these (Evans 1990, Passant 1990, Smith 1990).

PROMOTING HEALTHY NUTRITION

Good nutrition is basic to good health, at all ages, but is particularly important in later life. The nutritional needs of older people have not yet been fully differentiated, but it is known that there are specific nutritional problems in this age group. Furthermore, nutritional factors may well be important in the ageing process, so that careful attention to diet may well modify some features of ageing (Davies & Stewart 1987).

Certain points should be noted about nutrition in later life, since they modify advice. The four major principles of diet still apply, namely that food taken should be

- physiologically appropriate
- nutritionally balanced
- psychologically appealing
- socio-culturally acceptable.

However, changes in energy output in old age may modify calorific requirements. Alterations in the gastro-intestinal tract may affect chewing, swallowing and digestion (see Ch. 2). Co-existing disease and/or drug therapy may affect absorption and excretion and can cause nutritional deficits (see Davies & Stewart 1987).

Table 8.2 gives recommended allowances for major nutrients, describes major food sources and offers some comment pertinent to older persons' needs. However, it is important to bear in mind that, like all standardised tables, such details only apply to the older population in general, and hence will not always match individual requirements. Furthermore, as new research is undertaken, requirements undergo modification, ahead of official recommended allowances publications. Health promotion information will therefore have to be tailored to individuals or small groups, within these broad considerations.

Calorific and nutrients intake

An intake of 1800–2000 Kcal for women, and 2100–2400 Kcal for men, usually suffices. Factors to consider include metabolic rate and energy output; desirable body weight in relation to actual height, weight and build; climate and season; and any existing illness.

Protein requirements

As protein requirements remain relatively high, in order to maintain nitrogen balance and vital

Table 8.2 Some nutritional requirements and considerations in later life

Nutrient	Recommended daily amounts Men		Women		Comment	Major food source[a]
	65–74	75+	55–74	75+		
Energy (kcal)	2400	2150	1900	1680	Compiled from 10–12% protein; not more than 30% fat; balance from carbohydrate foods	
Fibre (g)	30	30	30	30	Provides bulk; prevents constipation; aids satiety; favourably affects colonic transit-timing	Whole-grain products; legumes; fresh fruit, vegetables
Protein (g)	60	54	47	42	Repairs cells. Maintains vital functions; enzymes. Is affected by prolonged heat (denatured)	Eggs; cheese; fish; legumes; milk; nuts; whole grains
Thiamine (Vitamin B_1) Also known as Aneurine (mg)	1.0	0.9	0.8	0.7	Facilitates energy release from CHO. Easily lost in cooking. Is water soluble	Eggs; fortified flour; milk; offal; whole grains and yeast products
Riboflavin (Vitamin B_2) (mg)	1.6	1.6	1.3	1.3	Maintains health of mucous membrane. Unstable in light and heat; water soluble	Eggs; liver; kidney; cheese; marmite; yeast products and potatoes in season
Nicotinic acid (Niacin) (Vitamin B_3) (mg)	18	18	15	15	Utilises food energy. Keeps nervous tissue healthy. Gross deficiency linked with dementia, digestive upsets and dermatoses	Cheese; eggs; fish; whole wheat grains; milk; some vegetables
Pyridoxine (Vitamin B_6) (mg)	2	2	2	2	Manufactures amino acids. Utilises essential fatty acids	Widespread in many protein foods. May be inactivated by certain drugs, e.g. Isoniazide, L-Dopa
Folate (folic acid) (μg)	300	300	300	300	Helps to prevent megaloblastic anaemia. May help to protect against dementia.	Bananas; bread; offal; oranges; whole grains; raw green leafy vegetables
Vitamin B_{12} (Cyanocobalamin) (μg)	3	3	3	3	Needed for cell division. Erythrocyte formation. Healthy nerves	Liver and other animal protein
Ascorbic acid (Vitamin C) (mg)	30	30	30	30	Oxidises rapidly. Water soluble. Easily lost in heat and in alkalis	Citrus fruits; blackcurrants; tomatoes; potatoes in season (NB: highest Aug–Sept; lowest March–May)
Vitamin A (μg) Retinol equivalent	750	750	750	750	Anti-infective action. Promotes healthy skin and epithelial tissue: Intake often inadequate: can be toxic	Fish liver oils; fortified margarines; eggs; liver; milk (variable amounts); cheese; carrots; green leafy vegetables; apricots

Table 8.2 Continued

Nutrient	Recommended daily amounts Men 65–74	Men 75+	Women 55–74	Women 75+	Comment	Major food source[a]
Vitamin D (Calciferol) (μg)	10	10	10	10	Needed for bone mineralisation. Thought to protect against osteoporosis; intakes often low. Produced by action of sunlight on ergosterol in skin, if exposed	Fatty fish; fish oils; fortified margarine; milk and dairy products; liver; Ovaltine
Vitamin E (Tocopherol) (international)	100	100	100	100	Acts on skin to aid elasticity and is thought to improve health of collagen. Thought to be an anti-ageing factor. Oxidises very rapidly	Vegetable fats; sunflower and sesame seeds; nuts; whole-grain cereals
Calcium (g)	1	1	1–2	1–2	Often inadequate intakes. Needed to prevent demineralisation and to metabolise Vitamin D and maintain healthy circulation.	Cheeses; whole or skimmed milk; eggs; yoghurt. All greens except spinach. Sardines; tofu.
Sodium (g)	4	4	4	4	Needed for many enzymes and for electrolyte balance. Often taken in excess in old age, due to sensory losses. Intakes should be reduced when water retention is present and may be restricted when hypertension is diagnosed/treated.	Added to many processed foods. Amounts not always quoted on labels. High amounts in bacon, butter, canned vegetables, cheese, some treated cereals, kippers and sausages. Often found in assocation with high sugar content of processed foods
Potassium (g or mmol)	2.5–6 g daily for all (= 65–200 mmol)				Intakes often very inadequate in old age. Deficiency leads to muscle weakness, poor grip, mental confusion and heart failure. May also be associated with depression (Davies 1981)	Fruit, especially bananas and oranges. Vegetables, especially potatoes. Marmite; herrings; legumes; offal; milk; tomatoes and tomato juice but note this is also high in sodium content
Iron	10–12 mg daily				Often inadequate intakes. Deficiency leads to energy loss, dizziness, dyspnoea, oedema of ankles	Dried/canned beans; cereals; whole wheat pasta; whole-grain breads; brown rice; liver; eggs; lentils; dark green leafy vegetables
Certain other trace elements are also very important for the elderly particularly:-						
Cobalt	Exact requirements not known at present				Needed for healthy blood and nerve cells to act with Vitamin B_{12}. May be deficient in Vegans, those without intrinsic factor and post-gastrectomy patients.	Present in liver; fish; cheese; egg; barmene

Table 8.2 Continued

Nutrient	Recommended daily amounts Men		Women		Comment	Major food source[a]
	65–74	75+	55–74	75+		
Iodine	Exact amounts not known				Required for healthy function of thyroid gland helps to prevent myxoedema	Sea food; vegetables grown in soil with iodine present; Iodised salt
Zinc	Exact amounts not known Thought may be 15 mg				Required for healthy enzyme functioning. Absorption is affected by a high fibre intake, so zinc intake adjusted accordingly	Present in most protein foods. Therefore increase protein intake for those on high-fibre diets
Water (pints)	3–4	3–4	3–4	3–4	Needed for body fluids and vital enzymes. Often inadequate intakes in later life and risk of dehydration	Water. Some in other foods such as fruits and some vegetables, but these amounts should be ignored in calculating intakes

[a]Major sources given represent those regarded as inexpensive in relation to food value. When advising on nutritional intakes for older people, consider cost in relation to benefit, choose foods in season, easy to obtain and prepare. Advise on storage and cooking, so that food values can be conserved as far as possible.
Table is based on data obtained from DHSS (1979b), Davies (1981), Ebersole & Hess (1985) and Davies & Stewart (1987).

processes, between 10% and 12% of daily energy intake should come from foods of high biological value. This can be met from such items as lean meat, poultry, offal, fish, cheese, eggs, milk, nuts, legumes and whole-grain cereals. With an increasing proportion of the population becoming less meat-oriented, it is necessary to be very flexible in advice. Where certain staple food items in a diet have limiting factors (that is, they do not contain all the essential amino acids), it is necessary to recommend complementing items.

The role of these essential amino acids is, as yet, insufficiently understood in gerontological nutrition, nevertheless preliminary research suggests that glycine and arginine supplements improve wound healing in older people; tyrosine may help to relieve depression, and tryptophan to promote better sleep (Ebersole & Hess 1985). Alerting signs of hypo-proteinaemia include pruritis, slow wound healing, fatigue, lethargy and oedema.

Other factors health visitors should consider in relation to the intake of high biological value foods, include:

- availability of appropriate foodstuffs
- cost in relation to value
- digestibility of such foods
- recipient's personal preferences
- any food intolerances or allergies.

Fats and fat-soluble vitamins

It is important to follow recent recommendations that fat intake should not exceed 30% of total body energy requirements daily, and that diet should include a higher proportion of polyunsaturated fatty acids to saturated ones (COMA 1984). For many older people this may mean both an overall reduction in their fat intake and an adjustment in its content. This may of course facilitate weight control as well as reduce the risk of cardiovascular disease (Smith & Jacobson 1988). However, a necessary safeguard is to encourage an adequate intake of the fat-soluble vitamins, especially for certain vulnerable groups.

Vitamin A continues to be required to meet demands on epithelial tissue, to aid body resistance against infection, and to maintain dark–light adaptation. Vitamin D is also needed to maintain the strength of bones and teeth, and to aid calcium metabolism. Although the chief source of Vitamin D is the action of ultraviolet light on the skin, it is important to appreciate that latitude, the angle of the sun during exposure, and the amount and duration of skin exposure, are limiting factors. Some elderly housebound persons have decreased opportunity for such skin exposure. In any case, ageing skin, together with the atrophy of sebaceous glands, probably affects ergosterol manufacture. Thus while it is important to encourage older people to take full advantage of sunlight, attention must be paid to dietary intake.

In practice this means encouraging older clients to eat fortified polyunsaturated margarines; fatty fish; fortified milks; and cold pressed oils such as sunflower and safflower seed oils. Eggs and cheese should also be taken in moderation, and eggs should be adequately cooked.

Unfortunately, some older people are fearful of the bones in fatty fish, or find some varieties of this, and liver, rather too strong in flavour for them. This calls for creative cookery to be discussed, and may mean a supplement should be recommended. Even so, it is necessary to bear in mind that fat-soluble vitamins can be toxic, and injudicious use is liable to be harmful.

Others regretfully cannot be bothered to shop or cook and tend to rely on packaged convenience foods which may contain additional preservatives, or lack the necessary vitamins. Those living alone, the depressed and those with poor appetites may be vulnerable to vitamin deficiency.

The high incidence of osteoporosis in older people is well known. Less well appreciated is the fact that osteomalacia is also a risk, being found in approximately 4% of all elderly admitted to hospital. Diets rich in Vitamin D and calcium may help to counteract both problems, but this should be given attention much earlier, particularly in middle age, as part of general health promotion action.

Carbohydrates, Vitamin B complex and associated nutrients

One of the main health promotion goals is to reduce the intake of refined, processed sugar, present in many tinned and convenience foods, and to increase the amount of complex carbohydrates consumed. Fibre-rich items, such as whole-grain cereals, bran, whole-meal bread, fruit and vegetables will help to prevent constipation and improve colonic transit time, thus possibly reducing the risk of diverticular and malignant bowel disease. An intake of 30 g of fibre daily is recommended (NACNE 1983, Wenlock 1984, Smith & Jacobson 1988). It may require the exercise of considerable ingenuity to persuade some older people to re-orient their eating habits in this way, but it is well worth trying. Eventually patterns of healthier eating in earlier life should pay dividends in healthier old age.

However, health visitors should be aware of the adverse effects of excess fibre, especially wheat bran, in the diets of some elderly people. The phytates present in the fibre content of wheat can inhibit calcium, iron, zinc and magnesium absorption. For the 'older old', encouragement should be given to including at least one green leafy vegetable in the diet every day to avoid this risk.

Older people should also be reminded of the need to ensure adequate intakes of the water-soluble vitamins, essential minerals and trace elements. There is some evidence to suggest they may be at risk of sub-deficiency states, especially in relation to thiamine, riboflavine, nicotinic acid, folic acid, ascorbic acid, iron, zinc, copper, chromium and selenium (DHSS 1979a, 1979b, Davies 1981; Davies & Stewart 1987).

As Vitamin B complex and Vitamin C are both heat and light sensitive as well as water soluble, prolonged or poor storage, and faulty cooking methods, can contribute to high wastage. Less mobile old people may have difficulty obtaining fresh foods, especially when they rely on small corner shops with slow turnover of stock. There is also a tendency for older males, especially those now living alone, who have been unaccustomed to preparing their own meals, to adopt 'tea and toast' regimes, to their cost. 'Widowers' scurvy' is a well-known, detrimental syndrome.

Minerals

Older persons should *not* increase their salt intake unduly, although altered taste often leads them to do so. Where others are responsible for cooking, they should be reminded of the need to control intake.

Potassium intakes are conversely often low. This is especially so in individuals who are receiving diuretics. Information about potassium-rich foods should always be provided in such circumstances. A useful way of maintaining a balance is to suggest the inclusion of a banana or an orange every day.

Iron deficiency is not uncommon, and significant anaemia has been reported as occurring in up to 7% of the elderly population, usually because of shortage of iron and/or folic acid and poor absorption of Vitamin B_{12}. The latter, of course, is indicted as a major factor in relation to pernicious anaemia, which is not uncommon in older people.

Nutritional intake and certain medical conditions

Certain other medical conditions in later life affect nutritional intake. For example almost all acute illness in old age appears to disturb vitamin levels, and in particular Vitamin C requirements can be increased by up to 1000 mg daily. Elderly diabetics may run the risk of chromium deficiency, and it is reported that supplements can be particularly beneficial when combined with diabetic diet. Persons suffering from leg ulcers may respond to increased intakes of Vitamin C (1–3 g daily), and 25–30 mg of elemental zinc, while those with increased thyroid activity often have increased demands for the B vitamins and trace minerals (Davies & Stewart 1987).

Fluid intake

The intake of fluid should also be monitored in later maturity, being maintained at about 4 pints daily, except in cases of medical restriction. Caffeine-containing beverages should be restricted to 3–4 per day and water and fruit juices encouraged.

Alcohol ingestion, too, should be tactfully determined. Not more than 30 g, or 3 units, per day being advised for men and 20 g (2 units) for women. It should be remembered that half a pint of beer, one measure of spirits, or one average glass of wine, port or sherry, provides approx 10 g of alcohol. Alcohol intake may have a particularly damaging effect on the metabolism of Vitamin B complex, magnesium and/or zinc. It may also interact with certain medications. In such cases encouragement to abstain is increasingly recommended.

Calorie restriction

Where obesity is present, diet is usually restricted to 1000 Kcal daily. However, nutrient requirements for protein, minerals and vitamins remain the same. Where these are lacking, a supplement may be recommended. Very-low-calorie diets are not recommended for older persons.

Assessing nutritional status

Assessing and monitoring nutritional status in later life is another important part of health promotion. Factors to consider when undertaking this include:

- client's knowledge of food values and sources
- levels of motivation towards food intake
- ethnic and cultural beliefs and practices concerning food
- socio-economic resources and specific client food budgets
- availability of foodstuffs, access to shops, markets, or food co-operatives
- freshness of supplies
- transport facilities for obtaining food, linked to levels of mobility
- means of food storage, preparation, cooking and the methods chosen
- lifetime and present patterns of eating and drinking, including the timing of meals in relation to body rhythms and activities
- degree of social contact — if meals are taken on a solitary basis or in company
- the degree of control older people can actually exert over the food they receive, especially when they are living with others, receiving meals-on-wheels, or attending luncheon clubs

- levels of physical, cognitive, emotional, social and spiritual health.

Measurement of individual nutritional status can be accomplished by noting height, weight, general appearance, colour, skin texture, muscle tone, mucous membranes and general vitality. Anthropometric measurements such as mid-arm circumference and skinfolds, either taken from the triceps of the non-dominant arm, or the tip of the scapula, are also helpful. For baseline comparison some authorities recommend supra-iliac and thigh measurements as well.

Such measurements must be accurate, but are quite quickly obtained. Skinfolds for arm and thigh are picked up in the vertical plane, the subscapular and supra-iliac measurements being taken at a slight angle. Skinfolds are usually measured three times and an average of the two closest readings used as the actual measure. Height and weight can be compared with standard tables such as that given in Table 8.3 and anthropometric data assessed against measurements given in Table 8.4. In cases where nutritional status appears compromised, biochemical assessments may also be made.

Table 8.3 A guide to desirable weights in late life[a]

Height (in bare feet)			*Weight (without clothes)*					
(ft)	(in)	(cm) (nearest equivalent)	(st.)	(lb)		(st.)	(lb)	(kg) (nearest equivalent)
Men								
5	0	152	8	4	—	9	1	53–58
5	1	155	8	7	—	9	4	54–59
5	2	157	8	10	—	9	7	55–60
5	3	160	8	13	—	9	10	57–62
5	4	162	9	2	—	9	13	58–63
5	5	165	9	5	—	10	2	60–65
5	6	168	9	8	—	10	5	61–66
5	7	170	9	11	—	10	8	62–67
5	8	173	10	0	—	10	11	64–69
5	9	175	10	3	—	11	0	65–70
5	10	178	10	6	—	11	3	66–71
5	11	180	10	9	—	11	6	68–73
6	0	183	10	12	—	11	9	69–74
6	1	185	11	1	—	11	12	70–75
6	2	188	11	4	—	12	1	72–77
6	3	191	11	7	—	12	4	73–78
Women								
4	9	142	7	0	—	7	11	44–49
4	10	145	7	3	—	8	0	46–51
4	11	147	7	7	—	8	4	48–53
5	0	151	7	10	—	8	7	49–54
5	1	152	7	13	—	8	10	50–55
5	2	155	8	2	—	8	13	52–57
5	3	157	8	5	—	9	8	53–58
5	4	160	8	8	—	9	5	54–59
5	5	164	8	11	—	9	8	56–61
5	6	165	9	0	—	9	11	57–62
5	7	168	9	3	—	10	0	50–64
5	8	170	9	7	—	10	3	60–65
5	9	173	9	10	—	10	6	62–66
5	10	175	9	13	—	10	9	63–68
5	11	178	10	2	—	10	12	64–69

[a] This weight range is for medium to large frames, as judged by shoe size. For small frames deduct 5–7 lb (2–3 kg) from medium weight. However, it is important to realise this is only a general guide which does not cater for specific individual factors.

Table 8.4 Anthropometric measurements in later life

Method of measurement	*Standard measurement*		*Usual range for older people*	
	Male	*Female*	*Male*	*Female*
Triceps skinfold thickness Measured over loosely hanging, non-dominant arm, by standard millimetre skinfold calipers, approx 1½ cm above mid-arm point. Gently lift skinfold and maintaining grasp read to nearest millimetre 2–3 seconds after releasing caliper extender. Usual to take average of 3 such readings. This estimates subcutaneous fat reserves.	12.5 mm	16.5 mm	7.4–11.5 mm	9.9–13.6 mm
Mid-arm circumference Measured at point midway between acromial process of scapula and olecranon process of elbow, on posterior aspect of arm. Use a non-stretchable tape; bend elbow to 90°; palm upwards. Read to nearest fraction of a centimetre, using no force. This estimates skeletal muscle mass (protein portion). Sometimes the mid-upper arm muscle circumference is measured as well or the subscapula skinfold.	29.3 cm	28.5 cm	17.4–26.3 cm	17–25.8 cm

Drawn from data from (i) Jellife D B 1966 The assessment of the nutritional status of the community. WHO, Geneva (ii) (ii) Ebersole P, Hess P 1985 Towards healthy ageing. Mosby, St Louis

Dietary assessment

For comprehensive dietary assessment the most systematic approach is to obtain a 7-day diary of what is eaten, when, where and how. It involves client willingness and active participation and can provide a basis for subsequent dietetic therapy. *However, it does not reveal why older people eat as they do, and these motivations are all-important.*

Where assessment reveals need for help with meals, efforts should be directed towards encouraging attendance at luncheon clubs, even if transport is required to get there. This is preferred to meals-on-wheels at home, since it caters for social contact and exercise as well as nutritional complementation. However, meals-on-wheels may of course be the only solution for some very frail, sick and housebound elderly people. It is necessary for those providing such a service to be well versed in nutrition education, and health visitors may find they are asked to participate in the in-service preparation of workers.

Nutrition education

Some may question if it is desirable or possible to attempt nutrition education with older people. However, Davies & Holdsworth (1982) and Holdsworth & Davies (1982) have shown from their research that profitable change *can* be brought about. This is supported by later work, including Davies & Stewart (1987).

For this reason health visitors should exploit

every opportunity afforded them to stress good dietary intake, suitable cooking and hygienic storage procedures. This is especially important when checking that those caring for older people are fully conversant with their nutritional requirements.

ORAL HEALTH PROMOTION

Fundamental to healthy nutrition and digestion, as well as to communication, socialising, the maintenance of self-esteem and general well-being, is oral health. It concerns the entire buccal cavity, teeth, lips, gums, tongue, salivary glands and mucous membranes. However, it is often a neglected basic need in later life.

Tooth loss is not entirely related to the ageing process, although age changes do occur (see Ch. 2). There is a tendency for teeth to become darker in colour, brittle, drier, worn down and uneven. Similarly, loss of tissue elasticity, atrophy of alveolar bone, decreased vascularity of gingivae and greater friability of buccal mucosa can lead to gum recession, periodental disorders and mouth ulcers. Many of the problems seen among older people represent an accumulation of faulty oral practices over many years. Hence oral health promotion for elderly people begins in utero and continues throughout life.

Where older people have preserved their own teeth they should be encouraged to conscientiously continue with regular oral hygiene and dental checks. Brushing correctly after meals, and using dental floss or toothpicks to remove the food debris that collects round teeth and soft tissue, should be followed by thorough rinsing. A soft, round-bristled tooth brush minimises the risk of gum trauma. Where there is difficulty with dexterity, some older people find it helpful to use a child's-size tooth brush. Alternatively one may try glueing a small soft rubber ball or handle-grip to an ordinary-size brush. Flossing should always include movements below the gum line for full efficiency.

Where it does not elicit a gag reflex the surface of the tongue should also be brushed. The type of dentifrice used is not important, but disclosing tablets or fluid are often helpful in demonstrating to older people or their carers whether plaque has been removed. Oral hydration is, of course, extremely important as part of dental health promotion.

Many older people are currently edentulous. Whenever possible they should have an oral assessment and be fitted correctly with dentures, for both masticatory, digestive, cosmetic and psychosocial reasons. Communication and articulation are always important, but never more so than in later life.

The same fastidious attention to hygiene that pertains to older persons with their own teeth, applies to those with dentures. These should be cleaned after each meal, and on any removal, using warm water and an appropriate denture cream. Regular re-appraisal is necessary to ensure correct adjustments, and it is wise to mark dentures on their under surface, indelibly, so that, should older clients be subsequently admitted to hospital or residential care, their dentures can be easily identified. The importance of oral care to the well-being of older people should be impressed on all caregivers, as it is an aspect which can be so easily overlooked (Ebersole & Hess 1985).

PROMOTING SAFETY

Safety education is an integral part of health promotion at any age, but its significance for older persons is highlighted in their mortality and morbidity statistics, which show accidents in the home to be a major factor (see Table 8.5 and Table 8.6).

Although the total number of accidental deaths for 1987, for all causes, was reduced by 7% over the previous year, and accidental deaths in the home, or residential accommodation, fell over 20% in the decade 1977–87, home accidents still accounted for *38% of all deaths*. Care must be taken in comparing and interpreting statistics which have been collected for different purposes, and hence use different bases. Nevertheless accidents constitute a serious concern among the very young and elderly people. Not unexpectedly, fatal cases prevail in those aged 75 years or more. The higher number of female deaths possibly reflects their greater longevity.

Table 8.5 Number and type of fatal and non-fatal accidents among persons aged 65 years or more occurring in the United Kingdom, 1985

FATAL

Fatal accidents in the home[a], UK 1985:

Accident type	*65–74* M	F	*75+* M	F	*Total*
Falls	201	257	661	1921	3040
Poisoning (inhalation & ingestion)	20	27	25	42	114
Burns (contact burns and scalds)	7	9	29	48	93
Burns (uncontrolled fire)	63	50	91	161	365
Cutting/piercing	1	1	0	2	4
Struck by object/person	2	3	9	8	22
Foreign body (mainly choking)	47	30	24	65	166
Electricity	2	1	1	0	4
Drowning	1	6	5	10	22
Other	10	8	6	22	46
Unknown	1	2	5	24	32
Total	355	394	856	2303	3908

[a] incl. residential institutions

NON-FATAL

Estimated annual numbers of non-fatal accidents in the home involving people aged 65+ in the UK

			Rate per 1000 Population 65+
Males	75 000	27%	21
Females	202 000	73%	38
Total	276 000	100%	31

Accident type	*Estimated frequency*	
Falls	180 000	65%
Cutting/piercing	28 000	10%
Struck by object person	25 000	9%
Burns	8 000	3%
Foreign body	5 000	2%
Other	8 000	3%
Unknown	21 000	8%
Total	276 000	100%

(Note: columns may not add exactly to the totals due to effects of rounding.)

Based on latest available figures at time of going to press from The Royal Society for the Prevention of Accidents.

Road traffic accidents

The rate for road users aged 60 years or upwards, killed or seriously injured, currently stands at 0.7 per 1000 (CSO 1989). This compares with 1.3 per 1000 over all ages, and 3.5 per 1000 for those aged 15–19 years. However, while older people constitute a reasonably safe group of motorists, slowed reaction times and sensory deficits do render them vulnerable to road traffic accidents, especially as cyclists or pedestrians. It is important for health visitors to reinforce the Highway Code, and to encourage older persons to wear light-coloured and/or protective clothing, especially at night.

Home accidents

Most home accidents are a combination of human error and environmental faults, but human frailty assumes even greater significance in later years. As both Tables 8.5 and 8.6 show, falls are by far the most frequent type of accident. They also account for most fatalities. Sex and advancing age appear to be significant factors, females being most at risk. However, this disparity is less marked in the highest age group.

In two community surveys of falls, tripping appeared to account for 50% of all causes, while 'dizziness', 'blackouts', or 'legs giving way' each accounted for approximately 7% of cases. In almost 20% of instances the elderly individuals were unable to offer explanations for their fall (Prudham & Evans 1981, Blake et al 1988).

Health visitors are, of course, aware of the different pathological causes of instability in older people. They are therefore particularly likely to counsel those in whom predisposing factors occur, especially those suffering from visual deficits, vertigo, basilar artery insufficiency, or proneness to postural hypotension.

Mobility is significantly impaired in those reporting falls, so sufferers from arthritis, neurological conditions, peripheral vascular disorders or the sequelae of 'strokes' are at particular risk. The side effects of certain drugs can also impair mobility. A significant association between falls and the use of hypnotics and antidepressants (though not antihypertensives or tranquilisers) was demonstrated by Blake et al (1988). Hence polypharmacy potentiates risk.

Discriminant analysis of selected medical and anthropometric variables indicated that poor handgrip strength in the dominant hand was predictive of falling, as was reported arthritis, giddiness or foot difficulty — points health visitors will wish to

Table 8.6 Number of home accidents treated in hospital in England and Wales, by age and sex, for 1987

	Age group										
	Males					*Females*					
	0–4	5–14	15–64	65–74	75 or over	0–4	5–14	15–64	65–74	75 or over	*All persons*
Type of accident (%)											
Falls	49.2	37.7	22.6	40.2	67.9	47.5	42.1	33.9	59.9	75.8	39.3
Cutting/piercing	6.1	16.2	30.0	25.7	8.7	5.2	12.2	21.0	11.9	4.1	17.2
Struck by object/person[a]	17.4	26.7	20.7	13.7	6.8	16.0	24.9	20.1	11.4	6.7	18.9
Burning	6.5	2.9	3.5	3.5	3.6	6.3	3.4	4.8	3.2	2.1	4.4
Foreign body	5.5	4.6	5.9	4.5	2.0	7.1	4.1	3.5	1.6	0.9	4.6
Poisoning	6.8	0.7	0.2	0.2	0.0	7.8	0.9	0.2	0.2	0.1	1.9
Over exertion	0.7	0.6	1.8	1.4	0.8	1.7	0.7	1.4	0.6	0.3	1.2
Other/unknown	7.7	10.8	15.4	10.8	10.2	8.2	11.7	15.2	11.3	10.0	12.6
Sample size (= 100%) (numbers)	14 015	8 686	25 863	1 988	1 659	10 877	7 019	26 752	3 546	6 177	107 253[b]

[a] Also falling object. [b] Includes 671 cases where age was unknown.
Source: Home Accident Surveillance System 1987, Consumer Safety Unit, Department of Trade and Industry
Based on data From CSO 1989 Social Trends No 19. HMSO, London. Crown Copyright.

note. Falls occur most frequently on steps, stairs and in living rooms. Attending to micturition at night appears a particular hazard.

Implications for health promotion

The primary health promotion aim is to encourage a combination of hazard-free surroundings and safe personal habits. Within the group context older persons should be encouraged to conduct comprehensive assessment of potential home and garden hazards, while they are active enough to remedy these.

Any necessary repositioning of shelves, window catches, door bolts or letter boxes should be carried out as soon after the event of retirement as possible. Waist-level shelves for milk deliveries are considered a good idea, avoiding the risk of sudden dizziness from stooping. 'Do-it-yourself' enthusiasts should make sure they are properly equipped. Regular visual checks should be encouraged and deficits in vision and hearing promptly corrected, since these are important risk factors for imbalance (Gerson at al 1989). Older persons and their carers should be reminded of the importance of good lighting, as life-long habits of frugality can cause them to economise by using low-wattage bulbs.

The use of walking aids and other safety equipment

Although some older people scorn the use of walking sticks, a stout umbrella or shooting stick can prove very useful. Gray & MacKenzie (1980) give a number of helpful tips about walking aids, including the use of a stick-strap to facilitate movement.

Bath aids, safety rails, firm banisters and raised toilet seats are among the many other devices for aiding safety. Some older people may prefer to come down stairs backwards; but whichever mode they choose, older clients should always check the number of steps and take special care when wearing bi-focal spectacles.

'Sway' is considered to be a contributory factor in falls among older females, so education about gait could be helpful (Mitchell 1984) (see also Ch. 2, p. 34).

The prevention of osteoporosis

The increase in fall frequency in later life is related to the number of fractures, especially fracture of the femur (Boyce & Vessey 1985). Osteoporosis and osteomalacia are indicted as causes. Prevention through adequate exercise has already been stressed. Other measures, such as avoidance or cessation of cigarette smoking, are recommended (Mellström 1982, WHO 1982). The use of calcium supplements is still regarded as debatable (Smith 1987). The evidence that oestrogens prevent bone loss, and thus reduce the fracture rate in post-menopausal women, is substantial (Riggs & Melton 1988). This has led many to advocate Hormone Replacement Therapy, especially for all premature, artificially-induced cases of menopause and those deemed 'at risk' of osteoporosis. A combination of oestrogen and sequential progestogen appears the preferred choice, although this too carries some risk of adverse effects. Fluoride is a further choice of preventive treatment. These drug approaches require medical decisions and mass screening for bone mass is not at present suggested. However, it has been recommended that those women who are below 65 years of age, who sustain a fracture in the hip or forearm, should receive hormone replacement therapy (Drugs and Therapeutic Bulletin 1989).

Action in the case of falls

Preparing for action in the unfortunate case of falls is another essential part of health promotion and safety education. Older people should be taught mat exercises, and shown how to rise if uninjured. They should be encouraged to work out a suitable alarm system beforehand, so that they can readily summon help in case of emergency. The danger of hypothermia following a fall should be explained and individuals encouraged to have safe, adequate house heating during the night in cold weather.

Where older group members have conditions which threaten consciousness, are taking specific drugs, or have known allergic responses, they should be recommended to wear a medic-alert bracelet, or to carry a card clearly stating the relevant information, to alert others.

Fire safety

It is always wise to reinforce teaching about fire hazards, especially if such dangers have been noted during home visiting. Safety suggestions include keeping fire-smothering blankets handy and positioning pan handles carefully, as well as taking care when using frying-pans, tea towels or oven-gloves.

Fireguards often become 'bones of contention', but they should be fitted. Older people who feel cold should be advised to use a light blanket over their legs when sitting close to the fire. All electrical wiring and appliances should be regularly checked. This can be difficult when older home-owners have limited income. Grants may sometimes be obtained from voluntary agencies to assist such replacements.

Particular attention should be paid to the fitting of smoke detectors, especially where older people are smokers, or where they tend to be forgetful and leave saucepans on stoves until they boil dry. Some advisors recommend the use of microwave ovens, to reduce this risk, but they have other disadvantages for older people unless their use is well understood.

Additional safety measures

All the important aspects of poisoning risks, which apply generally, also apply to older people. However, their higher incidence of sensory deficits, and increased use of drugs and medicines, renders them at greater risk of poisoning accidents. It is advisable to devise ways with the older client of checking whether medicines have been taken or not.

Protection against criminal damage and violence is also necessary. Older people have been shown to have marked psychological reactions to burglarly and physical assault. Clients should be advised about suitable security measures, such as door locks and window bolts, and should be cautioned not to admit unauthorised persons into their premises. They should not entertain persons who cannot produce accredited evidence of identity, and where possible should make a telephone check if in doubt.

Pocket alarms are helpful, if kept in good working order. Nevertheless it is important not to generate unnecessary fear in older people, so that their confidence is undermined and they become over-suspicious, or obsessive about security to the detriment of their safety or quality of life.

Further information on promoting safety, especially within the home, can be obtained from The Royal Society for the Prevention of Accidents (see Appendix 7).

Health promotion through prophylaxis

Vaccination and immunisation

Forming part of group activities within health promotion initiatives with older people, are several prophylactic measures. Since infections can create considerable morbidity, general information concerning personal and household hygiene and ways of raising resistance is frequently welcome. Immunisation, too, has a place in the care of older clients. Vaccination against known influenzal viruses should be offered, particularly to the more vulnerable elderly. Injections are best given in early autumn, and they must be repeated annually.

Active immunisation against tetanus should be regularly maintained (5-yearly intervals), especially as many older persons enjoy gardening and horticulture. For those holidaying abroad the usual recommended vaccinations against enteric disease apply, as does malarial prophylaxis.

Where older people are contemplating long-distance journeys by air, it is wise for them to check with their doctor that there are no contraindications. Those suffering from respiratory disorder may experience oxygen deficit at certain altitudes and so may need to ascertain whether their intended destinations are suitable for them.

Those suffering from circulatory disorders are often advised to arrange 'stop-overs' when travelling very long distances. To prevent undue 'pooling' and venous stasis, all older people should be advised to exercise their feet and legs during flights. Not only should they stretch their limbs and walk about the aircraft, but they should 'walk' for approximately 10 minutes in every hour while sitting still! This heel-to-toe mechanism activates the calf-muscle pump, so reducing the risk of oedema and thrombosis.

Promoting healthy stress management

Group techniques for the management of undue stress complement those available to individuals and provide useful items in the health promotion 'armoury'.

Older people have had long experience in learning to cope with life-events, but sometimes stress over prolonged periods can deplete adaptive capacity. This can then lead older persons into problems of maintaining homeostasis. The importance of stress as a direct or indirect cause of lowered levels of well-being was recognised by Selye (1976). Stress inventories were developed by Holmes & Rahe (1967) and Travis (1977). Though useful, they provide only generalised guidance and take little account of the wide range of individual differences found among older people.

Various techniques exist for reducing undue tension. One is to ensure healthy and restful sleep, since this is needed to provide organ respite, and to enable individuals to recover from fatigue and so restore energy.

The quality of sleep appears to reduce with advancing age; it appears more fragmented and is often a matter of concern. Health visitors will likely be familiar with the research on sleep (Morgan 1987). They appreciate that sleep consists of both orthodox and paradoxical type sleep. Orthodox sleep has four levels of deepening intensity, stage 4 being the most restorative physiological level. Dreaming is not generally a feature of this type.

Paradoxical sleep, however, is a very active phase, characterised by rapid eye movements and frequent, often vivid, dreams. This stage of sleep is considered crucial to mental and emotional balance, since much emotional material is discharged.

Although little is known about the effects of ageing on biorhythms, it is known that older persons tend to have less stage 4 orthodox sleep, and that they frequently pass direct from stage 2 to paradoxical sleep. Because they are in a lighter level of sleep when this happens, they tend to wake more easily, often before they have derived benefit from paradoxical sleep. Consequently they may be lethargic, complain of general malaise, and lack of 'refreshment' in sleep. Sleep patterns can be further disturbed when paradoxical sleep is affected by the administration of sedatives and/or hypnotics, or by repeated wakening. The latter may be due to excessive noise, nocturia, leg cramps, hunger or anxiety. Promoting healthier sleep means dealing with the underlying causes whenever possible. Simple measures which can be taught to older clients and their carers include:

- attention to bed-time rituals, to adequate warmth, quiet and ventilation
- the use of soothing measures, such as tapes, to induce sleep
- adequate mental and physical stimulation during the day, followed by a 'wind down' period prior to preparing for bed
- foot massage, which may have a soporific effect for some people
- the provision of beverages which contain the precursors of serotonin
- warm baths before retiring, which help some older people (but others find them stimulating).

Sleep apnoea may be increased in later life. If suspected it should always be investigated.

Relaxation techniques

Group relaxation activities can also help older people to reduce the effects of stress. One may use well-established approaches, such as The Alexander System, or simple muscle relaxation therapy, whereby group members are talked progressively through the relaxation of muscles beginning from the head and neck. This is usually accompanied by deep breathing exercises; it takes about 15–20 minutes to complete, and usually leaves members refreshed. Series of suitable exercises can be obtained from organisations such as Relaxation for Living, or from texts such as Pelletier (1983) and Doty (1987).

Biofeedback

Biofeedback is a method for controlling the autonomic nervous system. In this form of stress management, older group members are taught, through the use of small machines, to appreciate body–mind connectedness. Responses can then be controlled to lower blood pressure, reduce heart rate and relax muscle tension. Once learned the skills can be transferred to other stressful situations.

Autogenic training is a simpler method without using machines. Older persons can be taught to recognise the effects of stress, by recording their normal pulse rate and then monitoring the changes brought about when they encounter, or think about, highly stressful situations. Responses can then be controlled, through relaxation and breathing exercises. It has been successfully used to reduce pain, improve sleep, reduce tension, or control conditions such as irritable bowel syndrome, asthma or cardiac arrhythmias (Tennant 1981, Ebersole & Hess 1985).

Meditation

Meditation is another topic older people sometimes like to discuss. The techniques have been practised for many years and range from the Christian 'quiet time' through to transcendental meditation, which has gained recent popularity. Those who practise any form regularly for 15–20 minutes daily, have been shown to have reduced stress levels and lower levels of illness (Goleman 1976, Dytchwald 1983, Nash 1988).

Visualisation

Sometimes termed 'guided affective imagery', visualisation is a positive technique used as a form of self-healing through the ages. It has known a recent resurgence, being used both to control stress and as an adjunct therapy in treating various conditions, including cancer. Its use in group sessions, as well as with individuals, can aid relaxation and promote well-being (Samuels & Samuels 1975, Gollop 1983, Passant 1990). The use of therapeutic touch can also aid stress management in older people and is advocated by Smith (1990) and Sagar (1990).

Assertion education and self-advocacy

Empowering older people within the context of health promotion often involves improving their communication and self-presenting skills. Educating them in assertiveness and assisting them to present their aspirations and needs clearly is therefore pertinent. Exercises designed to effect these changes are given by Doty (1987) and are recommended to those wishing to develop this role with their older clients.

SUMMARY

This chapter has ranged through the principles affecting group health promotion in later life, and the factors to be considered when working with groups. It has briefly examined the impact of group dynamics on older adult learning and has explored social theory, self-efficacy and the health belief model in relation to health promotion strategies. The relevance of the health locus of control has also been considered, together with some of the implications for practice. In moving to look at some priority areas for health promotion in later life, attention has focused particularly on carers of older people in their crucial role. Topics of high concern for older adults have been identified and certain techniques suggested for dealing with these.

Health promotion in later maturity has thus been seen to be a dynamic and complex activity, presenting practitioners with great opportunity for satisfaction and feedback.

REFERENCES

Arber S, Gilbert G N, Evandrou M 1988 Gender, household composition, and receipt of domiciliary services by elderly disabled people. Journal of Social Policy 17(2): 153–175

Balter D, Daniels F, Finch J, Perkins E 1986 Training health visitors to work with community groups. University of Nottingham, Dept of Adult Education and Bassetlaw Health Education Unit, Nottingham

Bandura A 1977a Social Learning Theory. Prentice Hall, Englewood Cliffs, New Jersey

Bandura A 1977b Self-efficacy: towards a unifying theory of social change. Prentice Hall, Englewood Cliffs, New Jersey

Bandura A 1986 Social foundations of thought and action. Prentice Hall, Englewood Cliffs, New Jersey

Barr C et al 1985 The relationship of physical activity and exercise to mental health. Public Health Reports 100 (2): 195–202

Beaver M L 1983 Human services practice with the elderly. Prentice Hall, Englewood Cliffs, New Jersey

Becker M H (ed) 1974 The health belief model and personal health behaviour. Health Education Monograph 2: 336–353

Best J A 1975 Tailoring smoking withdrawal procedures to personality, and motivational differences. Journal of Consulting and Clinical Psychology 43: 1–8

Best J A, Steffy R A 1975 Smoking modification procedures for internal and external locus of control clients. Canadian Journal of Behavioural Science 7: 155–165

Bion W R 1968 Experiences in groups, and other papers. Tavistock Publications, London

Blake A J, Morgan K, Bendall M J, Dallosso H, Ebrahmim S B J, Arie T H D, Fentem P H, Bassey E J 1988 Falls by elderly people at home: prevalence and associated factors. Age and Ageing 17: 365–372

Blythway W R 1987 Informal care systems. An exploratory study of older steel workers in South Wales. Report to Joseph Rowntree Memorial Trust, University College of Swansea.

Bortz W 1982 Disuse and aging. Journal of the American Medical Association 248 (10): 1203–1208

Boyce W J, Vessey P M 1985 Rising incidence of fracture of the proximal femur. Lancet i: 150–151

Briggs A, Oliver J 1985 Caring: experiences of looking after disabled relatives. Routledge and Kegan Paul, London

Brown R 1988 Group processes: dynamics within and between groups. Basil Blackwell, Oxford

Burnside I 1983 Working with the elderly: group processes and techniques, 2nd edn. Duxbury Press, North Scituate, Massachusetts

Cartwright A, Henderson G 1986 More trouble with feet: a survey of the foot problems and chiropody needs of the elderly. DHSS, HMSO, London

Cartwright D, Zander A 1968 Group dynamics and theory, 3rd edn. Rome, Evanston, Illinois

Chamberlain J 1973 Validation of screening tests for unreported disability in the elderly. Unpublished research report. DHSS, London. Cited in Cartwright A, Henderson G 1986 op cit

Charlesworth A, Wilkin D, Durie A 1984 Carers and services: a comparison of men and women caring for dependent elderly people. Equal Opportunities Commission, Manchester

Ciba Foundation Symposium 134 1988 (Everard D, Whelan J eds) Research and the ageing population. Wiley, Chichester

COMA (Committee on Medical Aspects of Food Policy) 1984 Report of the Panel on diet in relation to cardio-vascular disease. Report on Health and Social Subjects 28. HMSO, London

Cornett S, Watson J 1984 Cardiac rehabilitation: an interdisciplinary team approach. Wiley, New York

Cotton E, Sharp G 1989 Rochdale Carers' Support Groups. Personal communication

CSO (Central Statistical Office) 1989 Social Trends No 19. HMSO, London

Dabbs J M, Kirshott J P 1971 Internal control and the taking of influenza shots. Psychological Reports 28: 959–962

Davies L 1981 Three score years and then? Heinemann, London

Davies L, Holdsworth D 1982 Pre-retirement education in a longitudinal survey, through periods of pre and post retirement. Gerontology Nutrition Unit, Queen Elizabeth College, London
Davies S, Stewart A 1987 Nutritional medicine. Pan Books, London
deVries H A 1975 Physiology of exercise and ageing. In: Woodruff D S, Birren J E (eds) Aging: scientific perspectives and social issues. Van Nostrand Reinhold, New York
DHSS (Department of Health and Social Security) 1979a Nutrition and health in old age. Reports on health and social subjects, No 16. HMSO, London
DHSS (Department of Health and Social Security) 1979b Recommended daily amounts of food, energy and nutrients, for groups of older people in the United Kingdom. Reports on health and social subjects, No 15. HMSO, London
DHSS (Department of Health and Social Security) 1984 Supporting the informal carers: fifty styles of caring. Social work service development group project. DHSS, London
Disability Alliance (ERA) 1989 Disability rights handbook, 14th edn (April). Disability Alliance (ERA), London
Doty L 1987 Communication and assertion skills for older persons. Hemisphere Publishing Corporation, Washington
Drennan V 1988a Health visitors and groups. Heinemann, London
Drennan V 1988b Celebrating age. Community Outlook (June)
Drugs and Therapeutic Bulletin 1989 (9th January). A 'Which' publication, Consumers' Association, Hertford
DSS (Department of Social Security) 1989 Caring for people: community Care in the next decade and beyond. Government White Paper, November. HMSO, London
Dytchwald K 1983 Overview: health promotion and disease prevention for elders. Generations 7: 5
Ebersole P, Hess P 1985 Towards healthier ageing, 2nd edn. Mosby, St Louis
Evans M 1990 Complementary therapies: reflex zone therapy for mothers. Nursing Times 86 (4) (24th January): 29–31
Everard D, Whelan J (eds) 1985 The value of preventive medicine: Ciba Foundation Symposium No 110. Pitman Medical, London
Gerson L W, Jarjoura D, McCord G 1989 Risk of imbalance in elderly people with impaired hearing or vision. Age and Ageing 18: 31–34
Getchell B, Anderson W 1982 Being fit: a personal guide. John Wiley, New York
Goleman D 1976 Meditation helps break the stress spiral. Psychology Today 9 (September): 82
Gollop S 1983 Pain and pain control. In: Wilson-Barnett J (ed) Recent advances in nursing series, No 6. Churchill Livingstone, Edinburgh
Graham M 1988 Keep moving, keep young: gentle yoga exercises for the elderly. Unwin Hyman, London
Gray M, MacKenzie H 1980 Take care of your elderly relative. Allen and Unwin, London
Gray Muir J A 1986 Prevention of disease in the elderly. Churchill Livingstone, Edinburgh
Gray Muir J A 1987 Physical fitness: the key to good health. Geriatric Medicine (June): 35–39
Green L W, Levine D M, Deeds S G 1975 Clinical trials of health education for hypertensive outpatients: design and base-line data. Preventive Medicine 4: 417–425
Groves D, Finch J (eds) 1983 A labour of love: women, work and caring. Routledge and Kegan Paul, London
Hicks C 1988 Who cares: looking after people at home. Virago Press, London
Holdsworth D, Davies L 1982 Nutrition education for the elderly. Human Nutrition, Applied Nutrition 36: 22–27
Holmes T, Rahe E 1967 The social readjustment rating scale. Journal of Psychosomatic Research 11: 213
Janz N K, Becker M H 1984 The health belief model, a decade later. Health Education Quarterly 11: 1–47
Jones C 1989 Personal communication
Jones D, Victor C, Vetter N 1983 Carers of the elderly in the community. Journal of the Royal College of General Practitioners 33: 707–710
King J 1984 The Health Belief Model. Nursing Times (24th Oct): 53–55
King's Fund 1989 A new deal for Carers. King's Fund Centre, London
Langlie J K 1977 Social networks, health beliefs and preventive health behaviour. Journal of Health and Social Behaviour 18: 244–260
Larson E B, Bruce R A 1987 Health benefits of exercise in an ageing society. Archives of Internal Medicine 147: 353–356
Litwack L, Litwack J, Ballou M 1980 Health counselling. Appleton-Century-Crofts, New York
Luker K A, Perkins E S 1987 The elderly at home: service needs and provisions. Journal of the Royal College of General Practitioners 37 (June): 248–250
MacHeath J 1984 Activity, health and fitness in old age. Croom Helm, London
Maiman L A, Backer M H 1974 The health belief model: origin and correlates in psychological theory. Health Education Monographs 2: 336–353
Marsiglio A, Holm K 1988 Physical conditioning in the aging adult. Nurse Practitioner (Sept): 33–41
Mellström D 1982 Tobacco smoking, ageing and health among the elderly. Age and Ageing 11: 45
Miller J, Solomon R 1979 The development of group services for the elderly. Columbia University Press, New York
Mitchell R G 1984 Falls in the elderly. Nursing Times (11th Jan): 51–53
Morgan K 1987 Sleep and ageing. Croom Helm, London
NACNE (National Advisory Committee on Nutrition) 1983 Proposals for nutritional guidelines for health education in Britain. Health Education Council, London
Nash W 1988 At ease with stress: the approach of wholeness. Darton, Longman, Todd, London
OPCS Office of Population, Censuses and Surveys 1988 Informal Carers. Report on a General Household Survey 1985 (GHS No 15), Supplement A (Green H). HMSO, London
Orr J 1985 The community dimension. In: Luker K A, Orr J (eds) Health visiting. Blackwell Scientific Publications, Oxford
Passant H 1990 A holistic approach in the ward: complementary therapies in the care of the elderly. Nursing Times 86 (4) (24th Jan): 26–28
Pelletier K 1983 Stress management: an approach to optimum health and longevity. Generations 7: 16

Phares E J 1976 Locus of control in personality. General Learning Press, Morristown
Prudham D, Grimley-Evans J 1981 Factors associated with falls in the elderly. Age and ageing 10: 141–6
Riggs B L, Melton L J 1988 Osteoporosis and age-related fracture syndromes. In: Everard D, Whelan J (eds) Ciba Foundation Symposium No 134: Research and the ageing population. Wiley, Chichester
Rochdale Carers Support Group 1988 Your lifeline to caring. Rochdale DHA/LASS Department: Community Health Education, Baillie Street, Rochdale
Rosenstock I M 1966 Why people use health services. Millbank Memorial Fund Quarterly 44: 94–124
Rosenstock I M 1974 Historical origins of the health belief model. Health Education Monographs 2: 328–335
Rosenstock I M, Strecher V J, Becker M H 1988 Social Learning Theory and the Health Belief Model. Health Education Quarterly 15 (2) (Summer): 175–183
Rotter J B 1954 Social learning and clinical psychology. Prentice Hall, New York
Rotter J B 1966 Generalized expectancies for internal versus external control of reinforcement. Psychological Monographs 80 (1)
Sagar E 1990 Therapeutic touch — a healing meditation. Nursing Practice 3 (2): 12–17
Sager K 1984 Exercises to activate seniors. The Physician and Sports Medicine 5: 144–151
Samuels M, Samuels N 1975 Seeing with the mind's eye. Random House, New York
Schunk D H, Carbonani J P 1984 Self-efficacy models. In: Matarazzo J D, Weiss S M, Herd J A, Miller N E, Weiss S M (eds) Behavioural health. Wiley, New York
Seeman M, Seeman T E 1983 Health behaviour and personal autonomy: a longitudinal study of the sense of control in illness. Journal of Health and Social Behaviour 24: 144–160
Selye H 1976 The stress of life (revised edn). McGraw Hill, New York
Shaw E E 1971 Group dynamics: the psychology of small group behaviour. McGraw Hill series in psychology. McGraw Hill, London
Sidney K, Shepherd R 1977 Maximal and submaximal exercise tests, in men and women in the seventh, eighth and ninth decades of life. Journal of Applied Physiology 43: 280–287
Siegrist J 1988 Models of health behaviour. European Heart Journal 9: 709–714
Smith A, Jacobson B (eds) 1988 The Nation's health: a strategy for the 1990s. A Report from an independent multi-disciplinary committee. King Edward's Hospital Fund for London, London
Smith E, Gilligan C 1983 Physical activity prescription for the older adult. The Physician and Sports Medicine 8: 9–10
Smith E, Serfass R (eds) 1981 Exercise and ageing: the scientific basis. Enslow Publishing, New York
Smith M 1990 Healing through touch. Nursing Times 86 (4) (24th January): 31–32
Smith P B 1980 Group processes and personality. Harper and Row, London
Smith R 1987 Osteoporosis: cause and management. British Medical Journal 294 (7th February): 329–332
Speake D L 1987 Health promotion activity in the well elderly. Health Values 11 (6) (Nov–Dec): 25–37
Strecher V J, DeVellis B M, Becker M H, Rosenstock I B 1986 The role of self-efficacy in achieving health behaviour change. Health Education Quarterly 13: 73–92
Svedin A M, Goroch-Tomlinson D 1984 They said we didn't exist! Social Work Today (2nd April): 14–15
Tennant R 1981 Identity awareness as a holistic approach to self-healing. Geriatric Nursing 2: 355
Tobias L L, MacDonald M L 1977 Internal Locus of Control and weight loss: an insufficient condition. Journal of Consulting Psychology 45: 647–653
Travis J W 1977 Wellness workbook for health professionals: a guide to attaining high level wellness. Wellness Resource Centre, Mill Valley, California
Ungerson C 1987 Policy is personal: a study in caring. Tavistock Publications, London
Wallston B S, Wallston K A 1978a Locus of control and health: a review of the literature. Health Education Monographs (Spring): 107–117
Wallston B S, Wallston K A, Kaplan G D, Maides S A 1976b Development and validation of the locus of control (HLC) Scale. J Consult Clin Psychol 44: 580–585
Wallston K A, Maides S, Wallston B S 1976a Health-related information seeking, as a function of health related Locus of Control and health values. Journal Res. Pers. 10: 215–222
Wallston K A, Wallston B S, DeVellis R 1978b Development of the multi-dimensional Health Locus of Control Scales. Health Education Monographs 6 (2): 160–171
Webster J A 1988 Key to healthy ageing: exercise. Journal of Gerontological Nursing 14 (12): 8–15
Weir F 1987 The Rochdale Carers' Charter. National Council for Carers and their Elderly Dependants, Rochdale
Wells N, Freer C (eds) 1988 The ageing population: burden or challenge? M Stockton Press, New York
Wenlock R W, Boss D H, Ageter L B 1984 New estimates of fibre in the diet in Britain. British Medical Journal 288: 1873
World Health Organization 1982 Epidemiological studies on social and medical conditions of the elderly. Euro Reports and Studies No 62. WHO, Copenhagen
Wright L 1986 Left alone to care. Gower, London

CHAPTER CONTENTS

9

Illness in old age

While undoubtedly the primary role of the health visitor is prevention of ill health, it is obvious that, in her work with old people, she will have to advise, manage or contain some situations which have gone beyond the tertiary preventive stage. Her role will become that of detector, carer, coordinator or even trouble shooter. It is therefore appropriate for Health Visitors to know both the ways in which illness in old people differs from that in younger people and to appreciate the causes and management of common medical problems in elderly people.

HOW ILLNESS DIFFERS BETWEEN YOUNG AND OLD

CASE STUDY

Mr P was an 80-year-old widower who lived alone. Gradually he did less and less for himself and eventually the house and garden became neglected. His appetite and weight deteriorated, his memory became blunted and he lost confidence in his ability to be self-caring. Depression set in. Arrangements were madé for him to have a home help, meals-on-wheels and a District Nurse. The opinion of a physician in geriatric medicine was sought when Mr P became virtually immobile and incontinent. Examination and investigation showed that the patient had Parkinsonism, myxoedema and osteoarthritis as well as suffering from polypharmacy.

He made a good recovery following physiotherapy and modification of his drug treatment. Later he had a successful home visit and returned to his home mobile and self-caring. Although no social services were required, the Health Visitor was asked to monitor progress.

Illness in the young often presents rapidly, the history is easy to obtain and symptoms frequently point to disease in one body system. However, the elderly, especially those over 75 years, often have multiple system disease, disorders or disabilities; the history is often difficult to obtain, the signs and symptoms are altered and the presentation of the disease is frequently non-specific. Often they are prescribed a multitude of drugs which cause problems with compliance as well as adverse drug reactions. In addition, the isolated, housebound and elderly confused person can present major management problems in community care.

Multiple diseases

It is classical medical teaching that a patient's signs and symptoms should be integrated into one disease entity. This approach frequently fails in the old elderly (over 75 years) who often have multiple acute or chronic disorders, e.g. chest infection with heart failure superimposed on long-standing features of arthritis, obesity, diabetes, leg ulceration and a stroke. Unfortunately, the signs and symptoms of new disorders and diseases may be wrongly attributed to existing conditions, e.g. the aches and pains of osteomalacia be attributed to osteoarthritis.

The history

Although it may be difficult to elicit, an accurate history of events leading up to the illness is absolutely vital, since it can strongly influence both treatment and management. The health visitor can be of considerable help as she can pass on to the doctors useful information from neighbours, friends, relatives, social workers, home help or meals-on-wheels supervisors.

Much can be learned from careful observation when visiting an elderly person, especially someone who is confused. For example a well-kept room suggests the person has been well until recently, or equally, has had effective backup help. Conversely an untidy house with an accumulation of newspapers or unopened milkbottles, stale food or unwashed dishes, suggests a longer-standing functional inability, confusion or self-neglect. Malodour suggests lack of cleanliness or incontinence. The presence of walking aids, raised toilet seats or chairs, a bed downstairs, a key hanging on a string inside the front door are all suggestive of mobility problems.

Signs and symptoms

It is perhaps not so well recognised that the pain threshold rises with age. Elderly people with an acute myocardial infarction, a perforated peptic ulcer, or even a fractured neck of femur may not complain of pain.

Fever is less common in the elderly, and a patient's temperature often cannot be used to assess progress of an illness. Indeed a potentially febrile illness may be associated with hypothermia.

Presentation of disease

Symptoms in the young are usually obvious, discrete and point to a specific disease process. Symptoms in the elderly, on the other hand, are often non-specific, vague and ill-defined. Common presentations include toxic confusional state, failure to thrive, or 'he's gone off his feet, and taken to bed' or 'collapse'. Direct questioning may not clarify the issue, but the health visitor, by discreet and systematic observation, can often establish the diagnosis or which body system is involved.

Adverse drug reactions

The elderly have benefited considerably from the vast increase in the range of drugs available for prescription, although it is now well recognised that the incidence of adverse drug reactions increases with age. This is mainly due to altered pharmacodynamics and pharmacokinetics as well as multiple prescribing and the effects of illness rather than age per se (Denham 1990). Since adverse drug reactions are such a potent cause of illness, health visitors should be alert to ways of preventing this form of iatrogenic ill health.

The frail elderly at home

Quite often the physically and mentally frail wish

to remain at home although they find it hard to manage and may be unrealistic about their capabilities. The recent White Paper on Community Care (1990) specifically encourages local authorities' social service departments to help older people to stay at home by offering them packages of care tailored to their specific needs. Even so, this support may be insufficient. The health visitor therefore has a vital role in monitoring the situation, ensuring that all necessary help is provided and quality of life is maintained. Relatives and neighbours who act as carers must also be supported and crisis situations prevented (see Chs 8 and 10).

COMMON ILLNESSES IN ELDERLY PEOPLE

Confusional states

CASE STUDY

Mrs W was a confused 83-year-old lady who was brought to the casualty department by the police. She had been found wandering in the street at night dressed only in her night clothes. She was hypothermic and, because of confusion, was quite unable to give any account of herself or her illness. No relatives or friends came with her. Later it became clear that until recently she had been quite well and capable of looking after herself. It seemed probable that she was suffering from toxic confusional state.

Confusion in old people may be due to a toxic confusional state or dementia or a combination of both. It is absolutely essential to distinguish between the two conditions since a toxic state is potentially treatable and reversible, while a dementing illness is usually irreversible and presents more as a management problem. Unfortunately there is a very regrettable tendency to equate confusion in the elderly with dementia, which results in failure to search for a treatable cause. It is lamentable, too, that another potentially treatable condition — depression — is frequently 'a missed diagnosis' because it can present as pseudo-dementia (see Ch. 10, p. 252–253).

Toxic confusional state (acute brain failure)

The history of the illness enables a toxic confusional state to be fairly readily distinguished from dementia; in the former there is a short history of sudden onset of mental changes, while in the latter there is a long history with slow onset. Old people with a toxic state may show fluctuations in their mental state, sometimes appearing lucid, sometimes very confused. They may be restless, aggressive or sleepy, with reversal of night/day sleeping patterns, and may experience visual hallucinations. Sometimes the client is not as confused as relatives allege. This discrepancy may result from a change in the level of tolerance of the carer. The degree of confusion can be assessed by using a mental test questionnaire (see the appendix at end of the chapter).

There are many causes of a toxic confusional state, the most common being:

- infections
- drugs
- heart failure
- metabolic disturbance, e.g. diabetes
- change of environment
- (constipation)
- (bereavement).

The health visitor may be able to recognise some of these by using her eyes intelligently. An infection is perhaps the most common cause. A chest infection is suggested by rapid breathing, associated with a cough productive of infected sputum — chest pain may not be a feature. Urinary infections may be suggested by a smell and a history of frequency. Dysuria per se may not be a symptom. Cellulitis, particularly of the skin of the legs will be seen as a reddened, hot area, which may be associated with blistering as in heart failure, or with pre-existing varicose or traumatic ulcers. Drugs are all too frequently a cause of confusion or hallucination. There is evidence that the ageing brain becomes increasingly sensitive to the effects of drugs which act upon it — therefore the health visitor should look particularly for the evidence of use of hypnotics, sedatives, tranquillisers, antidepressants and antiparkinsonian drugs. The fact that the person has taken the drug for a long time does not necessarily exclude it from consideration. Heart failure is suggested in a person who is becoming increasingly short of breath on exertion, has swelling of the ankles and also is unable to lie flat in bed. The diagnostic trap is that prolonged periods of immobility, as in sitting, can produce dependency oedema.

Other causes of confusion are less easily recognised, but knowing that the client is a diabetic can be helpful. Changes of environment or constipation can cause temporary confusion, but this occurs mainly in those patients whose mental reserve is already limited. Confusion after bereavement may not be a true reflection of the situation — the surviving spouse may have been supported by the one who has died, and who has successfully covered up or concealed the fact that the survivor's mental state was impaired. The treatment of toxic confusional state is the treatment of the precipitating cause, which in most cases is fairly straightforward and may be managed at home. Patients will need sympathetic handling, bright lights should be avoided and carers will need much patience. If patients have to be moved to hospital they must be given adequate explanations and friends should accompany them.

Dementia (chronic brain failure)

Clients with a dementing illness have a slow onset memory loss which is of long duration, usually over many months or years. Only a few cases can be treated and reversed; in the majority the best that can be done is to support both client and carer. The most common causes of dementia are:

- senile dementia of the Alzheimer type (50%)
- multi-infarct dementia (20%)
- mixed senile and multi-infarct dementia (20%)
- others, including:
  - Vitamin B_{12} deficiency
  - hypothyroidism
  - normal pressure hydrocephalus.

It is difficult to establish accurate prevalence statistics for dementia, because of diagnostic problems. However, at the age of 60 years, about 2% of the population are affected. The prevalence rises to 22% in those over 80 years, whose numbers will rise by about half a million by the year 2025. To health visitors, with their epidemiological approach, such disease statistics mean that more than half a million demented old people aged 60 and upwards are probably being cared for at home. Furthermore about 45% of affected men and 10% of affected women are living with their elderly spouse. Other family members give resident care to about 30% of sufferers, but the remainder live alone until their state has so deteriorated as to necessitate institutionalisation. Three out of four of those people who live alone in a demented state are supported by relatives, friends and/or neighbours, who may plead to the health visitor to do 'something' to relieve the socio-psychological problems produced by the elderly person. (Gilhooley 1984).

The aetiology of Alzheimer's disease, which affects more women than men, remains unknown. Many lines of enquiry are being followed (Deary & Whalley 1988). One of the most interesting is that middle-aged patients dying with Down's syndrome show brain changes indistinguishable from Alzheimer's Disease. Infective causes have been investigated since scrapie, a neurodegenerative disease of sheep, produces brain pathology like that of Alzheimer's disease. There is also interest in discovering a possible role for aluminium and other toxins.

The brain in Alzheimer's disease shows signs of atrophy with proliferation of senile plaques and neurofibrillary tangles, far more than are seen in the 'normal aged brain'. There is a marked degeneration of the cerebral cholinergic pathways involved in memory. Deficits are also found in other neuropeptides including somatostatin and corticotrophin-releasing hormones.

Mental deterioration is progressive with marked short-term memory loss, with some preservation of long-term memory. Those affected may try to cover up by confabulating. Abstract ideas become more difficult to understand, initiative and motivation are blunted, the capacity to make decisions is reduced and the person's previous personality is exaggerated with the client becoming more absent-minded and self-centred. Paranoid delusions can occur which can be most vexatious to relatives.

The person can become restless and start to wander, easily getting lost because of inability to remember her/his home address. The vocabulary becomes restricted, reduced in words and becomes simpler. Depression with anxiety and hypochondriasis may develop. Personal hygiene and care tend to deteriorate. Life expectancy for those who become dependent is said to be about 2 years, but skilled nursing can prolong life very considerably.

Multi-infarct dementia is more common in men and starts at an earlier age than senile dementia. It is caused by small multiple brain infarcts occurring over many years. The onset may be abrupt with clouding of consciousness caused by the infarcts. As this resolves, there is some degree of recovery until the next incident occurs, when further mental deterioration develops, but without full recovery. This produces the so-called stepwise deterioration in mental state. The personality is often well preserved and the patient can be all too well aware of the mental changes, thus becoming depressed. Emotional debility is common, and paranoia may develop.

A few causes of dementia, such as hypothyroidism and Vitamin B_{12} deficiency, are potentially reversible. These are easily detected by specific blood tests. Treatment can result in some improvement, particularly in those with Vitamin B_{12} deficiency. Normal pressure hydrocephalus is recognised clinically by an ataxia/apraxia of gait, incontinence and mental confusion. The diagnosis is easily confirmed by non-invasive computerised axial tomography (CAT scan). Treatment is by insertion of a shunt.

Many demented people can, for most of their lives, be managed at home where the surroundings are familiar. However, carers who have an elderly relative at home find their task very wearing, both physically and mentally, because of symptoms such as night wandering, incontinence, sleep disturbance, unaesthetic, bizarre or dangerous behaviour, gross disturbance of mood, and constant demands for attention. Indeed dementia often causes greater strain for the carers than does physical disability, thus leading to a breakdown of health and placing a strain on family and marital relationships, especially when children live in the household. However, where the elderly spouse is the carer there maybe a greater demonstration of acceptance. Clearly health visitors must be aware of the many problems posed by dementia so that they can intervene early in the situation and prevent the crisis when relatives will say 'enough is enough'. The features of the dementing illness particularly to watch for, since they make it so difficult to sustain the sufferer at home, are double incontinence, proneness to bad falls, gas or fire risks, especially in those living alone, persistent wanderers living alone, aggression towards other members of the family, and serious risk of neglect and financial exploitation by relatives and others.

It is important to realise that the closer the carer is in emotional terms to the sufferer, the more distressed he or she is likely to become with the personality disintegration of the loved one. Help may be needed to handle this emotional situation, especially when decisions about institutional care have to be made. Great comfort may be derived from attending support groups with those in similar situations and reading the publications of the Alzheimer's Disease Society.

It is essential that caring relatives and friends receive the maximum support from the primary health care team, hospital and social services as well as any monetary benefit to which they or the sufferer may be entitled, especially attendance allowance (see Ch. 7, p. 158 and Ch. 10, p. 246). They may benefit from meals-on-wheels, home help, care assistants, district nurse, community psychiatric nurse, luncheon clubs, attendance at a day centre or hospital, the continence service and intermittent respite care in hospital or residential home. Much useful information is available in the Health Education Authority publications *Who Cares* and *Taking a Break*. Drugs may be used to treat depression or reduce wandering, which is best prevented by ensuring that the client has an interesting daytime occupation which tires him or her out. No specific drug treatment for dementia exists at present. Permanent institutional care is reserved for those who cannot be managed at home. Those with minimal behaviour disturbance may be admitted to a residential establishment while the very disturbed may need admission to a psychogeriatric unit.

Communication techniques and very simple

reality orientation measures can help with the quality of life for demented elderly people. They can be encouraged to keep diaries up to date and helped to put dates and times within a meaningful context, e.g. 'today is Tuesday and Mrs Green is coming to tea' or 'As it is Thursday, you must be ready to go the Day Centre'. Other helpful measures include using photographs and mementos to aid reminiscence; labelling objects, doors and pictures clearly; and adopting simple colour-coding schemes. It is wise to suggest that the affected client wear an identity necklace or bracelet, giving the person's name, address or telephone number as a precautionary measure against wandering away from home.

Those who are confused may not bother or may be unable to manage their own financial affairs. Demands for payments of The Community Charge (poll tax), electricity, gas or telephone bills may be ignored and the person will be in danger of having all forms of power and heating cut off. Initially, if the person has a bank account, it may be possible to arrange payment by standing order or by payment of the small regular monthly amounts, and relatives may find it helpful to assume the Power of Attorney. This Power allows a person of normal testamental capacity to appoint someone else to manage his/her affairs. It can be quickly arranged through a local solicitor and may be very useful for the physically disabled. Until recently the Power was only valid while the person concerned was mentally capable. The Enduring Power of Attorney Act (1985) now makes it possible to appoint an attorney who will still have the power to act after the person becomes mentally incapable.

For the very confused it may be necessary to use the Court of Protection. Here relatives or social workers make an application to the court to take over the financial affairs of the client. The court will ask for a medical certificate confirming the mental state, and, if this is accepted, the court will take over the finances and appoint a relative to do the 'donkey work'. If a suitable person is not available, or is unwilling, the Official Solicitor will take over the function. The caring relative is responsible to the court for what he does, and, therefore, the mechanism is not a blank cheque for wild spending. The whole procedure can be reversed should the person's mental state improve. For clients in Scotland an approach should be made to the Quarter Sessions in Edinburgh.

Sometimes it may be necessary to arrange compulsory hospital admission of an elderly person. The Mental Health Act (1983) changed some of the previous regulations (1959). The Department of Health (1990) issued for parliamentary approval 'The Code of Practice' which gives details of practical procedural advice for those who have to apply the Mental Health Act. However, the current situation is as follows:

Section 2. Admission for assessment (previously Section 25). The maximum period of detention is 28 days. The criteria are:

a. the patient is suffering from a mental disorder of a nature or degree which warrants his detention in hospital for assessment and subsequent treatment as necessary, and
b. he ought to be detained in the interests of his own health and safety or with a view to the protection of others.

Application is made by an approved social worker or nearest relative, based on the written application of two registered medical practitioners who must state that the current criteria for assessment are satisfied. One of the practitioners must be approved by the Secretary of State for Health as having special experience with diagnosis and treatment of mental disorders.

Section 3. Admission for treatment (previously Section 26). The maximum period of detention is 6 months, renewable for a further 6 months and then for periods of 6 months at a time. The criteria are:

a. a patient suffering from mental illness which makes it appropriate for him to receive medical treatment in hospital to alleviate or prevent deterioration of the condition
b. for the patient's health and safety and the protection of others.

Applications and recommendations involve two registered medical practitioners (similar to section 2), and an approved social worker or nearest relative.

Section 4. Admission for assessment in cases of

emergency (previously Section 29). The maximum period of detention is 72 hours. The criteria are that it is of urgent necessity for the patient to be detained, and compliance with the provision for admission for assessment would involve undesirable delay. The procedure involves recommendation by one medical practitioner (e.g. a general practitioner), who must have seen the patient within 24 hours prior to admission, and an application by an approved social worker or nearest relative.

On occasion the health visitor may face the situation where an elderly patient is quite unrealistic about his or her capabilities of managing at home even with maximal community and social service support. This may be a suitable occasion for the use of Sections 7–10 of the 1983 Mental Health Act — Reception into Guardianship (previously Sections 33, 34). The criteria are (a) the person should be suffering from mental illness or severe mental impairment and (b) it is in that person's interest or for the protection of others that he or she be received into guardianship. The procedure involves two registered medical practitioners and an application by an approved social worker or nearest relative. The effect is that the guardian now has the power to require the patient to live in a specific place or to attend specified places for treatment. The maximum period of detention is 6 months, extending for a further 6, and then for period of 1 year at a time.

Self-neglect

CASE STUDY

Mrs E M, aged 68 years, was admitted with a history of increasing weakness, anorexia and loss of weight for several weeks. She had become a recluse since the death of her husband 15 years earlier and had never invited anyone into her house until she became ill. It was found to be exceedingly dirty, with thick layers of dust on all flat surfaces. Some 30 to 40 full milk bottles lined the wall of the front hall and there were piles of paper in the hall and in other rooms of the house. In the bedroom clothes were dropped when discarded and were never picked up; consequently it was necessary to walk on a layer of clothing to get to the bedside.

The condition of self-neglect is now increasingly recognised and the features are well described (Clarke et al 1975). Characteristically these clients of the health visitor are often of above-average intelligence but are unkempt, dirty and often incontinent. They live in what others consider to be squalid surroundings (Fig. 9.1) and are often well known to social services. Their clothing and bed linen have usually not been cleaned for a long time. The house is dirty, and items, particularly newspapers, are kept never to be discarded. Poverty is not usually a problem although the client may appear to be penniless. They tend to feed themselves out of tins or to live on tea and biscuits and may thus suffer from malnutrition. Social workers and others find that trying to help these people can be very time-consuming and frustrating. Neighbours often demand that something be done — implying that the client should be 'put away'. However, admission to hospital is usually associated with a high mortality rate, probably because the person concerned has become so unwell and can no longer resist well-meaning persuasion.

Two other groups of people who may neglect themselves are chronic alcoholics and paraphrenics. Chronic alcoholics are unable to control the amount they drink, which can lead to malnutrition, vitamin deficiencies, paranoia and dementia. Alcoholism is developing when clients tell lies about their alcohol intake, avoid the topic, take drink earlier and earlier in the day and give ex-

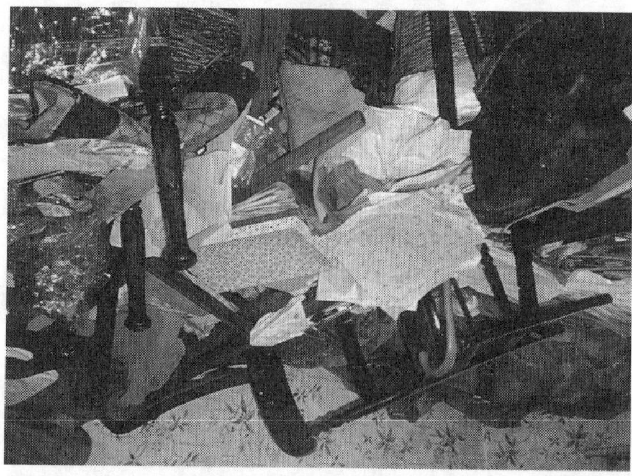

Fig. 9.1 Typical appearance of living-room of a patient with Diogenes syndrome (self-neglect).

cuses to explain the situation. Paraphrenia is late-onset schizophrenia which classically occurs in elderly isolated females. Such a client is often suspicious of close neighbours and fears they are spying on her. Thinking is disordered and difficult to follow. Some clients may be mute while others are hyperactive and show incongruity between feelings and experience.

Caring relatives and neighbours can find it very difficult trying to help those who neglect themselves, particularly if the person is 'awkward minded', eccentric and cantankerous. Goodwill is soon lost and a crisis situation will soon develop, particularly if some illness intervenes or support is withdrawn.

Health visitors can be faced with difficult ethical and management problems since the person appears ill, is failing to thrive and is clearly not coping but equally refuses admission either to an old people's home or to hospital. If the person is mentally clear and is adamant that admission is unacceptable, then it is reasonable to continue to care for that person at home with as much care as can be given and readily accepted. Unfortunately, if death occurs at home, there is often much ill-informed criticism of the caring services, when they have often done their best to help within the limits that the patient will allow.

There may be situations, however, when although the person is mentally clear, compulsory admission is considered necessary. This involves the use of Section 47 of the National Assistance Act of 1948 or the 1951 Amendment. This allows the Director of Public Health, or equivalent, together with the general practitioner or geriatrician, to move the person in need of care and attention from his or her home, if it is in the interest of the patient or would prevent injury to health of, or serious injury to, other people. A person 'in need of care and attention' within the meaning of the act is 'one suffering from grave chronic illness . . . or being aged, infirm or physically handicapped living in insanitary conditions and unable to devote to him or herself, or is not receiving from others, proper care and attention'. The 1948 Act requires an application to a magistrates' court with 7 days notice being given to the patients. The 1951 Amendment allows direct application to a magistrate and removal of a patient without delay. Accommodation in hospital or in a home must be available. Discharge of these patients can be a problem. Neighbours may resist, because they have found a new situation more acceptable. Much depends on the attitude of the old person. If he or she is pleasant, there will doubtless be willingness to try again.

Falls

The incidence of falls rises steeply with age and is more common in woman (see Ch. 8, pp. 198–201). However it is often not appreciated how frequent falls are in the elderly. It is calculated that in the United Kingdom 3 million falls occur in old people in the community in a year. While less than 2% result in actual injury, this will include 30 000 cases of fractured neck of femurs. Unfortunately, about 3000 deaths occur as a result of falls. Many elderly people lie on the floor for several hours before they are found and about half of these patients will die within 6 months. Most falls occur in the daytime inside the home, especially the living room and on the stairs. They are particularly common amongst those living alone, the socially isolated and the depressed and the demented. Though falls may not result in injury, they frequently induce a fear of falls in the person concerned, who loses confidence and refuses to leave the house or even to walk at all.

The health visitor should try to find why a person has fallen. The causes include:

- environmental factors, e.g. loose mats, poor lighting, polished floors
- physiological/ageing processes, e.g. reduction of balance control
- medical disease
  - cardiovascular system, e.g. postural hypotension, cardiac arrhythmias
  - central nervous system, e.g. Parkinsonism, stroke, poor eyesight
  - locomotor system, e.g. arthritis
  - early phase of acute illness
- drugs
- local causes, e.g. painful feet.

Some of the causes are quite easily prevented or

treatable. Unfortunately, it is often difficult to obtain a clear, accurate history or to obtain a very useful witness, but it must be remembered that the falls can be a non-specific indicator of ill health and therefore the causes must be identified if at all possible.

Environmental problems cause almost half of accidental falls. The elderly may trip over loose carpets or wires, slip on well-polished floors, or fall on steep stairs without adequate handrails or lighting. Poor eyesight and ill-fitting footwear will compound the situation.

Postural control deteriorates with age, because of cerebellar degeneration and impaired proprioception, and results in delayed assimilation of postural information, and increasing body sway. Reaction times increase, and an elderly person who stumbles may not be able to correct the situation quickly enough. General ill health and inability to concentrate compound the situation.

Cardiovascular disease is a potent cause of falls. Normally the tendency for the blood pressure to fall when the person moves from the horizontal to a vertical position is very rapidly corrected. This self-correcting mechanism may be impaired in the elderly and produce postural hypotension. It can be aggravated by drugs which affect blood pressure, e.g. antihypertensive agents, L-dopa, tricyclic antidepressants, phenothiazines and diuretics. Cardiac arrhythmias, particularly bradycardia or tachycardia, are important causes of falls. Often the diagnosis can be made with a 24-hour ambulatory ECG. Some falls are due to vertebrobasilar insufficiency, which produces impairment of blood supply to the brain when the head is tilted sharply upwards or twisted sideways.

Central nervous system diseases frequently impair mobility, which can affect balance. Thus patients with Parkinsonism or a stroke may find it difficult to make sudden or quick alterations in the direction of walking, and, when these are attempted, falls are the result. Diseases of the labyrinth of the ear or its central connections are not uncommon in the elderly, and can cause vertigo and resulting falls.

Arthritis and muscular weakness will also make it difficult for the elderly to maintain proper balance. The situation may be compounded by painful conditions such as corns and ingrowing toenails and by the early phase of an acute illness.

Drugs which cause postural hypotension or excessive sedation can easily cause falls. The hangover effect of some hypnotics is well known. Alcohol can also blunt postural control, while long-acting hypoglycaemic drugs such as chlorpropamide can cause falls because of low blood sugar levels.

The health visitor can help in management/prevention by noting how, when and where the falls tend to occur. She can note the number and type of drugs which have been prescribed and can check the files. She can check for evidence of impaired mobility, painful feet and environmental problems. She will be able to advise about lighting, positioning of furniture and carpets, and avoidance of polished floors. It may be helpful to bring the bed downstairs and have a bedside commode. Ramps over steps might be needed or extra handrails on the stair. The domiciliary physiotherapist may be able to give 'mat' exercise to restore the patient's confidence in getting off the floor without assistance. The local authority may be able to fit an alarm system to bring assistance when required.

Many of the factors which cause falls also produce poor mobility. Their recognition is important since inability to move about the house or get out of it can seriously impair the quality of life.

Hypothermia

Hypothermia, a core body temperature of less than 35°C, has only been relatively recently recognised as a problem in the elderly. It occurs when heat production, generated by the conversion of food to energy, is exceeded by heat loss from skin and expired air. It usually occurs in elderly people who are not in good health. It is difficult to be sure how many older people actually die because of hypothermia. In 1984 it was predicted that about 20 000 to 100 000 deaths might occur in the elderly in the United Kingdom from this cause. While it is accepted that there is a high seasonal mortality in the elderly associated with cold weather, statistical evidence from death certification currently suggests that death from hypothermia is comparatively rare, amounting to about 1% of total excess winter deaths (Collins 1989).

Hypothermia results from

- cold environment
- impaired thermoregulation with age
- secondary precipitating factors, e.g. infections, poor mobility, fractures, endocrine disorders, diabetes, uraemia, drug side effects, previous episodes of hypothermia, dementia or depression.

A recent study of people aged over 65 years living at home showed that three quarters had a room temperature of less than 65°F, which is the minimum temperature recommended by the Parker Morris report on Council Housing and less than the recommended 70°F suggested by the DHSS. Thus hypothermia can easily develop if an elderly person, clad only in night attire, falls to the floor at night and is not found for many hours.

Increasing age is associated with reduced efficiency of thermoregulation: the shivering action is muted, the basal metabolic rate does not rise with cooling, the loss of body subcutaneous fat reduces insulation and there is defective venous constriction (see Ch. 2). In addition the elderly are less aware of temperature changes and have reduced sensitivity to cold. Young people can detect mean temperature differences of about 0.8°C, whereas the elderly can only differentiate between mean temperature differences of 2.5°C while some can only perceive differences of 5°C. Consequently, old people may wear inadequate clothing and have inadequate heating or room insulation. Lack of finances may be a contributory factor.

There are many secondary precipitating factors for hypothermia. Any severe illness caused, for example, by infections or heart failure, which can result in a toxic confusional state, or lack of an awareness of surroundings, may result in a fall in body temperature, especially if the environment is cold. Any disability, or disease of the brain, cardiovascular, or locomotor systems, which limits mobility or precipitates falls is a potential risk factor. Drugs which impair mobility (sedatives or tranquillisers), impair consciousness (hypnotics), or impair shivering (e.g. phenothiazines) are potentially dangerous to the elderly. Falls and inability to get up are risk factors. Patients who are demented or depressed may not realise that the room temperature is low. Those people who have had a previous episode of hypothermia are particularly at risk. Hypothermia is easily diagnosed once diagnosis is suspected. A quick test is to assess the anterior abdominal wall temperature. If this feels cold to the hand, then the person is cold. A rectal temperature will confirm the situation. A hypothermic patient often looks myxoedemic. The face is pale and puffy, cerebration is slow and the voice husky. Consciousness is impaired below 32°C, and patients are usually unconscious when the temperature is less than 27°C. Tone of the muscles is increased and the reflexes are depressed and relaxed. The pulse is slow and the blood pressure low. The abdomen may look distended. The lower the temperature, the greater the risk of cardiac arrest.

The health visitor will not necessarily be involved with the treatment of hypothermia. However, admission should be considered for patients with a temperature of less than 35°C, though some patients with a temperature of about 35°C can be managed at home, provided adequate precautions are taken. All hypothermic patients should be removed from the cold environment and then allowed to warm up slowly, usually by being wrapped in a 'space blanket'. Rapid external warming in the elderly can cause an afterdrop of temperature and circulatory collapse. Rapid intense warming by cardiac bypass or rebreathing techniques is not often used in older people.

The health visitor is mainly concerned with preventing hypothermia. She must be able to identify those 'at risk', e.g. those living alone, the frail, the housebound, the depressed and confused. She can help to ensure that her clients maintain adequate environmental temperature, giving advice on reducing draughts and heat loss by insulating lofts and hot water tanks. It may be possible to obtain suitable local authority financial heating and insulating grants and to have the advice of gas and electricity board adviser teams as well as the local branch of Age Concern. However, an old person may need to live in one heated room to save fuel (see also Ch. 7, p. 159–162). Advice about avoiding falls and the use of adequate clothing may be necessary.

INCONTINENCE

Incontinence of urine has been defined as the unintentional and involuntary passing of urine in an inappropriate place or at an inappropriate time twice or more in the past month. It may be minimal, slight, moderate or severe, which can be defined as:

- minimal — no extra laundry; no pads or expenses; no restriction on activities
- slight — very small amounts of extra laundry; pads worn only occasionally; no restrictional activities
- moderate — extra laundry or pads and/or expenses; some restriction of activity
- severe — considerable extra laundry — or pads or expenses; activities restricted; requires assistance from others.

Incontinence can be a major problem in the care of the elderly, and may be 'the final straw which breaks the camel's back'. It is an illness or a symptom of illness which, if not curable, can often be improved, and certainly the management can be made much more satisfactory. The incidence varies with the population studied. A community study (Thomas et al 1980) showed that 6.9% of men and 11.6% of women over the age of 65 were incontinent. One in five of those who were incontinent were moderately or severely affected. Not surprisingly the incidence is over 50% in long-stay institutions.

Physiology of micturition

Normal micturition control depends on several intact levels of nerve function (Fig. 9.2) At the lowest level is the local parasympathetic reflex arc which connects the bladder to the spinal cord (sacral centre). At higher levels there are centres in the pons, midbrain and posterior hypothalamus which are necessary for complete bladder emptying and are responsible for the correct functioning and integrity of the bladder detrusor muscle, trigone and urethral sphincter. The highest centre

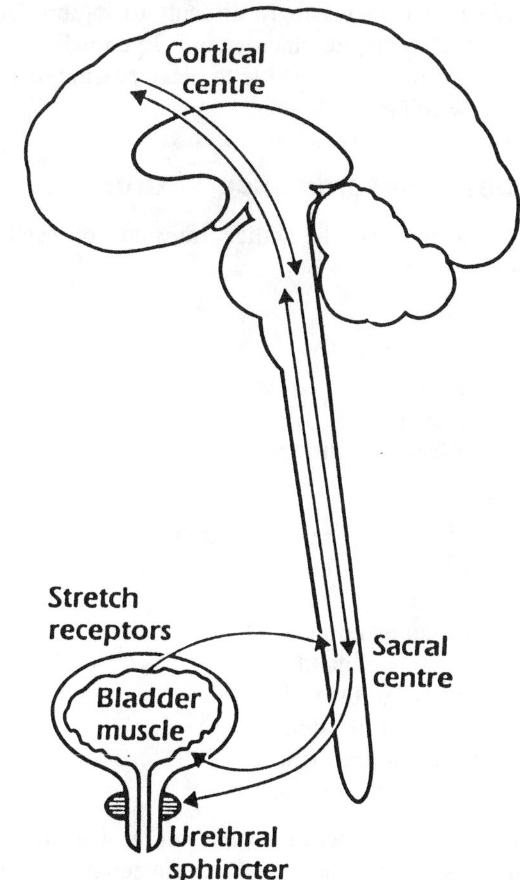

Fig. 9.2 Representation of nerve control of micturition.

for control of micturition is the frontal lobe, which enables a person to be aware of the state of fullness of the bladder and to inhibit emptying until a suitable moment. As the bladder fills, sensory impulses pass from the stretch receptors along the reflex arc to the spinal cord where impulses pass to the higher centres and to the motor fibres of the reflex arc, which controls, with the help of return impulses from the higher centres, the bladder detrusor muscle, causing it to contract, while relaxing the muscles on the external sphincter and the pelvic floor. The desire to pass urine is usually felt when a bladder contains 250–300 ml, but micturition can be inhibited by voluntary will exerted from the frontal cortex.

Increasing age is associated with functional changes which affect bladder function. Elderly people find it increasingly difficult to inhibit the reflex and postpone micturition. Eventually the old person may only be able to delay passing urine for a few minutes.

Types of incontinence of urine

Incontinence may be either transient or established:

1. Transient
   - acute illness
   - drugs
   - constipation
   - infection of urine;
2. Established
   - disorders of nervous pathways
     a. uninhibited bladder (neurogenic bladder)
     b. autonomous bladder
     c. atonic bladder
     d. reflex bladder
   - detrusor instability
   - stress incontinence
   - overflow incontinence.

Transient incontinence may occur as part of an acute illness such as a toxic confusional state or acute cerebrovascular accident, especially if the patient is admitted to the strange environment of a hospital. Drugs are a potent cause of temporary incontinence: e.g. loop diuretics, such as frusemide, given to patients with poor mobility, or hypnotic drugs which impair sensory input to the frontal cortex. Drugs with an anticholinergic action such as the antidepressants may cause retention of urine which can be potentiated by constipation. Temporary incontinence can result from constipation or when increased sensory input to the sacral reflex arcs occurs, e.g. from cystitis, atrophic urethritis associated with atrophic vaginitis, or local lesions of the bladder such as with a stone or tumour.

A person has established incontinence when the problem persists after acute conditions have been treated. The cause may be disorders of the nervous pathways to the brain or bladder. Various types of neurogenic incontinence are described, of which the most common type in old age is the neurogenic bladder. In this situation, damage to the frontal cortex, as in dementia, results in loss of ability to inhibit reflex bladder contraction. There may be urge incontinence when the person's desire to pass urine is almost immediately followed by the passage of urine. The other types of neurogenic incontinence are less common in the elderly: autonomous, when there is destruction of the 2nd to 4th sacral segments in the corda equine, as in spinal cord tumour, causing ineffective bladder contraction; atonic, when the afferent part of the reflex arc is damaged as in diabetes, causing retention with overflow; and reflex, when the connections between the reflex arc and the frontal cortex are severed, as in spinal injury, causing an unstable bladder which empties reflexly.

Bladder disorders may cause incontinence. The commonest problem in the elderly is detrusor instability, which is characterised by uninhibited bladder contractions occurring at any stage of bladder filling and can follow coughing, laughing, getting out of bed or standing up, resulting in total bladder emptying. Elderly people with unstable bladders have frequency, nocturia and urgency, but are not always incontinent. However, they are predisposed to urge incontinence, nocturnal incontinence and stress incontinence. In men obstruction to urinary outflow, due to an enlarged prostate, can cause outflow obstruction.

Stress incontinence is a different condition and separate from detrusor instability. The history in both has similarities, but in stress incontinence a small amount of urine is squeezed out of the bladder because of an increase in intra-abdominal pressure and an ineffective urethral closing mechanism. It is most common in multiparous women and those with uterine prolapse but can occur in younger persons as well.

Management of incontinence of urine

The health visitor may be asked to advise relatives of clients with persistent established incontinence. There are many ways in which she can help. Attention to the following management points is essential:

1. encouragement of optimism
2. charting of urinary output, and details of both continence and incontinence
3. habit training and avoiding constipation
4. odour
5. care of the skin
6. clothing
7. physiotherapy
8. appliances
9. access to toilet/commode
10. drugs
11. catheter.

Above all, she must be optimistic, since much can be done to improve the patient's quality of life and self-esteem. She must treat her client — not just the wet bed. Initially it is useful for the time of micturition and incontinence to be charted, since it can help to establish the type of incontinence, timing of habit training and can indicate the most suitable appliance. Habit training can be a successful technique, which not only involves the client being taken to the toilet regularly, even when not requested, but also means trying to help the client understand the mechanism of the disturbance of bladder function. The bladder fills at the rate of about 100 ml/hour during the day and if the client cannot hold more than 250 ml of urine before micturition the right time for toileting is every 2 hours. Over a period of time it will generally be possible to extend the time of visit to the toilet.

An accurately completed continence chart will help to establish the appropriate frequency of toileting for that particular person. However, great patience is required, especially with those people who pass urine just after visiting the toilet. Regular toileting fails when the bladder's capacity is so small that it is exceeded if the urine is allowed to collect for only 2 hours. At night urine formation is reduced in volume, which will help control incontinence, but fluid restriction after 6 p.m. may still be needed. Naturally all clients should be advised to avoid constipation.

Probably nothing is more disturbing to the client's morale than the smell of stale urine. This problem can be reduced by changing soiled linen and placing it in a bucket containing disinfectant; preventing the urine becoming concentrated by ensuring adequate fluid intake; rapid treatment of urinary tract infection; and cleaning carpets as soon as they are soiled. Proprietary aerosol or solid block room deodorisers are often extremely helpful.

Care of the skin is helped by preventing it being in prolonged contact with urine and ensuring that it is kept clean and dry. Clients should be advised to wear indoor clothing during the day, and all clothing should be machine washable. Various types of specialised clothing are available (see Disabled Living Foundation — address in Appendix 7).

Physiotherapy can help to improve mobility to and from the toilet and improve pelvic floor tone. Exercises to improve pelvic muscle power are given in three stages and need to be practised conscientiously for 6 months. Stage 1 involves the client, sitting or standing, pretending that she is trying to avoid diarrhoea by tightening the ring of muscle around the anus. Stage 2 involves sitting on the toilet, passing urine and attempting to stop the flow in midstream by contracting the muscles around the urethra. Stage 3 involves the client, sitting or standing, tightening the muscles around the anus, then the urethral muscles and then both together. All exercises should be practised several times a day. If there is any doubt about how these exercises should be carried out the opinion of a qualified physiotherapist should be obtained.

The health visitor should also look for difficulties experienced by clients reaching the toilet in time. If the toilet is upstairs and the patient is slow, a downstairs commode may be necessary. Male urinal bottles, especially with non-slip valves, can be helpful. Alternatively, extra rails for the stairs and a raised toilet seat may be needed. Clients may also experience problems when looking for public toilets if they don't know where they are; they may need to plan shopping to ensure they are always near a toilet.

Incontinent clients may be prescribed drugs which suppress bladder contractions, e.g. terodilene or a tricyclic antidepressant. However, they are not always effective and are not without troublesome side-effects. Oestrogen replacement therapy is usually prescribed for elderly incontinent women with atropic vaginitis.

Relatives will often need advice about absorbent appliances, which are usually of two types: insert pads and sheets or underpads. Unless overloaded, all absorb fluid without becoming wet. The time an appliance will last depends on its absorbance capacity and the rate of urine formation. If a person forms 100 ml per hour during the day it will take 3 hours to saturate a 300 ml capacity pad. Oversaturated pads can disintegrate and/or cause skin rashes. Insert pads are worn between the legs and are held in position by pants or retained in special pants by a pouch either inside or outside the pants. Most protect against mild or occasional incontinence and are usually not recommended for night use, although some (Molnlycke pants) can be used over the 24-hour period. Most types hold 250 ml urine and therefore 2-hourly changing is usually necessary. The retaining pants may be disposable or reusable and may be plastic, elastic netting, or paper.

Absorbent appliances for beds or chairs are of two main types: thin underpads or large sheets. The thin disposable underpads have limited absorbent capacity — 350 or 650 ml depending on the size. They tend to disintegrate when wet and are best for clients who have only mild incontinence. Alternatively, washable absorbent draw sheets can absorb up to 3 litres of fluid without soaking the bed. These sheets are comfortable to lie on, are economical to use, the surface remains dry and there is no disposable problem. However, there is a high initial purchase cost, they become heavy when wet and are unsuitable for households without laundry facilities. At least three sheets are required per person: one in use, one in the wash, one drying.

Ultimately catheter drainage may be suggested for those where all other methods fail. Used with discretion it can alleviate much discomfort and improve morale. The drainage bag should be concealed as a leg bag or in a sporran bag, rather than be carried for all to see. The health visitor must be sure that the client or the relatives are able to empty the catheter bag. Unfortunately catheters are associated with urinary tract infections and can be pulled out.

Many health districts now have continence advisers. They represent a valuable practical source of up-to-date information and knowledge of many aspects of incontinence. Their opinion should be sought whenever necessary. They complement rather than usurp the function of health visitors and community nurses.

Faecal incontinence

Though faecal incontinence is less common than urinary incontinence, it, too, can cause a crisis situation. It is found in 22 people per 1000 population over 65 and many of them receive no health or community services. There are three principal causes: faecal impaction, neurological disease and diarrhoea.

Faecal impaction

This is a consequence of constipation, where there is a slowing of the passage of intestinal contents which allows time for excessive removal of fluid. The hardened faeces impact in the rectum and colon and are lubricated by excessive mucus secretion. The patient becomes unaware of the mass in the rectum and loses the sensation of 'call to stool'. The faeces above the impaction become liquified by bacterial action and pass around it, presenting at the rectum as spurious diarrhoea. If the situation is allowed to continue, especially if antidiarrhoeal preparations are given, the patient becomes more constipated, resulting in anorexia and vomiting, and even restless behaviour. Pressure of the distended rectum on the bladder neck can precipitate urinary incontinence. The condition is easily diagnosed by rectal examination.

Treatment may require manual removal of faeces; suppositories; or enemas. The bowel will require re-education by ensuring that the diet contains adequate fibre as in fruit or bran. The effect varies with the size of the fibre particle — the larger the particle, the greater the faecal weight, due to water retention. A side-effect of bran is flatulence. Patients may be given fibogel, a colloid agent which makes the motion easy to pass;

senokot a muscle stimulant of the large bowel; or bisacodyl, which causes large-bowel peristasis.

The elderly require re-eduction about the use of laxatives, to avoid abuse leading to diarrhoea, dehydration and severe electrolyte upset. Excessive laxatives in the presence of obstructive bowel pathology can result in perforation. Excessive use of liquid paraffin can result in leakage of fluid faeces from the rectum, malabsorption of Vitamin D and, if small amounts are retained in the pharynx, spill-over can occur into the lungs, causing pneumonia. It is not really necessary to arrange a weekly bowel clearance as the Victorians seemed to think.

Neurological causes

The neurological causes may be local or central. Local neuronal degeneration with myopathic changes can occur in the large bowel and may be secondary to chronic constipation. Diabetes mellitus can be associated with degeneration of the autonomic nerves to the bowel, which can also affect gut low motility.

More important is central causation, where faecal incontinence can result from lack of inhibition of the normal 'gastro-colic' reflex. Formed motions are passed involuntarily, sometimes into clothes or bedding. The situation is usually treated by planned routine of regular evacuation of the bowels.

Diarrhoea

Patients with severe diarrhoea, which can follow from purgative abuse, may temporarily loose adequate sphincter control, with resulting incontinence. The treatment will be that of the cause, with possible use of constipating agents. Spurious diarrhoea is found in patients with carcinoma of the rectum or proctocolitis.

ABUSE OF THE ELDERLY

This problem is increasingly coming to medical attention. It is fully discussed in Chapter 10, but the following case studies illustrate how it may present.

CASE STUDIES

Mrs D, a 75-year-old, was severely incapacitated by extensive rheumatoid arthritis. She frequently refused to come into hospital to give relatives relief, since she feared being abandoned. Eventually she did agree and she was then abandoned. She literally turned her face to the wall and died within 3 days.

Mr M was 83 years old, cantankerous, confused and frequently liable to hit out at or scratch those who cared for him. One day the caring nurse threatened to break his arm if he struck her again. He did, so she did.

Mrs H, an 84-year-old, lived in the small front bedroom of a house belonging to her daughter and son-in-law. She was admitted to hospital with a stroke and made a total recovery within 3 weeks. The relatives refused to have her back again and eventually she was found accommodation in a warden-controlled flat, to which all her furniture was moved. It later transpired that she and her son-in-law, though living in the same house, had not spoken to each other for 10 years.

MEDICATION FOR THE ELDERLY

Though drugs have brought great benefit to old people, adverse drug reactions are important causes of illness in the elderly. Not only are the elderly prescribed proportionately more drugs than younger people, but studies in the UK and the USA have shown that the incidence of adverse drug reaction rises with age (Fig. 9.3). A survey of admissions to geriatric units in the UK showed that 1 in 10 were admitted solely or partly because of adverse drug reactions (Williamson & Chopin 1980). Not all the patients recovered — indeed mortality due to drugs rises with age. Two groups of drugs caused two-thirds of all reactions: those which act on the cardiovascular system (e.g. digoxin, diuretics and hypotensive drugs) and those which act on the central nervous system (e.g. hypnotics, tranquillisers, antidepressants and antiparkinsonian drugs).

Adverse drug reactions arise from excessive prescribing, coupled with inadequate review of long-term medication, inadequate clinical assessment, altered drug metabolism (pharmacokinetics)

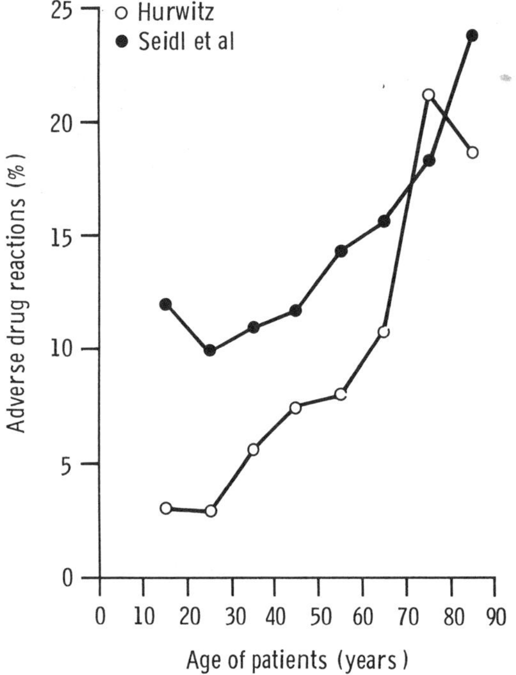

Fig. 9.3 Incidence of adverse drug reactions, by age of patient (after Hurwitz 1969, Seidl et al 1966).

and altered drug sensitivity (pharmacodynamics) which occur in old age, and impaired compliance. Perhaps the most important factor is excessive prescribing. Doctors are keen to treat disabilities which affect people, but this may result in an old person's being prescribed 10 to 12 different drugs, which makes it difficult for the patient to remember how and when to take the medicine.

An additional problem is that drugs prescribed during an acute phase of an illness may no longer be needed in the later convalescent phase. However, to stop drugs which have already been prescribed requires a time-consuming routine to reassess current requirements. It is often quicker for the doctor to complete a new prescription form. Inadequate clinical assessment can occur when symptoms are treated rather than the disease because history taking and examination are very difficult and time-consuming. Dependency oedema of the feet on account of immobility may be incorrectly assumed to be the result of congestive cardiac failure. If diuretics are given, incontinence can result.

There is now ample evidence that the way drugs are handled/metabolised in the elderly is less efficient than in younger people. The principal factors are a decrease in renal function, and impaired liver function (Ch. 2). Consequently drugs are less efficiently detoxicated and excreted. Thus a standard adult dose of a drug will last longer and be more effective in the older person. An additional factor is that the ratio of fat to lean body mass increases with age, thus prolonging the action of fat-soluble drugs if dosage is not altered appropriately. Drug absorption in the gut does not greatly change with age, although food can modify uptake (Viswanathan & Welling 1984).

The effect of altered pharmacodynamics is evidenced by the ageing brain, which is more sensitive to drugs which act upon it, compared with the brain of younger people. Consequently hangover effects of hypnotic drugs and minor tranquillisers are more prominent, and confusion following the use of antidepressants and antiparkinsonian drugs is quite common.

Impaired drug compliance is a major problem in old people: as many as three-quarters of elderly people make errors in their prescriptions, a quarter of which are potentially dangerous. There are three main causes. First, the person may take a positive decision to stop taking medication because of the absence, or persistence, of symptoms; early response to treatment, or side effects. In addition, those with impaired eyesight may not be able to read the label, while the confused elderly may fail to remember how and when to take the tablets. Second, the doctor or the nursing staff may give inadequate explanations about how to take the medication, e.g. nearly half of a group of patients failed to take off the wrapping from suppositories before insertion. The doctor is also responsible for completing adequately the prescription form which the patient will take to the chemist for dispensing. Inadequately completed forms may result in the chemist putting the instructions 'to be taken as directed' on the bottle. One ill elderly patient seen recently had a bottle of 0.25 mg of digoxin tablets which were 'to be taken as directed'. She was taking them three times a day. The third factor in compliance is the actual medication and its container. Drugs which are un-

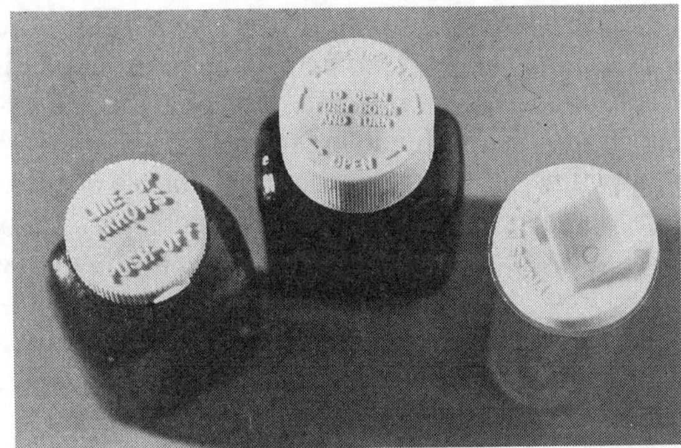

Fig. 9.4 Child-resistant containers pose problems for older persons at times.

pleasant to take, cause side-effects, or are difficult to swallow may not be taken. People may have difficulty in opening drug bottles, especially the child-resistant containers, e.g. the clicloc, pop loc, and snap safe (Fig. 9.4). Blister or bubble packs also cause problems.

Patients who do not comply accurately with their medication are likely to keep or hoard the medicines. Recent DUMP (Disposal of Unwanted Medicines and Poisons) campaigns have shown the size of the problem: for instance, 2$\frac{1}{4}$ tons of medicines were returned in Glasgow. In 1977 one-third of a million tablets and capsules were returned in Birmingham, but this was considered to represent only 3% of the potential total (Harris et al 1979). Over 70% of the drugs were more than 1 year old. Another DUMP campaign in 1984 in Cornwall resulted in the collection of enough poison to kill more than 200 000 people!

The dangers of hoarding are that drugs will be shared or used inappropriately. New supplies of medicine may be confused with older stocks already in the house (Fig. 9.5). Although most drugs have a long shelf life, some do not: e.g. trinitrin tablets deteriorate within about 2 months.

Health visitors must be aware of the need for accurate prescribing, compliance and regular reassessment so that they can take advantage of their close and understanding relationship with their clients and help as necessary. They should be alert to the problems of overdose and adverse effects on the one hand, and those of inadequate therapeutic effect or lack of compliance on the other. They

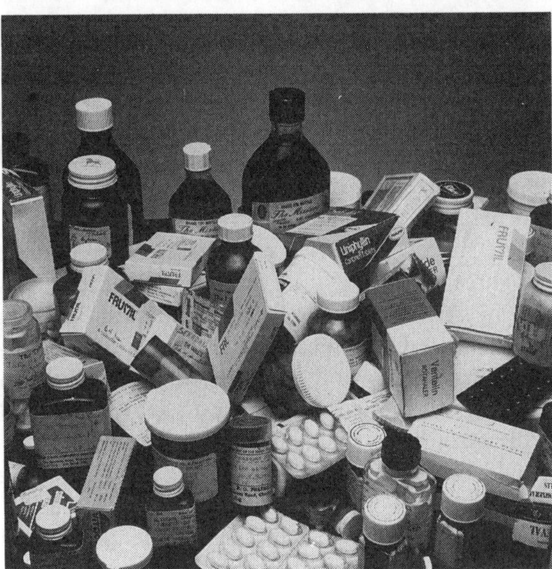

Fig. 9.5 Examples of some hoarded drugs.

should be able to improve compliance by reinforcing verbal instructions using written instruction cards and medication aids. They should ensure that the labels on drug containers are legible, the directions are understood and the patient can open the bottle.

PATIENTS WITH SPECIAL MEDICAL NEEDS

Health visitors may be asked to advise not only their elderly clients with special problems or needs but also their caring relatives, friends and neighbours. The post-myocardial-infarction patient; those whose mobility is limited by a stroke, Parkinsonism, or chronic obstructive airways disease; and the elderly diabetic are among those who commonly seek advice.

Post-mycocardial-infarction patients

Patients discharged home following a myocardial infarction may still be worried and fearful about their future, even when counselled by hospital staff. While there is no doubt that a heart attack is a serious illness, the long-term survival of the elderly infarct patient is better, relative to their natural expected mortality, than younger patients. Furthermore many people are able subsequently to lead an active life. The greater the degree of independence the person achieves after the event, the better the life expectancy. Therefore clients should be encouraged to be optimistic about the future and persuaded to lead as normal a life as possible.

The client can take many simple pragmatic measures himself. Since excessive weight causes the heart to work unnecessarily hard, weight should be reduced sensibly and slowly to the normal range. Fats and sugar should be taken in moderation. If a diet is advised, to lower the blood cholesterol level, it should be adhered to. Alcohol should be taken in moderation. Cigarette smoking should cease — abrupt cessation is probably easier than long-drawn-out reduction in the number of cigarettes smoked. Exercise is clearly important. Going for walks is good and should be started 4 to 6 weeks after infarct; however, care should be taken to avoid sudden, severe exertion in the early days. The client is the best judge of his or her capabilities and time will show what can be achieved. Some clients may not find it physically easy to cope at home. Here the health visitor must be able to assess the situation and call in what extra help is needed. She should also ensure that those clients who are on medication know how and when it is to be taken. Advice about when to resume sexual activity may also have to be given: it is usual to wait 4 to 8 weeks after the infarct. Driving a car should not be undertaken for 2 months.

The bronchitic patient

The physical problems of chronic bronchitis and emphysema will be well established and irreversible by the time patients become elderly. Indeed few patients with chronic obstructive airways disease survive to become aged. The disease is due almost entirely to cigarette smoking, especially cigarettes with high tar content, with the possible contributory factors of air pollution or dusty atmosphere. The disease results in bronchial narrowing, dyspnoea, excessive grey or white sputum, and a persistent cough. The lung tissue itself is damaged, impairing blood oxygenation.

Health visitors must help the client to get the best quality of life possible. Cigarette smoking should stop, unless it is the only pleasure the patient has. Clients should be warned of the dangers of crowded public areas where the chance of picking up a chest infection is increased. The advisability of an anti-flu vaccination should be considered. Excess weight serves no useful purpose and should be reduced. Unfortunately there is no alternative to willpower in adhering to a diet. Clients should always take as much exercise as possible and try to keep fit. A physiotherapist may help, particularly with the exercises and improved controlled breathing during periods of dyspnoea.

Clients who are very dyspnoeic may require additional help/advice from a home help, occupational therapist, or social worker. Rehousing on the ground floor may be necessary. Health visitors should ensure that clients understand their medication. Domiciliary oxygen or an oxygen concentrator may be needed by those who require oxygen for long periods each day. Room temperatures should be maintained at even levels and sudden changes in temperature avoided, as this can precipitate bouts of coughing.

The stroke patient

The incidence of strokes rises rapidly with age, particularly over the age of 60 years. Each year 2 new cases occur for every thousand of the population. Approximately one-fifth die within the first month, although there is some evidence that mortality is declining, two-fifths are left disabled, and the remaining two-fifths return to normal or near normal. Stroke is the third commonest cause of death after ischaemic heart disease and cancer. Although approximately four-fifths of all strokes are due to cerebral infarction, the occlusion of the cerebral blood vessels can be caused by a variety of factors such as atheroma, blood disorders and small artery disease. This heterogeneity of causation makes it difficult to plan primary preventive measures, but treating hypertension and stopping smoking are to be strongly supported. Transient ischaemic attacks, which carry a 5% risk of becoming a full stroke within 12 months, should be treated with 300 mg of aspirin a day — a treatment not entirely without side-effects but which reduces the risk of stroke, myocardial infarction and death by about 30% (Warlow 1987).

The health visitor can do much to relieve the worry, anxiety and/or depression which are not uncommon features after strokes, as when the active member of the household, or the wage earner suddenly finds him or herself depending on others perhaps for the first time. The health visitor must encourage her client to be optimistic and try to be as independent of others as possible. The patient should be 'stretched' to make the maximum use of his/her capabilities. The specialised advice and help of the physiotherapist, occupational therapist and speech therapist can be a great help in this situation. The clients should be able to express their thoughts and to avoid suppressing feelings which can cause frustration. Relatives, too, will require patience, understanding and encouragement, as well as specialist advice about financial allowances which may be relevant. Both client and relatives may find it helpful to join a stroke club. The Chest, Heart and Stroke Association publishes useful leaflets (see Appendix 7 for address).

Clients may also worry about a recurrence of stroke. This is a possibility, but clients can help themselves by ceasing to smoke, reducing weight to normal and taking correctly any prescribed drugs. Optimism for the future should be maintained and clients should be encouraged to enjoy life without a fear of a possible future event.

The Parkinsonian patient

Unfortunately the cause of this disease is largely unknown, although some cases result from the use of phenothiazines or virus infections. The incidence increases with age, with a prevalence in those over 60 years greater than 1000 per 100 000 population. Since the introduction of L-dopa both the expectation and quality of life for the Parkinsonian patient has greatly increased.

The health visitor should be aware that, although the clinical features of the disease in the elderly are similar to those in younger patients, there are two exceptions. Classically patients have an impassive facial expression and a moderately flexed body posture with a slowness of movement and absence of arm swinging, leading to a shuffling gait with the short steps associated with difficulty in initiating movement. This, together with postural hypotension due to autonomic dysfunction, can result in frequent falls. However elderly patients frequently do not have the classical pill-rolling tremor of the hands, while some have impaired cognitive function typical of patients with Alzheimer's disease.

Treatment with physiotherapy and drugs is reserved for those with symptoms. Physiotherapy helps to build on improvements made by drugs, and restore confidence particularly after falls. Elderly patients, unlike younger ones, are usually started on L-dopa (usually in combination with a decarboxylase inhibitor). Other drugs such as bromocriptine, selegiline, amantidine and even anticholinergic drugs may be added later according to the patient's needs.

In 1982 the first brain transplants in the treatment of Parkinsonism were performed using adrenal medullary autografts since they produce large amounts of catecholamines. Many surgeons have not found the technique successful and 5% to 10% of patients have suffered serious side-effects. Consequently, foetal brain tissue transplant has been used instead. Initial results have shown some promise but the work is experimental and several problems need to be resolved (Lindwall 1988). Stereotactic thalamotomy for Parkinsonism is no longer performed because of serious late side-effects.

Health visitors have a valid role in monitoring the drug compliance and recognising adverse drug reaction. L-dopa, for example, can cause nausea, vomiting, postural hypotension, hallucinations and dyskinesia. Anticholinergic drugs frequently cause confusion.

Health visitors must be able to advise on general health, well-being, and diet. The latter should contain roughage to combat constipation. Frequent small helpings of food may overcome problems of chewing and swallowing. Clients should avoid becoming overweight, should take regular exercise to stretch stiff muscles but avoid becoming overtired. The health visitor must encourage optimism and motivation in order to help ward off depression. She should be prepared to ask the occupational therapist to advise when there are problems with the activities of daily living. Writing may become difficult, and it can be helpful to suggest the use of felt-tipped pens which can be lifted between each letter to make writing more legible. The speech therapist can offer valuable advice for those with speaking or swallowing difficulties (Bramble 1981). The Parkinson's Disease Society (see Appendix 7) has done much to help those suffering this disorder. It has established local support groups, and patients should be advised to make contact with one.

The elderly diabetic

These patients can present many problems for the health visitor, such as poor control of the disease due to illness, infections, or problems with diet and drug compliance, and the need for special care of the feet on account of peripheral vascular disease and neurological problems. Good diabetic control helps to restore the risk of complications, particularly those involving the nervous system.

Many elderly people with diabetes require only to adhere to a special diet, but this can require considerable self-discipline. An unnecessarily large intake of carbohydrate has to be avoided, although adequate amounts of fat, proteins, vitamins and fibre in the diet are required. Clients should maintain an ideal body weight, and obesity should be controlled or reduced. Adequate exercise is useful to help maintain good health and fitness, reduce weight and improve metabolic control.

Some elderly patients require additional oral antidiabetic drugs. Health visitors should help to maintain good drug compliance and they should be aware of side-effects. Chlorpropramide, for example, has a long duration of action and can produce non-specific symptoms of hypoglycaemia, such as confusion, disturbed consciousness and drowsiness. Drugs with a short duration action such as tolbutamide and glipizide are to be preferred.

A few elderly diabetics will need insulin. The health visitor should ensure that her client knows how, when, where and in what dosage the drug should be given. She should be sure that the patient can see and identify marks with a syringe. She and the client must be able to recognise the signs and symptoms of hypo- and hyperglycaemia.

Health visitors may be involved in monitoring diabetic control. Urine tests are least informative in the elderly, because of a raised renal threshold. Blood tests are more reliable, but measuring blood glucose by strip, read by eye or meter, though simple, requires accurate technique. The use of glycosylated HbA, to assess diabetic control during the previous month, is not yet widely available.

Elderly diabetics must be warned to take care of their toenails and the skin of their feet, especially if there is evidence of peripheral vascular disease. Comfortable shoes should be worn, the skin kept dry and clean, and any infection treated promptly. Smoking should be discouraged. Sore lesions on the feet may not be noticed until late if peripheral neuropathy is present with consequent reduction in pain sensation.

Visual impairment can occur in the elderly diabetic because of cataracts, retinopathy or other non-diabetic cause (see Ch. 10). Cataract is probably no more common in the elderly diabetic than non-diabetics, although *severe* cataracts requiring surgery are five times more common. Retinopathy is as frequent in the elderly as in younger diabetics, although 'malignant' retinopathy is less frequent. Unfortunately there is little evidence that good control of diabetes in the elderly improves the prognosis of diabetic retinopathy.

The osteo-arthritic client

It is well known that the incidence of osteo-arthritis increases with age, but fortunately many of those with a radiological evidence of arthritis do not have symptoms.

Osteo-arthritis is considered an exaggeration of ageing changes in the joints, particularly those which take the body weight, such as the hips, and osteo-arthritis of the knees can be associated with lateral instability due to disorganisation of the joint and laxity of the knee ligaments. Other joints, such as the shoulders, elbows and wrists may be involved, particularly if a person tends, for long periods of time, to lean heavily on a walking aid, thus putting much of the body weight through the shoulder joint.

The health visitor can assist in the management of clients with osteo-arthritis in three ways. First, she can help to ensure that the person gets adequate pain relief. Often an analgesic therapy is only taken irregularly, with resulting limited effectiveness. What is required is regular therapy to break the vicious cycle of pain — a fact which the health visitor can emphasise. Aspirin and paracetamol are often quite effective for mild pain but other non-steroidal anti-inflammatory drugs (NSAIDs) or even indomethacin may be used for moderate to severe pain. Gastric ulceration and gastrointestinal bleeding can follow the use of NSAIDs, so the health visitor should be alert for symptoms of indigestion and/or anaemia. Second, she can suggest physiotherapy to improve joint movement and muscle strength. Third, she may be able to assist the client's motivation to reach a normal weight. Clearly, excessive weight can only exacerbate arthritic joint problems, and removal of unnecessary pounds or stones cannot but be advantageous. Unfortunately, losing weight is easier said than done — as many know! If these measures fail and the patient is in such pain that it impairs quality of life and mobility, then referral for possible surgery has to be considered. In such cases the health visitor has the supportive role pre-operatively and may be involved in some supervision and aftercare convalescence. Close liaison with district nurses is also necessary.

Hospital treatment and aftercare

An increasing number of older people are being admitted to hospital for treatment in various specialties. Health visitors therefore have an increasing part to play in pre- and post-hospital visiting. When admission is planned, it is helpful if a home visit can be paid to prepare the person, deal with any questions of anxieties and provide them with appropriate information. There is much evidence to suggest that those receiving adequate information beforehand benefit and are more likely to do well. Furthermore, comprehensive assessment of personal and social conditions can also prove helpful to hospital staff, assisting their decision making and outpatient care. However, it is the post-discharge period which is so important, since the health visitor can often monitor progress and so facilitate client rehabilitation. Not all clients require clinical nurse care but may benefit from health education and encouragement, guidance and supervision. Through evaluating client and carer needs and taking action to meet these, it is often possible to prevent readmission.

A number of geriatric units already have liaison schemes in operation, but the follow-up of older persons from other specialties is less likely to be routine. It is particularly helpful for a health visitor to scrutinise the attendance of older people at accident and emergency departments, (see Ch. 6, p. 139–140). Not only can they help to follow up such clients, they may often be able to identify precipitating causes, especially for accidents or social situations which need exploration and action. This is an area ripe for professional development. Expansion of a post-discharge health visiting service is likely to increase demands dramatically, but may well be justified in terms of improved quality of life and the possible reduction in the number of elderly people readmitted to hospital. Collaboration within general practice teams can make such a service feasible and can weld hospital and community staffs together in the care of the clients.

SUMMARY

This chapter has reviewed the important ways in which illness can present in the elderly. The differences between disease in the young and the old have been explained. Keen observation by the health visitor can frequently identify the cause of a non-specific illness. She can also, by early intervention, prevent situations developing into crises.

APPENDIX

Mental test questionnaire

It would be very useful to assess a client's mental state. A simple test of memory and orientation can reveal gross impairment in those who may superficially pass for normal. An example is given below (Denham & Jefferys 1972).

- What is your name?

- What is your age?
- What is your address?
- What is your marital status?
- What was your previous job or what did you do before your marriage?
- What year is it now?
- I would like you to try to remember an address for me. I will repeat it twice, and then I will ask you what it is in a minute: 74 Columbia Road.
- In what years did the Second World War start and finish?
- Who were the British Prime Ministers at the beginning and during that war?
- What is the name of the present Prime Minister?
- What is the Queen's name?
- What is the name of the Prince of Wales?
- Where is Belfast?
- What is happening there?
- What was the address I have just given you?

These are 16 questions which do not take long to ask and do not usually lose a person's concentration. The key questions are the person's name and where he or she lives. If the client is a mobile wanderer, he/she can easily get lost once away from familiar local environment.

The test enables progress of a confusional state to be monitored, but it does *not* distinguish a toxic confusional state from a dementing process, it only indicates impairment of cognitive function. Scores correlate well with incontinence/continence and rehabilitation potential. Low scorers tend to be incontinent and take a long time to rehabilitate, because of lack of understanding (Denham & Jefferys 1972). False or misleading low scores occur in patients who are deaf, dysphasic or depressed. Clearly, many questions cannot be appropriately applied to those of non-British background.

REFERENCES

Bramble M G 1981 Dysphagia in Parkinsons Disease — another manifestation of dopamine–acetyl choline imbalance. In: Clifford Rose C and Capildeo R (eds) Research progress in Parkinsons Disease. Pitman Medical, Edinburgh

Clarke A N G, Manakakar G D, Gray I 1975 Diogenes Syndrome: a clinical study of gross neglect in old age. Lancet 1: 366–368

Collins K J 1989 Hypothermia in seasonal mortality in the elderly. Care of the elderly 1: 257–259

Deary I J, Whalley L J 1988 Recent research on the causes of Alzheimer's disease. British Medical Journal 297: 807–809

Denham M J 1990 Adverse drug reactions. In: Denham M J, George C F (eds) Drugs in old age: new perspectives. Churchill Livingstone, Edinburgh

Denham M J, Jefferys P M 1972 Routine mental testing in the elderly. Modern Geriatrics 2: 275–278

Gilhooley L M 1984 Social dimensions of dementia. In: Hanley I, Hodge J (eds) Psychological approaches to the care of the elderly. Croom Helm, London

Harris D W, Karandikas D S, Spencer M G et al 1979 Returned medicines campaign in Birmingham in 1977. Lancet 1: 599

Hurwitz N 1969 Predisposing factors in adverse reactions to drugs. British Medical Journal 1: 536–539

Lindwall O 1988 Brain implant — clinical aspects. In: Chemistry or Surgery, a symposium organised by Parkinson's Disease Society

Seidl L A, Thornton G F, Smith J W, Cluff L E 1966 Studies of the epidemiology of adverse drug reactions. Bulletin of the Johns Hopkins Hospital 119: 299–315

Thomas T M, Plymat K R, Blannin J, Meade T W 1980 Prevalence of urinary incontinence. British Medical Journal 281: 1243–1245

Viswanathan C T, Welling P G 1984 Food effects on drug absorption in the elderly. In: Roe D A (ed) Drugs and nutrition in the geriatric patient. Churchill Livingstone, Edinburgh

Warlow C 1987 Anti-thrombotic drugs and the prevalence of stroke. In: Verstraete M, Vermylen J, Lijnen H R, Arnout J (eds) Thrombosis and haemostasis. International Society on Thrombosis and Haemostasis. Leuven University Press, Leuven

Williamson J, Chopin J M 1980 Adverse reactions to prescribed drugs in the elderly: a multicentre investigation. Age & Ageing 9: 73–80

CHAPTER CONTENTS

10

Caring for older people with special needs

All older people undergo some decrement; hence they experience varying degrees of loss, whether related to functional capacity or social contact. However, for some older people, disability, social isolation, deprivation or discrimination can take a heavy toll, creating particular difficulties and hence special needs.

In this chapter we review some of these difficulties and needs, with particular reference to the health visiting role, and consider services which can be mobilised to help affected and vulnerable older clients or their families.

The particular groups examined include those older people who are

- physically impaired, disabled or handicapped
- sensorily disabled, or
- psychologically disturbed.

We also consider the special needs of older people in ethnic minority groups, as well as the elderly abused.

Although the promotion of the health of carers is considered in Chapter 8, the particular needs of those looking after disabled, deprived, or disturbed adults cannot be divorced from those of their dependants; hence they are mentioned here. If this creates some overlap we offer no apology, since it is unlikely that the needs of carers will thereby be over-estimated.

OLDER PEOPLE WHO ARE PHYSICALLY IMPAIRED, DISABLED, OR HANDICAPPED

The last two decades have seen growing international interest in the welfare of physically impaired persons. Events which have fuelled this interest include:

1. the Alma Ata declaration, setting out the goal of 'Health for all by the year 2000' (WHO 1978)
2. the Report of the Working Group on the prevention of disability in the elderly (WHO 1981a)
3. the International Year of the Disabled Person, 1981
4. the First International Conference on Health Promotion, Ottawa, Canada (1986)
5. the Report on The Health of the Elderly (WHO 1989).

A stride forward in the epidemiology of disability came with the publication by WHO (1980) of The International Classification of Impairments, Disabilities and Handicaps (ICIDH). This made it possible to compare data between countries, hence highlighting similarities or differences in incidence and prevalence. It also clarified nomenclature, defining:

- impairment, . . . as any loss or abnormality of psychological, physiological, or anatomical structure or function
- disability, . . . as any restriction or lack of ability (resulting from an impairment) to perform an activity in the manner, or within the range, considered normal for a human being
- handicap, . . . as any disadvantage for a given individual, resulting from an impairment or a disability, that limits or prevents the fulfilment of a role that is normal (depending on age, social and/or cultural factors) for that individual.

The significance of these definitions is that, although impairments can arise from several causes (viz hereditary disorder or acquired injury or disease), which may, or may not, be preventable, they need *not* proceed to disability, and they certainly *need not* constitute handicap. Grasping this important concept allows action to be directed towards stopping progression at any one stage. Thus, while the introduction of certain health practices may limit subsequent disability among older people, as research shows (Branch 1985), the improvement of the organisation of health and social services for those at risk of being disabled could make a major contribution to their quality of life (Royal College of Physicians 1986).

PREVALENCE STUDIES OF IMPAIRMENT AND DISABILITY IN BRITAIN

To adequately understand the needs of older disabled persons, one must first locate them within the total context of disability. In Britain the most recent prevalence studies of disability were undertaken in 1985–8 (OPCS 1988a). The findings of this research were eagerly awaited, because no national survey had been undertaken since the Harris study 1969–1971 (Harris 1971). This earlier study had focused on impairments among the adult population only, whereas the 1985–8 survey covered disabled children as well, and compared those living in private households with those in communal establishments. It also examined the problems of disabled persons in a more extensive way, thus it provided more realistic estimates. The objectives of the study were:

- to provide comprehensive estimates of disability by age, severity and type of disability
- to derive information about the social and financial consequences of disability, sources and levels of income, and the effects of disability on mobility and employment
- to examine the use of, and need for, health and social services.

In line with the ICIDH the 1985–8 survey defined disability as

> a restriction or lack of ability to perform normal activity, which has resulted from the impairment of a structure, or function of body or mind.
>
> (OPCS Report 1 1988a)

Hence the survey focused on the *results* of an impairment — at what persons could *not do*, in terms of everyday activity, rather than on the precise nature of their disabilities.

Viewing disability as a continuum, ranging from slight to severe, a threshold was determined, below which persons with certain impairments were excluded from the study. These included persons who, because of the use of medications, aids or appliances, were able to restrict the extent to which disability affected their lives: e.g. controlled diabetics, or epileptics. Such decisions raised contradictory criticism. Official reaction argued that the threshold was set too low. Conversely, disablement groups protested that under-estimation occurred, because:

- Northern Ireland was excluded from the study — an important omission
- the threshold excluded persons who nevertheless incur considerable disability-related expenditure
- the methods used (large scale structured interviews) were an insensitive way of eliciting disability-related expenditure
- the survey assumed that it is possible to assign a strict monetary value to all the extra costs associated with disability. This assumption, it is argued, ignored the difficulties disabled persons have in isolating 'normal' from 'extra' expenditure on items such as heating, lighting and food; did not take account of the limitations on costs for those disabled on low income; and disregarded the hidden costs of 'lost' opportunities in employment, mobility, bargain hunting, or 'shopping around'.

Nevertheless, in spite of these varied objections, the 1985–8 study provided valuable information. For instance, it identified ten main areas of disability: namely, Behaviour, Communication, Continence, Dexterity, Hearing, Intellectual functioning, Locomotion, Personal care, Reaching and stretching, Seeing. It also identified, through a complex system of scoring, and comparison within and between groups, ten categories of severity, where Category 1 = least severe disablement; Category 10 = most severe disablement. Overall prevalence estimates were then deduced.

DISABILITY PREVALENCE ESTIMATES

There are an estimated *6.2 million* disabled adults in Great Britain — that is, 14% of the total adult population. 5.8 million of these live in private households and one-third of these are in the higher severity categories (Fig. 10.1). By contrast, the 422 000 disabled adults living in communal establishments are almost all classified as severely disabled.

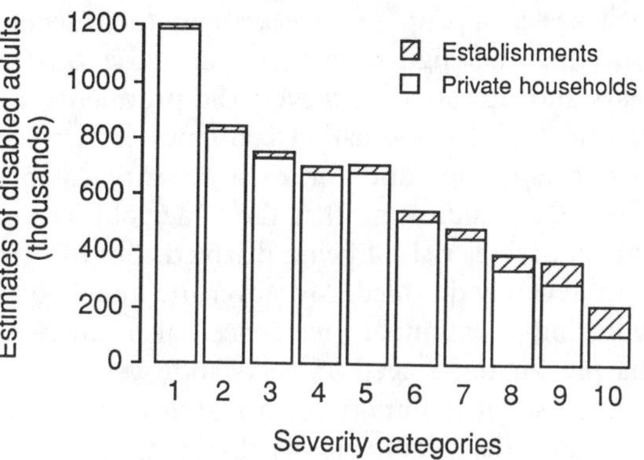

Fig. 10.1 Estimates of numbers of disabled adults, in private households, and in communal establishments, shown by severity category. (Source: OPCS 1988a; Crown Copyright.)

Ageing and disability

The relationship between disability and age, noted by Harris, was confirmed in the 1985–8 study. *69% of all disabled adults were 60 years or over (4.2 million persons).* The absolute numbers increase in

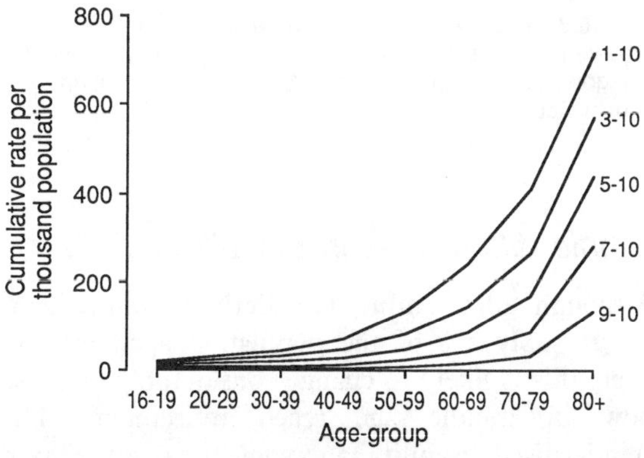

Fig. 10.2 Age and disability: estimates of prevalence of disability among adults in Great Britain, by age and severity category. (Source: OPCS 1988a; Crown Copyright.)

each age group up to 79 years and then decline, reflecting the higher mortality in those aged 80 years and upwards. However, the prevalence rate per 1000 of the population continues to rise with each age group, and for each severity category (Fig. 10.2), indicating that the 'older old' are not only at greater risk of being disabled, but of being more severely disabled. Moreover the likelihood of requiring communal residence also increases sharply for those aged 85 years and over.

Even so, it is important to realise that the majority of older people are *not* disabled.

Sex disparity in disability

There are more disabled women than men (3.5 million women compared with 2.5 million men) (Fig. 10.3). This disparity is due to the preponderance of women in older age groups, especially those aged 75 years and over (see Ch. 1, pp. 5–6).

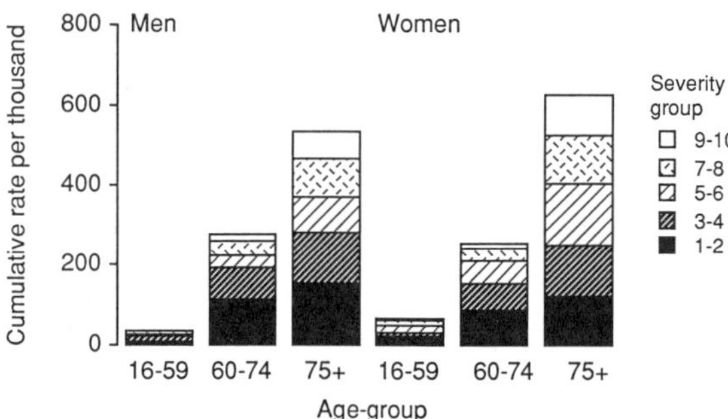

Fig. 10.3 Age, sex and disability: estimates of prevalence of disability among adults, by age and severity category, for men and women. (Source: OPCS 1988a; Crown Copyright.)

Ethnic differences in disability

Although ethnic minority elderly currently contribute only 4% of the population aged 60 and over, this is likely to change considerably as those now in middle age reach retirement. The standardised disability rates show the risk variation for each group:

- Whites 137 per 1000 population
- Asians 126 per 1000 population
- Afro-Caribbeans 151 per 1000 population,

indicating vulnerability which health visitors will wish to note.

Social class differences in disability prevalence

Various studies demonstrate a social class relationship with disability — a preponderance occurring in lower socio-economic groups, irrespective of downward social mobility as a consequence of disability (The Black Report, DHSS 1980, Townsend & Davidson 1982).

Regional variation in disability prevalence

There is considerable regional variation in disability prevalence. Standardised rates show that Northern England, Wales, Yorkshire and Humberside have higher levels than do the South, East, South-East and South-West of England. Scotland has high absolute numbers, because of a higher elderly population, but the standardised rates are around the mean (see Table 10.1).

Implications for practice

Health visitors will note the need for further research, as highlighted by these sex, ethnic, social class and regional variations. They will also be aware of the challenge posed by an older disabled population, weighted to females. Practitioners can expect to find two-fifths of their older clients with some form of disability, with this proportion rising among the 'oldest old'. This is important when considering assessment, because older persons tend to attribute their difficulties to 'old age', and hence may not mention their limitations. Such an attitude needs to be dispelled when treatment and help is available.

Of further interest is the grading of disabilities by type. The six main types found in the Prevalence Survey were:

- locomotor difficulties (affecting 4 million adults of all ages)

Table 10.1 Estimates of prevalence of disability among adults, by region and severity category, (cumulative rate per thousand population)

Severity Category	North	Yorks and Humberside	North West	East Midlands	West Midlands	East Anglia	GLC	South East	South West	Wales	Scotland	Great Britain
	In private households (cumulative rate per thousand)											
10	2	2	3	2	3	0	2	2	4	5	2	2
9–10	10	9	10	8	9	8	7	8	9	14	10	9
8–10	17	18	16	14	18	15	17	15	18	22	18	17
7–10	31	27	25	23	31	27	27	24	31	34	28	27
6–10	45	39	37	35	43	36	37	35	41	53	40	39
5–10	64	58	52	50	59	51	51	50	56	71	58	55
4–10	83	74	70	65	75	61	61	65	73	93	76	71
3–10	108	92	88	81	91	81	76	79	91	114	94	88
2–10	130	114	105	99	112	100	94	95	110	138	116	107
1–10	162	148	130	128	135	127	117	124	135	164	147	135
1–10 standardised for age	162	148	131	131	141	123	119	123	124	160	131	135
	Total population (cumulative rate per thousand)											
10	4	4	6	6	4	1	4	5	7	8	4	5
9–10	13	13	15	14	12	10	11	13	15	19	12	13
8–10	21	23	23	21	22	18	22	21	25	27	21	22
7–10	35	33	32	31	35	30	33	31	39	41	31	33
6–10	50	46	45	44	48	39	44	43	50	60	44	46
5–10	69	65	60	60	64	55	58	58	65	77	61	62
4–10	87	82	79	76	80	65	69	73	83	100	80	78
3–10	112	100	96	91	96	85	84	87	101	121	98	95
2–10	134	122	113	109	116	104	102	104	121	145	120	114
1–10	166	156	139	138	139	130	125	132	145	170	151	142

Source: OPCS 1988a; Crown Copyright.

- hearing problems (affecting some 2.5 million)
- personal care difficulties (affecting some 2.5 million)
- dexterity difficulties
- seeing problems and reaching and stretching difficulties
- continence and communication difficulties.

Older persons followed this general pattern. It will be readily appreciated that many persons have multiple difficulties.

Such a list serves to highlight the type of problems with which clients and carers have to cope, as well as the knowledge areas with which workers must be familiar.

Major conditions causing disability

Differentiated from the types of difficulties were the conditions causing disability. These followed a similar pattern to the Harris survey 16 years earlier, viz:

- arthritis and rheumatism (all forms)
- circulatory disorders
- ear conditions (mainly deafness)
- eye conditions (mainly cataract and senile macular degeneration)
- neurological disorders (especially stroke, Parkinson's disease and epilepsy)
- respiratory disorder, chiefly bronchitis and or emphysema.

This list also serves as a guide to practitioners, concerning the knowledge areas they will be required to utilise most often. It also indicates areas for further research.

Disabled adults living alone

All disabilities which restrict mobility and flexibil-

Table 10.2 Percentage of older disabled adults living alone, in each age group, shown by sex distribution

Disabled persons	*Age groups* 65–74	75+
Men	16%	26%
Women	41%	58%

Based on data from OPCS 1988a; Crown copyright

ity can create problems in the activities of living, but clearly these are of greater significance for those living alone (see Table 10.2).

Both the Harris study (1971) and the Prevalence of Disability Study (OPCS 1988a) showed that 30% of all disabled adults live alone, 11% of these being in severity category 9 or 10. This proportion is exceeded for disabled older women. The OPCS survey showed that 16% of disabled men and 19% of disabled women, aged 75 years or more, living alone, were also housebound. Their vulnerability is thus demonstrated.

The informal carers of disabled adults

In all, some 4 million informal helpers were found, in the survey, to be involved in the care of disabled adults, living in private households; 1.25 million of these were identified as '**main carers**', and 40% of these were 65 years or more. This reinforces the point that it is often the elderly who care for the old. Even so, it is estimated that 44% of all disabled adults have no identified carer.

Although there may be slight variation in the findings between this study and the General Household Survey of Informal Carers, mentioned in Chapter 8, taken together the figures provide a more comprehensive picture than was previously available.

- Approximately 75% of the informal carers of disabled adults are relatives (OPCS 1989). Over 1 million reported that they give 'personal care' to their relative, in addition to their other caring duties.
- 42% of 'main carers' spend all day and periods at night caring for their dependant, 12% having done so for 15 or more years.

This reinforces the all-pervasive nature of disability, although statistics cannot capture the full essence of this.

The case studies of Mr Day and Miss Brown may convey something of the pressures encountered by sufferers and carers alike.

CASE STUDIES

Mr Peter Day was 66 years old when he developed spastic paralysis and became immobile. Due to an associated arteriosclerotic dementia he gradually became unable to communicate, had great difficulty in swallowing, was doubly incontinent and had bouts of uncontrollable shouting. His wife Louisa, herself a pensioner, cared devotedly for him for 7 years.

Apart from general practitioner services, she received limited other help. During this time she had no holidays, was not offered respite care, and was rarely able to go out for personal purposes. She had to shop at a nearby corner store, with a limited range of goods.

Finally worn out by disturbed nights, constant lifting of her husband and frequent washing of incontinent laundry, she consented to Peter's hospital admission. However, when Mr Day died 3 weeks later, his wife was stricken with remorse and suffered guilt and depression for some time.

Miss Emily Brown, aged 82 years, housebound and severely crippled from arthritis, lived alone in a ground floor flat. She had great difficulty washing herself, cooking, or carrying out domestic cleaning. Her married niece, who had five young children to care for, travelled 90 miles each fortnight to undertake her aunt's washing, major cleaning and 'stand-by' cooking. Even though her niece's husband complained that these trips detracted attention from the family, Miss Brown's niece felt it 'was her duty' to continue to visit regularly. This placed considerable strain on marital relationships.

THE HEALTH VISITING ROLE IN RELATION TO DISABILITY

Primary prevention

The major part of the health visitor's role in disability lies in the area of primary prevention. Therefore the longer-term reduction of problems among older people must begin with disability prevention in the earlier years. By encouraging optimum pre-conceptual and antenatal care; promoting healthy growth and development in infancy and childhood, adolescence and young adulthood; contributing to accident prevention and inculcating healthy lifestyles, health visitors can help to prevent disabling conditions. The health visiting principles of stimulating an awareness of health needs and facilitating health-enhancing activities, are paramount (see Ch. 4, p. 69).

Secondary prevention

Where primary preventive efforts have failed to eliminate predisposing conditions and impairment has occurred, early detection, prompt treatment and ongoing surveillance are required. The value of epidemiological studies and prevalence data is that they indicate who is at risk of developing more serious problems, when, where and, often, why. They thus help health visitors to apply the concept of vulnerability, through the exercise of case-finding and surveillance skills.

Considerable health education may have to be undertaken before clients are convinced of the need to take action on pre-symptomatic conditions, or before harmful lifestyles are discarded. However, it is only by teaching, persuasion and encouragement that health promotion is 'marketed', and the conditions causing disability can be controlled.

Tertiary prevention

Although tertiary prevention is not the major part of health visiting work with disabled persons, in the context of this chapter it receives more detailed attention. It is the level of activity engaged in when frank disablement has occurred, and it seeks to reduce the effects by providing amelioration, support and rehabilitation.

To function effectively in this aspect of their role, health visitors endeavour to

- appreciate the effects of disability from their clients' and client-carers' perspective
- assess clients' and carers' needs, offering guidance on ways of meeting these, and providing information and marshalling services as necessary
- ascertain clients' and carers' coping strategies, strengthening these so that optimum functioning is maintained. Supplementary strategies are activated as indicated.

Appreciating the physical effects of impairment and disability

Whereas minor impairments are frequently well tolerated and sufferers may regard them as challenges, severe disabling states impose greater limitations, frequently causing immobility. In turn every body system is then affected. Practitioners require a comprehensive grasp of the pathophysiological processes involved, so that they can offer appropriate information and empathetic guidance. This may include information on the modification of exercise, guidance on the most effective forms of moving and the postural, breathing, nutritional and hygiene measures necessary to prevent stasis and infection.

Impact is clearly related to both the severity of the disability and its extent. Hence there is a need to consider the nature and the course of disorders. Some conditions, such as stroke, occur with devastating suddenness, but the initial effects may subsequently improve. Other conditions may be progressively deteriorating. Some have an insidious onset, allowing time for gradual adjustment. Others may be superimposed on existing disorders, creating multiple problems. A few conditions may be terminal. Because of these variations, reactions will accordingly differ. Individual differences in pre-morbid personality and sociocultural attitudes and expectations, will also colour responses. They need to be taken fully into account when endeavouring to understand client perspectives.

The physical effects of dependency on older carers should also be considered. Gross fatigue, or muscular and joint damage arising from strain or faulty lifting, are common. These call for teaching and demonstrating skills, and the location of suitable aids to avoid injury. Moreover, it is important to realise that the physical restrictions imposed by the disability often create the distressing psychosocial concomitants. Hence, enabling clients to reduce the physical effects of disability and maximise movement and independence will likely have multiple benefit.

Understanding and appreciating the psychosocial effects of physical disability

For many older persons the emotional and social effects of physical disability are profound. Chronic pain, altered body-image, restriction of movement, and/or enforced dependence, can cause biographic disruption and a sense of loss of self (Bury 1982, Charmaz 1983, Nichols 1984, Wade et al 1985, Twining 1988).

Cherished plans may have to be abandoned and notions of reciprocal support reviewed. Roles often have to be reversed and lifestyles drastically reconstructed. In consequence, self-esteem may be lowered, or ego-identity distorted, depending partly on the nature of the disability and partly on the reactions it provokes from others. Because drives and expectations are forcibly altered, older disabled adults often feel hurt or distressed. Then reactions such as grief, anxiety, despair, apathy, regression or hostility are not uncommon.

On a social level, enforced isolation can generate suspicion, although many disabled people have high resilience and adapt, philosophically. Nevertheless, research studies support a strong association between physical handicap and psychological morbidity.

Helping older disabled persons to ventilate feelings

Health visitors will realise that unless affected older people are given opportunity to ventilate their feelings in a safe, confidential, non-emotive relationship, and mourn for the abilities they have lost, they will not be able to constructively apply themselves to problem-solving. Then the rehabilitative approaches of health visitors and others will pass unheeded. Appropriate counselling needs to be available to facilitate adjustment and prevent undue dwelling on negative perceptions (Twining 1988).

Assessment of needs and resources

Assessment begins where the client is. This is vital when deciding how best to proceed. While it follows general principles, certain specifics should be noted. Subjective data are highly relevant, since they convey clients' and carers' perceptions and expectations. Objective data are best obtained unobtrusively, to provide as accurate and distortion-free a picture as possible. The model chosen will guide the format of the assessment — directing planning. Thus if mobility, flexibility and dexterity are major problems, goals set will likely focus on maximising functional ability. Then the Activities of Living Model may be selected (see Ch. 5, pp. 387–388). If self-care is the major purpose, then it may be preferable to use Orem's model (see Appendix 3). This model requires that the abilities of older disabled adults are identified, deficits in self-care determined, and decisions taken with client as to the action needed to bridge the gap (Orem 1980). If stress-adaptation is considered a major goal, then Roy's adaptation model, or The Neuman Model, may be preferred (see Ch. 5, pp. 388–389 and Appendix 3). Nevertheless, whichever, model is chosen, the following points need to be observed.

Gait, posture and locomotion

Practitioners should note the ability of older disabled adults to change position, sit, stand, and/or walk with or without help; balance, bend, carry, climb stairs, handle prescribed aids, kneel, pick up objects and return to position. The range of joint movements possible, the presence of crepitus, pain, tremor, gait abnormalities, or inco-ordination should be noted. Especially is this necessary in connection with actions requiring flexibility and dexterity.

Discovering client-perceptions concerning their body-image may reveal how far these are distorted by pain, postural problems, or the use of appliances. The comprehensive information gained from careful analysis of such data will highlight the type and nature of teaching and help required.

Eating and drinking

In order to meet clients' individual needs, and deal with specific problems, practitioners need to determine the older disabled adult's ability to chew, taste, swallow, and retain substances. How far the client can handle crockery and cutlery, cut up food, safely shop for and prepare meals, or cook, should be ascertained. In addition the ability of any informal carer to prepare, serve and adequately supervise meals, should be noted.

Eliminating

Problems of elimination, met with in ageing, are often exacerbated when disability is present. Although the focus is on promoting maximum independence, assisted independence, using aids, may be the achieved level.

Identifying problems is a sensitive issue, but it is necessary to obtain accurate and detailed information about how clients' and carers' manage the disabled person's toilet arrangements and if problems such as constipation, incontinence, or retention are being experienced. Assessment of skin condition, and associated information on skin care, is clearly related.

Care must be taken to ascertain available resources, such as washing machines or tumble dryers. In ascertaining clients' and carers' coping mechanisms, it is necessary to discover how *they think they can best be helped*. Information on incontinent laundry services, and/or the provision of protective devices, may be welcomed. In this connection, in the recent Disability Prevalence Survey, *10%* of disabled adults said they did not know where to find information on any services, and a further *8%* were unaware of how to obtain laundry services; *2%* considered they required an incontinent laundry service which they were not receiving.

Personal hygiene and dressing

As part of the general assessment of disabled adults, attention should be directed towards clients' ability to wash, bath, shower, shave, brush and comb hair, cope with oral hygiene, undertake foot and nail care and apply make-up if used.

Similarly it is necessary to observe the ability of clients to dress independently, manage fastenings, cope with hosiery and footwear, or put on special appliances such as elastic stockings, supports or prostheses. Frequently benefit is lost because prescribed aids or appliances cannot be fitted properly, especially when clients live alone.

Because multiple disabilities are common, it is important to note that even when dexterity and flexibility are present, poor sight may restrict personal hygiene, dressing and other activities.

Maintaining safety

While all the accident prevention measures outlined in Chapter 8 apply equally to older disabled adults, certain safety features are crucial. They include discovering

- how immobile clients, especially those living alone, could escape in the event of fire, flood or similar disaster
- the degree of vulnerability of different disabled adults to criminal attack
- what alarm systems are available to attract attention in the case of any accident
- what hazard control measures are available in relation to movement about the home, such as by wheelchair, or on foot using aids.

Similarly one should ascertain what measures are used to prevent/reduce risks to the older disabled adult when entering or leaving cars; using public transport; or obtaining access to public buildings.

Environmental and domestic hygiene

The ability of older disabled adults to adequately clean their domestic settings, dispose effectively of food debris, or other waste products, and manage personal and household laundry, should also be noted. This should be judged in the light of available amenities, and may prove a crucial point when client carers are themselves elderly and frail.

Communicating

The extent to which disabled older persons can interact and communicate can affect the quality of their entire life. Hence it is necessary to determine levels of sight, hearing and speech, as well as the capacity for touch, writing, using a telephone, and/or any other technical assistance available.

Patient-operated selector mechanisms are becoming increasingly sophisticated, so it is necessary to make sure older disabled persons who are issued with such equipment are competent in operating it.

Furthermore it is important to assess with whom, and with how many persons, clients interact; the quality and perceived value of such contact; and the personal perceptions disabled clients have of their social support systems. Such networks appear vital in promoting positive attitudes and may be highly relevant in view of the proportion of elderly disabled persons who live alone (see Table 10.2), and the 11% of these who are also housebound.

Helpful insights on the centrality of communication in human experience are provided by MacLeod Clark (1985), Le May & Redfern (1987) and Redfern (1989).

Expressing sexuality

Because of the constraints posed by specific impairments, there may be particular, associated sexual difficulties. The Association for Sexual Problems of The Disabled (SPOD) is always willing to give personal advice (see Appendix 7 for their address).

By appraising gender awareness, and relating this to observed behaviour and communications from the client and/or carer, practitioners can determine the ability of older disabled adults to maintain satisfying and appropriate emotional, social and sexual relationships (see Lewis 1985).

Sleeping routines

Although all the points about promoting healthy sleep apply equally to older disabled adults (see Ch. 8, pp. 202–203) sleep disorders may be more common for them. Such difficulties can prove a source of anxiety to clients and may create problems for carers. It is therefore always necessary to ascertain the type and amount of sleep obtained, preferred sleeping positions in relation to the underlying disorder, and usual rest routines. Medications should be particularly noted, along with the effects they have upon sleep patterns.

Other factors

Assessment should also include consideration of client coping mechanisms and the efforts taken to overcome the effects of disability. This is where determining levels of self-efficacy, and ascertaining client beliefs and the health locus of control, may be particularly useful in guiding rehabilitative strategies (Ch. 8, pp. 178–181). Following assessment a full report is necessary, to establish a baseline for planning purposes. This enables relevant and feasible goals to be selected, strategies to be defined, progress to be monitored and evaluation undertaken.

Others can use the documentation, within the limits of confidentiality, to gain an awareness of client needs and to determine the rationale of care. The degree of the disabled client's and his/her carer's participation in assessment and subsequent planning, as well as the practitioner's accountability, should be well differentiated.

Intervention following assessment

Intervention is, as always, multi-focused, with practitioners working at individual, group and community level.

Individual level

Here action is directed towards facilitating adjustment, and helping client and carer overcome the effects of disability as far as possible, through enhancing residual ability. Inculcating positive attitudes, providing practical guidance, and strengthening adaptive coping mechanisms form the mainstay of interventions. Raising client self-esteem, assisting clients to acquire compensatory skills, and mobilising practical aid and appropriate services, are undertaken as indicated.

The desirable goal is of course *'renormalisation'*. This allows older disabled adults to adjust to physical changes, modify their activity, work through their reactions to grief and loss, and accept dependency and the help of others where appropriate.

Sometimes older disabled adults slow their pace inappropriately and become over-dependent. This can sometimes be encouraged by over-solicitous carers, requiring health visitors to use tact and skill in guiding both client and carer to modify behaviour. While recognising the right of older disabled clients to choose passivity if they so wish, encouraging an attitude of 'non-acceptance' may halt regressive tendencies and thus enable clients to fight back.

Guidance may be provided by maximising functional capacity, such as maintaining independence in dressing through modification to clothing. Front-opening garments, velcro fasteners, wrap-round skirts and drop-front trousers may enable some disabled persons to cope alone.

Other helpful items include clip-on braces; ready-made ties or bows on elastic; capes rather than sleeved coats; elastic shoe laces; dressing sticks; hosiery tongs; long-handled pickup sticks; and zip aids.

Information may be given on aids such as sponges or hairbrushes on long or angled sticks; loofahs on straps; or long roller towels fixed to walls on flexible rubber rails, to facilitate drying.

Some older disabled adults become adept at preparing their own food if provided with raised-edge or spiked boards, utensils with suction-cup bases, or non-slip mats. Adapted can openers can be found, while metal sieves or steamers obviate the need to strain cooked vegetables, so reducing the risk of scalding.

Other ways of enhancing remaining ability include teapot pouring stands; devices on taps to aid turning; split level hobs to enable wheelchairs to be used during cooking; and the use of oven-to-table ware.

Where disabled older adults have problems in manipulation, thick rubber tubing can build up handles on cutlery or other implements. Velcro straps can attach cutlery to frail wrists; flexible angled straws facilitate drinking; small walking trolleys or shoppers-on-wheels enable some disabled elderly persons to transport things from room to room. Ramps may replace steps; while household goods may be stored in swing-out baskets, to make them more accessible. Stair lifts may be fitted, enabling greater mobility and independence.

Interventions at group level

At group level, techniques may change. Within groups, instigating and initiating skills and stimulating awareness may come to the fore, as practitioners unobtrusively activate groups of disabled adults towards self-help. Raising their consciousness about what is available, or can be achieved, may be more affective than taking overt action oneself.

The range of self-help groups is extensive. A comprehensive guide is provided by Knight & Gann (1988). Specific health promotion measures are often best introduced on a group basis, as peer-support can prove very effective in reinforcing effort.

Intervention at community level

At the community level it is necessary to create an awareness of the needs of disabled people, and their helpers, so that a caring, supportive environment prevails. Enabling community members to appraise and develop resources for older disabled persons is a very worthwhile task. It involves working closely with voluntary organisations and community groups, co-operating in joint ventures to benefit disabled people, and acting as a resource for those who wish to introduce community initiatives.

The influence principle is thus strongly utilised, with practitioners adopting an advocacy role.

Co-operating with other workers

Occupational therapists

Among their many functions these paramedical

Table 10.3 Proportion of disabled adults who had seen different health professionals in the year prior to the Disability Survey interview, by severity category and age: adults living in private households

Health professional seen	*Age 16–49*						*Age 50–64*					
	Severity category					All disabled adults	Severity category					All disabled adults
	1–2	3–4	5–6	7–8	9–10		1–2	3–4	5–6	7–8	9–10	
	Percentage of disabled adults who had seen each health professional											
Consultant or hospital doctor	45	50	55	58	64	51	45	51	56	63	64	51
Hospital nurse	18	19	22	32	30	22	19	22	20	25	33	21
Physiotherapist	10	12	12	17	16	12	7	13	16	20	33	13
Occupational therapist[a]	2	3	6	9	14	5	1	2	3	7	17	3
Radiologist[b]	14	14	16	19	16	16	18	22	21	24	25	20
Dietician	4	4	5	7	6	5	4	5	8	7	12	6
Speech therapist	0	0	0	2	2	1	0	0	0	2	4	1
Hearing therapist[c]	4	3	1	2	2	2	3	2	2	3	2	2
Optician or oculist	2	2	2	4	6	2	3	3	2	5	6	3
Hospital social worker	2	3	5	6	9	4	1	1	2	6	10	2
Artificial limb/appliance fitter	2	3	2	3	3	2	1	2	3	4	9	2
Psychologist/psychotherapist	5	8	8	7	7	7	2	1	3	2	4	2
General practitioner	70	75	78	81	77		80	84	86	90	90	84
Chiropodist	1	1	2	4	7	2	2	3	6	10	20	5
Health visitor	2	5	7	11	12	6	1	2	4	8	20	3
Community nurse	4	7	10	15	30	9	4	7	9	15	46	9
Osteopath/homeopath[d]	5	5	7	8	9	6	4	4	5	9	4	5
Any of the above	78	84	88	89	93	84	84	90	93	95	97	89
Base:	*621*	*476*	*424*	*248*	*101*	*1870*	*964*	*635*	*454*	*256*	*108*	*2417*
	Age 65–74						*Age 75 and over*					
Consultant or hospital doctor	38	45	47	64	58	45	29	38	42	41	58	39
Hospital nurse	15	19	24	29	34	20	13	16	19	22	28	18
Physiotherapist	6	8	12	18	28	10	3	5	8	11	19	8
Occupational therapist[a]	1	1	2	8	7	2	0	0	2	4	7	2
Radiologist[b]	14	19	22	25	18	18	10	13	12	14	16	12
Dietician	3	4	4	6	8	4	1	2	2	3	6	2
Speech therapist	–	0	1	2	3	1	—	—	0	1	1	0
Hearing therapist[c]	3	3	2	5	1	3	3	2	2	4	7	3
Optician or oculist	4	5	5	10	2	5	7	7	6	5	2	6
Hospital social worker	1	2	2	3	7	2	1	1	1	3	6	2
Artificial limb/appliance fitter	1	3	2	4	3	2	0	1	1	1	3	1
Psychologist/psychotherapist	1	1	2	1	1	1	—	0	1	0	1	0
General practitioner	77	82	88	88	95	82	76	84	82	90	92	84
Chiropodist	6	8	12	17	21	10	9	19	26	33	32	22
Health visitor	3	5	8	14	20	7	5	7	11	13	19	10
Community nurse	6	9	18	27	56	14	9	18	26	42	64	26
Osteopath/homeopath[d]	3	3	3	7	3	3	2	2	2	2	2	2
Any of the above	83	88	94	96	99	89	84	'90	92	95	98	90
Base:	*1017*	*622*	*462*	*288*	*144*	*2533*	*864*	*719*	*715*	*566*	*317*	*3181*

[a] Occupational therapists may have been described as social workers, community nurses or health visitors
[b] Radiologist includes radiographers and radiotherapists
[c] Hearing therapist includes audiologists and hearing technicians
[d] Osteopath/homeopath includes acupuncturist, chiropractor and reflexologist
Source: OPCS 1989; Crown Copyright.

workers are skilled in determining the most appropriate aids and gadgets for different individuals. Their professional advice should be sought so that assistive equipment is not inappropriately offered.

It is noteworthy that in the recent disability survey, *less than* 5% of all older disabled adults had received occupational therapy services in the year prior to the study (see Table 10.3).

Physiotherapists

While not every older client requires regular physiotherapy, many do benefit. Collaboration with these professional workers is thus a valuable strategy when assisting clients to maximise their abilities. However, as Table 10.3 shows, only 1 in 10 disabled adults in the recent Disability Survey (OPCS 1989) had received physiotherapy services in the year prior to the study.

Speech therapists

The importance of communication has already been stressed. The relevance of speech in overcoming some forms of disability is obvious, yet a number of elderly disabled persons who might benefit from these skilled professionals appear not always to receive such help (Table 10.3). Health visitors can help to redress such situations by prompt referrals and by seeking advice on how best to complement speech therapy, in the home.

Literature

There is a wide range of literature on measures for overcoming disability. Examples include Gray & MacKenzie (1980), The Consumers' Association's Annual publications on Coping with Disablement, Blackburn (1988), and the comprehensive directory by Saunders (1989).

The British Red Cross Society publish a catalogue of Aids and Appliances and mount a permanent exhibition of equipment for disabled persons, as does The Disabled Living Foundation. The latter has also an advisory service, and extensive publications.

A telephone enquiry service specifically for disabled persons is provided by DIAL UK; and The Health Information Service, based at The Lister Hospital, Stevenage, operates a national service, being an NHS-recognised help-line. Addresses and telephone numbers are given in Appendix 7. Many self-help groups also offer specific information and hints on overcoming particular disabilities (see Knight & Gann 1988).

MOBILISING SERVICES

Mobilising the statutory and voluntary services in order to supplement self- and lay-care, is a frequent health visiting activity.

Health services

Like other groups, physically disabled persons are entitled to the full range of primary and secondary health services provided under the NHS (see Ch. 6, pp. 117–124). Clearly much help is channelled through the primary health care team. A large input is contributed by district nurses, especially in relation to older adults in the higher severity categories (see Table 10.3). Health visitors and district nurses have to determine whom each will visit, and when, so that specific skills are most effectively deployed, overlap avoided, and gaps in care prevented. This is greatly assisted if a neighbourhood nursing scheme is in operation (Ch. 6, pp. 119).

Additionally the complex nature of many conditions frequently requires disabled persons to receive hospital and specialist services, as well as paramedical services just described. Day Hospitals, short-stay admissions and respite care are much in demand. A few places offer night centres for respite, which are much appreciated. Nevertheless, as Tables 10.3 and 10.4 show, only a relatively few persons receive any forms of help. Age and severity of disability understandably appear to be major influencing factors. Although a high proportion of disabled adults saw their GPs in the year prior to the study, only 1 in 5 saw a health visitor, although a further 6% considered they required health visiting services. This figure rose to 10% in respect of district nursing services, and 34% for chiropody. The latter service would seem to be highly relevant in helping disabled persons to remain mobile.

Personally prescribed aids, such as wheelchairs, artificial limbs and prostheses, are usually supplied through Department of Health Appliance Centres. It is important for health visitors to collaborate with personnel responsible for advising and fitting aids, in order to ensure their correct use.

Loans and equipment

Most DHAs operate a loans service for nursing equipment, ranging from walking aids, commodes, cradles and back-rests, through to wheelchairs, special beds and mattresses. Incontinence aids are another feature. However, in the recent Disability Survey (OPCS 1989), *25% of older disabled adults were not using any form of equipment.* This may have been because it was not needed, but might mean that they were unaware it was available.

Night nursing services

These are frequently a boon to the severely disabled, especially where there are elderly carers. However, not all DHAs provide these or night-sitter services, and their future provision appears closely related to financial policies.

Social services

Possibly the closest liaison which health visitors and social workers achieve, comes through their joint concern for deprived or disabled elderly people. Local Authorities through their Social Services Committees (LASS), are empowered to provide a range of services for disabled persons. However, not all of these are obligatory, so care varies between authorities.

The relevant legislation currently comprises

1. The National Assistance Act 1948
2. The Health Services and Public Health Act 1968
3. The Chronically Sick and Disabled Persons' Act 1970
4. The Disabled Persons' (services, consultation and representation) Act 1986.

Additionally, major legislative changes are pending, in respect of the NHS and Community Care Bill (DSS 1989).

Under the National Assistance Act, 1948, Local Authorities were given power to provide for the welfare of persons who are: blind, deaf and/or dumb, or substantially or permanently handicapped by illness, injury or congenital disability.

Services permitted but not made compulsory, included:

- advice on available services, and guidance on how to overcome the effects of disability
- the provision of residential homes, hostels, or centres, where needed
- the establishment of Workshops for handicapped persons, and help to market goods
- recreational and social facilities
- maintenance of a register of handicapped persons
- ability to contribute to the funds of voluntary agencies/or use them as agencies.

The Health Services and Public Health Act, 1968

This legislation widened the remit for professional workers, allowing them to offer care in settings other than the disabled person's own home. It also provided for housing to be adapted and gadgets fitted, to enable persons to overcome their disability.

The Chronically Sick and Disabled Persons Act, 1970

This Act contained both obligatory and permissive powers, although it was intended that all the powers would eventually become mandatory, thus acting as a charter for disabled people. However, due largely to economic stringencies, only partial implementation has occurred.

Existing mandatory arrangements include a requirement for LASS Departments to maintain a register of all disabled persons in their area, and to ascertain their needs.

However, it should be noted that there is no similar obligation on the part of disabled persons so to register. Many in fact do not do so, either because of a lack of awareness of any benefits from such registration, or indifference, or a fear of stigma.

Furthermore, since there are no national standardised criteria concerning 'needs', most local authorities have imposed their own. Inevitably this has led to great variation between authorities. The issue has assumed greater importance with subsequent amending legislation, which places responsibility on LASS Departments to undertake a full assessment of the needs of disabled persons registered with them, if requested by the disabled person to do so. However, disabled persons are often unaware of the onus placed on them or their representative to request an assessment of their needs; hence they do not apply. Empowering older disabled persons means acquainting them of their rights and of the necessary steps for action.

Permissive legislation includes powers to enable disabled persons to

- obtain practical help in the home
- obtain recreational facilities and transport to get to these
- adapt their home in order to secure greater comfort, safety and convenience
- obtain holidays, meals in the home or elsewhere, and telephones or other equipment required to use them.

Additionally LASS were empowered to

- require access to be made available in public places, and facilities to be provided in public places for disabled persons
- provide parking concessions for disabled persons, through the issue of orange badges and the designation of certain sites
- provide special housing for disabled persons in certain circumstances.

The Disabled Persons Act, 1986

This provided for

- an authorised representative to be appointed for each disabled person, with the right to request welfare services and to accompany the person to any meeting or interview held to consider services for them
- mentally disordered persons, leaving hospital, to be notified to the LASS, so that their needs can be assessed
- co-option to committees of persons representing disabled persons' interests
- each LASS to provide the Secretary of State with information annually to enable him to provide an Annual Report on the community care of mentally disordered persons.

More detailed accounts of these important legislative provisions can be found in Darnborough & Kinrade (1988).

The realities of practice

In spite of these various provisions, the realities for the disabled may present health visitors with a very different picture in their practice. Facilities available rarely satisfy demands. The recent OPCS Disability Survey revealed that only 10% of older disabled adults had attended Day Centres in the year prior to the study; 16% had attended social clubs; overall 4% had received respite care, though this rose to 16% for those in the most severe categories; and 45% had had a holiday, although this fell to 22% for the most severely disabled.

Of course not all disabled persons require all these services, or wish to attend; nevertheless others who do cannot find places. Recent financial stringencies have entailed that sharper criteria have rendered some ineligible for services such as telephones, a point to be borne in mind when caring for older people living alone, for whom a telephone constitutes a useful means of contact and surveillance.

The Disability Survey also revealed the proportion of disabled adults who received various social services in the year prior to interview (see Table 10.4). Although age and severity of disablement have some influence on provision of services, it appears that household situation also determines who receives help. Those living alone seem more likely to be assisted. The fact that the presence of an elderly carer may preclude help, should be

Table 10.4 Proportion of disabled adults who received different services in the year prior to the Disability Survey interview, by severity category and age: adults living in private households

Type of service received	Severity category					All disabled adults
	1–2	3–4	5–6	7–8	9–10	
	Percentage of disabled adults who received each service					
Age 16 to 49						
LA home help	0	1	4	6	8	2
Meals on wheels	—	—	0	0	—	0
Laundry service	0	—	0	—	1	0
Incontinence service	—	0	0	1	3	0
Night sitting service	0	—	—	—	—	0
Mobility/technical officer for the blind	—	—	0	1	1	0
Social worker	3	6	16	18	33	10
Voluntary services	0	0	1	2	3	1
Visiting service	—	0	—	0	1	0
Private domestic help	1	1	3	3	2	2
Private nursing help	—	—	—	—	1	0
Other services	0	0	1	2	1	1
Any of the above	4	8	23	26	42	14
Base:	*621*	*476*	*425*	*248*	*101*	*1870*
Age 50 to 64						
LA home help	2	3	6	12	14	4
Meals on wheels	0	1	2	4	1	1
Laundry service	0	0	0	2	1	0
Incontinence service	0	—	0	0	4	0
Night sitting service	—	—	—	0	—	0
Mobility/technical officer for the blind	0	0	0	0	1	0
Social worker	2	5	9	13	23	6
Voluntary services	0	0	1	1	2	0
Visiting service	0	—	—	0	2	0
Private domestic help	2	1	2	4	7	2
Private nursing help	—	0	0	—	—	0
Other services	0	1	2	1	1	1
Any of the above	5	9	18	28	42	12
Base:	*964*	*635*	*454*	*256*	*108*	*2417*
Age 65 to 74						
LA home help	6	8	20	20	28	12
Meals on wheels	0	2	2	5	2	2
Laundry service	0	1	0	1	4	1
Incontinence service	0	0	1	1	4	1
Night sitting service	—	—	—	—	1	0
Mobility/technical officer for the blind	—	0	0	1	1	0
Social worker	2	3	8	12	22	6
Voluntary services	1	1	1	2	2	1
Visiting service	0	0	1	1	1	0
Private domestic help	3	3	3	4	4	3
Private nursing help	0	—	0	—	2	0
Other services	1	1	1	2	3	1
Any of the above	12	15	29	36	55	21
Base:	*1017*	*622*	*462*	*288*	*144*	*2533*
Age 75 and over						
LA home help	17	28	41	43	30	31
Meals on wheels	5	6	11	17	11	9
Laundry service	—	1	2	2	5	1
Incontinence service	—	—	1	2	5	1
Night sitting service	—	—	0	1	1	0
Mobility/technical officer for the blind	—	1	1	0	3	0
Social worker	2	4	7	10	12	6
Voluntary services	1	2	2	2	—	1
Visiting service	0	0	0	1	—	0
Private domestic help	6	7	7	7	4	7
Private nursing help	0	—	1	2	3	1
Other services	0	1	1	2	2	1
Any of the above	27	38	51	58	50	42
Base:	*864*	*719*	*715*	*566*	*317*	*3181*

Source: OPCS 1989; Crown Copyright.

noted in view of the heavy toll which caring exerts (Charlesworth et al 1983, MacLean 1989).

Unlike health services, many social services are means-tested; notwithstanding this older disabled adults' identified unmet needs. 21% considered they required but were not receiving home help services; 10% requested social worker services; while incontinence laundry services and night sitters were most requested by those in severity Category 10. For these and other reasons a reform of community care has been considered necessary.

COMMUNITY CARE IN THE NEXT DECADE AND BEYOND

Government proposals on community care are currently before Parliament (DSS 1989).

The White Paper contains six key objectives:

1. to promote domiciliary and respite services which will enable persons to live in their own homes, whenever feasible and sensible
2. to ensure that practical help for carers is made a high priority
3. to make proper assessment of need and good case-management, the cornerstone of high-quality care; (packages of care should be designed in line with individual needs/preferences)
4. to promote a flourishing independent sector alongside good public provision
5. to clarify agency responsibility and accountability
6. to secure better value for money and introduce new funding for social care.

The proposals make LASS responsible for assessing need, designing care and securing its delivery. They will be required to encourage the development of private and voluntary services and will be in charge of financial support for those entering residential establishments in future.

LASS are also required to set up inspection and registration mechanisms to monitor standards, and to establish a complaints procedure. A new specific grant will be paid from Regional Health Authorities to LASS, to promote social care for seriously mentally ill persons discharged from hospital.

The introduction of an 'internal market' for services, between LASS, DHAs and District Authorities, will be a new development.

Implications for health visitors

These proposals contain implications for health visitors and other health workers. In particular they will be required to participate in

- assessment procedures on a multi-disciplinary basis
- providing community nursing advice where necessary, on the development of individual care arrangements; (this may mean staff acting as 'Key workers' for some clients)
- providing care once 'packages' have been agreed with clients and carers
- participating in monitoring and evaluation of care services.

The intention to strengthen the role of voluntary agencies may also require health visitors to modify aspects of their practice.

Voluntary organisations

Britain has a tradition of partnership between statutory and voluntary services. Voluntary bodies have frequently pioneered services, which have then been taken over by the state. Some offer a complementary service.

There are distinct advantages for voluntary bodies. They are often able to respond more flexibly to need than are statutory authorities, who are bound by legislation. Staff are dedicated, often unpaid or low-paid, so that costs tend to be lower. Services are frequently locally based, generating community interest and support.

Against this must be set the confusion that can arise from a plethora of small, often highly specialised associations, sometimes providing overlapping services. This makes it difficult to coordinate care; clients become bewildered, and effort can be duplicated. Furthermore some older clients feel reluctant to share their needs with volunteers who live locally and whom they may know in other capacities. Agency and staff attitudes may sometimes be patronising, and clients may resent being regarded as recipients of charity.

Some of these difficulties can be obviated by improved education and training, and by the action of such bodies as Councils of Voluntary Services.

It is necessary for health visitors to familiarise themselves with the organisations operating in their locality, their aims and objectives, the constraints imposed upon them, by their charter, constitution, or their charitable status.

Some bodies are mainly fund-raising and disbursing agencies; others promote research into specific conditions and offer particular welfare services. Almost all offer an advisory service and some give practical help. The Crossroads Home Care Attendance Scheme, The British Red Cross Society, and The St John Ambulance Brigade are particularly relevant in the care of disabled persons. (National addresses of various organisations can be found in Appendix 7.)

STATE BENEFITS FOR DISABLED OLDER PEOPLE

Apart from any entitlement to contributory or non-contributory Retirement Benefit, and/or Income Support, older disabled persons may be eligible for alternative Benefits.

Severe Disablement Allowance

As mentioned in Chapter 7 (p. 158) a few older disabled persons, with an 80% or more disability, may have been in receipt of SDA before reaching 60/65 years. It is usually advantageous for them to opt to receive this, rather than Retirement Benefit, as it carries small tax advantages and avoids the overlapping Benefits Regulations. However, it is worth noting that less than 16% of disabled pensioners were found to be in receipt of any form of disability-related maintenance benefits in the recent Survey (OPCS 1988b).

Attendance Allowance

This Benefit may be available to

> persons who require frequent or prolonged attention throughout the day and/or night, in connection with bodily functions, or if they need continual supervision throughout the day and/or night, in order to avoid substantial danger to themselves or others.

Attendance Allowance (AA) is paid to the affected person, and is non-taxable and non-means-tested.

However, regulations are stringent. There are residential qualifications, and in most instances care must have been required for at least 6 months before the application is made. Furthermore those living alone are often ruled out, because although they require help to assist them to function in personal activities, they may not be able to receive '*prolonged attention*', or '*continuing supervision*'. Consequently their condition may deteriorate, making it necessary for them to have additional professional help.

Health visitors may wish to note that, in the recent Disability Survey, only *4%* of all disabled pensioners were in receipt of higher rate AA, while *5% only* received the lower rate. Within severity category 10, (the category in which it is likely most persons would be eligible), the proportions were *50%* and *23%* respectively. When questioned, *45%* of all those not receiving benefit said 'they had never heard of the allowance' (OPCS 1988b).

Apart from acquainting older sick or disabled persons of this Allowance, and assisting them with their claim procedures, health visitors may sometimes be asked to provide supportive evidence. They may also assist in preparing appeals. Clients can also receive advice from organisations such as The Disability Alliance, Welfare Rights Associations, or Citizens' Advice Bureaux.

Mobility Allowance

Mobility Allowance (MA) is a non-means-tested Benefit, designed to help severely disabled persons to become more mobile. It appears highly relevant when so many disabled persons have locomotion difficulties. Furthermore the allowance is non-taxable and is disregarded for purposes of Attendance Allowance, Income Support, or War Pension. It therefore makes a useful contribution towards transport costs for the disabled housebound.

Unfortunately older disabled persons are only eligible for MA if they can claim *before they are 66 years of age and could satisfy the criteria before they were 65*. Qualifying criteria include inability, or virtual inability, to walk, because of a physical condition likely to last for at least 1 year. Those qualifying for MA may retain it until they are 75 years of age.

The regulations have been criticised as harsh, ageist and discriminatory. In the recent Disability

Survey only *2%* of disabled pensioners were in receipt of MA.

All benefits are regularly uprated, at, or just below, inflation levels (Disability Alliance Briefings 1989).

A Disability Benefits Review

Because of the findings of the recent Survey, showing that the incomes of many disabled persons are substantially below those of the general population, a Benefits Review has been mooted. No pronouncement has yet been made. Overall 35% of all disabled persons were found to have incomes *50% below the average manual wage*.

Disabled pensioners had incomes approximately 69% of the average national wage, and were thus deemed to be in receipt of an income similar to non-disabled pensioners, reflecting the low level incomes of many retired persons. However, this does not take account of the disability-related expenditure, determined in the Survey. Amounts given below reflect 1988 prices.

- 2 million disabled persons assessed spending £5 per week, or more
- 1 million, £10 per week or more
- 0.5 million, £15 per week or more.

Even so, disablement groups have protested that these amounts are unrealistically low.

When assessing the financial circumstances of disabled older clients, health visitors may wish to bear these points in mind. They may also wish to note the campaign, which is currently intensifying, for a national disablement income benefit.

CARING FOR OLDER PEOPLE WITH SENSORY IMPAIRMENTS

VISUAL IMPAIRMENTS AND DISABILITIES

Vision is one of the most valued senses; hence age-related changes affecting sight are likely to impinge sharply upon the quality of life. The conservation of vision and the prevention of impairment, and hence disability, are thus essential parts of the health visiting role at all ages. Nevertheless, in the older adult it is imperative to detect defects early, and to institute prompt treatment.

Major causes of visual impairment or disability

Apart from visual impairment resulting from congenital disorders, or acquired from disease or injury in early life, most people develop visual problems after 65 years of age. Major causes include:

- glaucoma
- diabetic retinopathy
- senile macular degeneration (SMD)
- cataract.

Glaucoma

The technical difficulty of screening population aggregates was discussed in Chapter 6. However, family history, and the concomitant presence of vascular disease, are two high-risk factors which should alert health visitors to the need for further investigation. Likewise the early recognition of potential symptoms, such as the perception of 'halos' around objects, is important. There appears to be some ethnic differences in incidence, with Afro-Caribbeans being at increased risk (WHO 1989).

Diabetic retinopathy

The prevention of diabetic retinopathy is essentially a matter of controlling obesity as a possible predisposing factor in the onset of maturity-type diabetes, and in the effective management of all diabetic states. An associated vascular condition indicates increased risk.

Senile macular degeneration

In SMD, as with glaucoma, genetic factors have been implicated. Although it is a complex matter, a significant correlation has been noted with blue irises. The postulation is that non-brown irises transmit more light than the more heavily pigmented ones. If this hypothesis is found to be correct, a more effective preventive measure would be available. (Weale 1989). Pending further research, studies are continuing into the effects of photo-coagulation and laser therapy, as measures of treating SMD in its earlier stages (WHO 1989).

Cataract

Excessive and prolonged exposure to light, without adequate visual protection, is also cited as one of the many environmental factors thought to be associated with cataract (Zigman 1981; WHO 1989). Diabetes is a known predisposing factor. Research also shows a possible association with frequent and severe bouts of childhood diarrhoea (Minassian et al 1984).

Myopia in earlier life is also correlated with later onset of cataract. The problems of reducing risk to older people by taking preventive action in childhood myopia are discussed by Weale (1989). Meantime, for established cases of cataract, surgery offers highly effective treatment. The comparatively recent technique of lens implant offers a more acceptable operative procedure to many older persons than the thick 'cataract lens', which formerly provided external lens substitute for most sufferers.

In each of these causes the preventive and case-finding functions and health promoting skills of health visitors appear to be relevant. Neverthless, however effectively health promotion measures and/or screening techniques are deployed, there will remain a proportion of older people who are blind or partially-sighted. Consequently they require ameliorative, supportive and rehabilitative services.

The prevalence of visual impairment

There are currently about 93 000 registered blind persons, and a further 53 000 registered partially-sighted persons, aged 65 years or more, in Great Britain. This contrasts sharply with the 1 137 000 disabled persons aged 60 years and over, reporting a 'seeing disability', in the recent Disability Prevalence Survey (OPCS 1988a). This indicates how few persons actually register.

Among all groups there is a preponderance of females, especially in the group 80 years and upwards. These facts highlight the need for improved assessment of the visual health of all older people, as well as the dissemination of comprehensive information.

Registration

Registration for both blindness and partial sight is voluntary on the part of the client; those who fail to register probably do so because they are unaware of the process or do not perceive any advantage. However, there are mandatory legislative provisions as outlined above, regarding both health and social services. Many of these apply only to the blind. To obtain such services, registration must be made with the LASS, but the ophthalmic condition must be certified by a registered medical practitioner with additional qualifications in ophthalmology.

Services and benefits

Services available include the provision of specially qualified social workers, able to give home teaching on the best ways of overcoming visual disability. Only a few older persons who acquire their blindness later in life actually learn to use embossed type, but for those who do, both Moon and Braille are available. Social workers can arrange for braille dials to be fitted on watches, cookers and certain household appliances. There is also a range of specially adapted household items and safety devices available.

Holidays can be arranged for visually impaired older persons, and their families, and clubs and recreational activities are arranged to help such older people find new interests and release for their emotions.

Many partially sighted persons enjoy the large-print books, and there is a range of embossed playing cards and games which some use.

Voluntary organisations for the visually disabled

There are many voluntary organisations for the visually impaired or disabled, including the Royal National Institute for the Blind (RNIB). Talking books are available through this agency, and there is a music library. Radios can be supplied for those in need, through The Wireless for the Blind Fund.

Mobility training can be offered, particularly assisted by The Association for Guide Dogs for the Blind, although the very old can rarely benefit from this service. Health visitors will realise that older people sometimes take longer to adapt to changed circumstances, and some of the provisions which younger persons can utilise are inappropriate for them, unless they were introduced earlier in life.

Monetary benefits for the visually disabled

Older visually impaired/disabled persons, with appropriate contribution records, are entitled to State Retirement Benefit, and in certain circumstances may be entitled to Invalidity Benefit or Severe Disablement Allowance, for which they have opted. Those on very low incomes may qualify for Income Support. If they do, blind persons may obtain the Higher Pensioner Premium, from age 60 (see Ch. 7, pp. 158–159).

Provided they fulfil the eligibility criteria, visually impaired persons may be able to claim Attendance Allowance, and if they have an associated mobility problem they may be eligible for Mobility Allowance. Entitlement to Housing Benefit of course is also theirs if they fulfil criteria.

Those registered as blind are also entitled to some income tax concessions; to reduced-cost TV licences; free postage on Talking Books cassettes; they may also obtain some travel concessions from British Rail.

Where necessary those requiring residential accommodation may receive some help towards the cost of their fees, and, in future, additional services may be provided under community care reform proposals.

Reducing the physical effects of visual impairment

Health visitors can make a useful contribution in reducing the physical effects of visual impairment or disability, through recognising its impact on locomotion and balance, as well as the restriction it can place on mobility. Older visually impaired persons face difficulties associated with space, orientation, and with hazard control. They thus require help to manipulate the environmental variables of light, size and contrast, to maximum advantage. This can be achieved through placing light in such ways as to improve contrast perception and reduce dazzle.

Safety education is vital. It includes assessing and arranging internal environments so that the risk of falls is reduced and orientation is facilitated. Attention should also be paid to external environments, so that garden or traffic accidents are minimised. Clients may also welcome information concerning any prescribed treatments, such as medications or drops.

Practitioners will recognise there is need for close liaison with social workers, GPs, ophthalmic specialists and opticians. They should also familiarise themselves with any District Low Vision Service (Royal College of Physicians 1986).

The Disabled Living Foundation has developed a special pack for community health nurses, concerned with the visually impaired, designed to help staff enhance remaining ability and strengthen coping mechanisms.

Reducing the psychological aspects of visual impairment or disability.

Understandably, psychological reactions are strong and related to the meaning visually disabled persons attribute to their condition. Stages of the adjustment process have been identified by Allen (1989), who found from her research that whereas pre-impact stages were accorded little significance, this changed sharply when the nature of the visual, threat was recognised. Then fear, shock, disbelief, anger and depression were displayed in varying degrees. A profound sense of loss was not only related to visual ability, but to opportunity to carry out valued tasks. Informants found it most difficult to ask for help; to accept the inability to recognise friends and acquaintances, to recognise time, and to protect themselves and their property. The factors most helpful in adjustment, were social support, maintenance of reciprocity, and the knowledge or belief that one might retain some vision.

These factors clearly inform health visitors, who will also note that unhelpful factors were found to include lack of information, lack of support, the presence of other health problems, perceived unhelpful or negative attitudes of others, and labelling.

Help should therefore be directed towards building on existing coping strategies, providing opportunities to talk with others who have successfully adjusted to visual impairment, in supporting individuals as they learn new ways and in listening to them as they talk out their feelings. Ongoing reassessment, monitoring of causative conditions, preventing deterioration where possible and maintaining hope, are all helpful activities. Time facilitates adjustment, as does the possession of internal sources of strength, such as spiritual belief, and the assurance of personal worth.

The deaf-blind

Approximately 2% of those on The Blind Persons Register are elderly deaf-blind. A few have been affected from birth, and are mute as well. Some will have acquired their conditions from illness or injury in childhood or earlier adulthood, but the majority develop both impairments in later maturity. They require special aids and one-to-one teaching, as well as particular empathy, and psychosocial support. Focus must be on quality of life. Such older persons should be referred promptly to LASS for specialised care, and should also be given information about the Deaf/Blind Association. They are of course eligible for the services and monetary benefits for both blind and deaf persons, but cannot always utilise these so readily, because of their dual and sometimes triple handicap.

HEARING IMPAIRMENT

The prevalence of hearing impairment among elderly people has been variously estimated. In one community-based survey using audiometric techniques, a prevalence rate of 600 per 1000 of the population aged 65 years and over was estimated (Herbst & Humphrey 1980).

This means over 4.5 million older adults have some noticeable hearing loss — a far greater number than previously ascertained. It is of course related to the precise nature of the investigation, and contrasts with the 2 032 000 persons aged 60 and over who, in the recent Survey, were regarded as 'disabled' by their hearing impairments (OPCS 1988a).

However, only 60 000 elderly hearing-impaired adults are currently registered with LASS departments, 20% as deaf and 80% as 'hard of hearing'. Such discrepancy again demonstrates considerable under-registering, resulting from either ignorance, indifference or dissatisfaction with service provisions. Nevertheless this highlights the need for health visitors to carry out case-finding and surveillance, and to disseminate information and carry out health promotion activities.

The categories of hearing impairment are:

- those deaf without speech
- those deaf with speech
- those deemed hard of hearing.

The majority of older adults fall into the last category, the next highest being those deaf with speech. Thus most older adults with reasonable vision can communicate via lip-reading and oral speech, especially when this is amplified.

As with other groups of disabled older adults the full range of health and social services is available to the hearing impaired. Audiometrists and Otologists are available through the NHS, and aids can be supplied free of charge, when prescribed. However, while many people readily wear spectacles, not all hearing-impaired persons wish to wear a hearing aid. This relates to a fear of stigma and to the unsatisfactory nature of some of the appliances offered. This is an area ripe for health promotion.

Most LASS employ specialised case-workers to help older deaf persons overcome their disabilities;

some also have interpreters. Specific social and recreational clubs are available; while some colleges arrange lip-reading classes. Aids to daily living, such as flashing door bells and television or telephone amplifiers, are also useful. Some guide dogs for the deaf have been used very successfully.

Spiritual facilities are available through the Diocesean Missioners for the deaf, who provide special counselling services, run Church services using a combination of speech and sign language, and provide family support. It is of course helpful if health visitors can learn sign language, to assist them in communicating with their deaf clients.

Although hearing impairment does not necessarily have serious physical effects, some older people do have associated vertigo, or attacks of vomiting as in Meniere's disease. Tinnitus can prove very handicapping, and some older clients respond to 'masking' in this condition, while others find it fatiguing. Referral to the Tinnitus Association can prove helpful (see Appendix 7 for address).

The psychosocial needs of hearing-impaired older adults

Above all other needs, the psychosocial aspects of those disabled by hearing difficulties predominate. Several studies show significant relationship between deafness and depression, social isolation and withdrawal, independent of age or socioeconomic circumstances (Herbst & Humphrey 1980, Twining 1989). This indicates which areas health visitors might profitably explore with older clients. It also calls for effective and sustained social support; opportunities to participate and contribute; a wide range of alternative interests; and chance to ventilate feelings freely. All these aid adjustment.

Regular monitoring, re-assessment and review of client situations should be undertaken, in the light of current research. In this way health visitors can help to bring creative insights into their work with hearing-impaired older adults.

THE NEEDS OF PSYCHOLOGICALLY IMPAIRED CLIENTS

Measuring psychological and psychiatric morbidity among older clients is a complex task, for three reasons:

1. the difficulties in differentiating normal psychological age changes and responses, from pathological ones
2. the difficulties in applying precise diagnostic criteria; hence problems in comparing data
3. the intertwining of causative events, especially those associated with physical illness, impairment and disability; socio-economic problems; and/or social isolation, loss and bereavement.

Overall marked psychiatric disturbance occurs in approx 7% of all older adults. A further *10%* exhibit moderate symptoms, and up to *13%* mild ones. Nevertheless, contrary to common stereotypes, and in spite of the high bed occupancy rate in psychogeriatric units, *almost 60% of older adults are without any psychological impairment.* This should be constantly borne in mind when undertaking community mental health programmes. However, while some older adults are at risk of various forms of mental disorder, particularly dementia, they are particularly prone to depression.

DEPRESSION

This affective disorder is characterised by sadness of mood, a sense of emptiness, detachment, and often raised anxiety levels. Symptoms are frequently masked, simulating physical illness. Such symptoms are frequently non-specific, such as anorexia, weight changes, constipation, tachycardia, or generalised or localised pain, particularly backache. There is often a lack of energy, or interest. This is frequently attributed to 'old age' and regarded as 'inevitable'. The various symptoms may be under-valued, or labelled as hypochondriasis (Stanhope & Lancaster 1988).

The prevalence of depression

Not surprisingly, in view of the range of potential symptoms, the prevalence of depression has been variously estimated. According to Murphy (1982, 1983), who carried out community-based research, 29% of older adults living in private households were frank, or borderline, depressives.

From the Nottingham studies, Arie (1988), reported 10% in each age group, from 60 years up to 80 years. Other researchers have, however, suggested levels as high as 40%. It is important to be aware of these various figures and of the frequency of depression, since unfortunately the condition is often not diagnosed until it is too late — suicide being a consequence. The incidence of successful suicide is high among older people, especially men. Rates increase generally in the spring.

Suicide for this reason constitutes a tragedy, since treatment for depression can be most successful. Hence the situation calls for greater awareness and the effective deployment of assessment and case-finding skills. The reduction of suicide and parasuicide rates forms one of the WHO targets mentioned in Chapter 6.

Types of depression

There are two main forms of depression: reactive and endogenous types. Although difficult to differentiate in older people, the majority of cases appear to be of the reactive type. Features include fatigue (often lasting all day and worse in the evening), with problems in getting off to sleep at night. This contrasts with the endogenous type, which occurs independently of environmental and social circumstances, is worse in the morning, with classic early waking.

Causes

Exact causes of depression are still largely speculative. Research findings suggest a range across biological and psychosocial dimensions. Such theories include:

- constitutional predispositions, familial tendencies, and personality structure (Kline 1976, Post 1981)
- reactions to impairment, disability, or painful and chronic illness such as cancer (Blumenthal 1980, Petty & Sensky 1987, Arie 1988)
- early serious life-events, or disruptive life-events (Brown & Harris 1978, Hall & Zwemer 1979, Murphy 1982)
- loss, attack, restraint and/or threat (Hanley & Baikie 1984, Jenkins 1985)
- stress (Blumenthal 1980, Nash 1988, Stanhope & Lancaster 1988)
- iatrogenic factors (Blumenthal 1980)
- social and economic factors; lack of a confidante (Murphy 1983)
- loneliness (Ingham & Miller 1982, Arie 1988, Scrutton 1989)
- poverty (Arie 1988)
- nutritional factors and/or food sensitivities, vitamin deficiencies, mineral or trace element deficiencies, or high copper levels (Davies & Stewart 1987, Petty & Sensky 1987)
- acute infections, mostly viral (Petty & Sensky 1987)
- Hormonal imbalance (Scrutton 1989).

The recognition of depression

Because many elderly people who experience low-level wellness do not necessarily emphasise their lowered spirits and flattened affect, it is important that they are observed and systematically assessed. Significant points include lessened interest in personal or environmental hygiene; indecisiveness; self-absorption, self-deprecation and self-reproach; and diffuse pessimism. Additionally clients may be restless, retarded or confused. They may sometimes experience hallucinations. Hence recognition of the condition is often difficult. However, a personal or family history of depression can be a pointer, emphasising how necessary it is to obtain a full health history, consult past records and take account of significant and/or recent distressing events, when making an assessment.

Medical management of depression

It has been argued that depression is frequently 'medicalised', to the detriment of recognising it as an emotional and social problem. This can reduce the need for persons to look at the causes of their depression and foster the inner resources needed to deal with it. It is therefore important to offer counselling alongside any medical treatment, in order to reduce dependence on medication and focus on developing effective personal coping strategies (Scrutton 1989). Nevertheless the care of depressed older persons includes a medical component.

In reactive states, persons can be helped if the precipitating cause can be discovered and alleviated. Hospital admission may be helpful in some cases. Restoration of self-respect and provision of non-specific care can effect some improvement. Some psychiatrists feel therapy is of limited value if it does not include an attack on the mood disorder at the central nervous system level. Hence tricyclic drugs, such as in imipramine, are often prescribed. Tetracyclic antidepressive drugs and monoamine oxidase inhibitors are rarely used with older persons.

Electroconvulsive therapy may be employed, although the ethics of its use are hotly debated. Where it is used clients and carers need information and explanation to help them decide whether to accept treatment. If they affirm this, they need support and encouragement to continue. Memory is sometimes temporarily disturbed, but longer-term benefit is claimed.

Monitoring drug compliance, reactions and interactions

The forgetfulness of elderly depressed persons treated outside hospital often renders drug compliance problematic. Carers should be alerted to the need for accurate, regular administration of medicines. Possible side-effects of tricyclic drugs include dry mouth, postural hypotension, confusion, or retention of urine in men.

Liaison with community psychiatric nurses can be very helpful in monitoring therapy.

Psychological treatment

Psychological treatment includes both cognitive and behavioural therapy as well as psychotherapy. Demand far exceeds supply and, apart from private treatment, one-to-one intervention is rare. Group therapy is more common and is thought to be more effective.

Counselling

From the counselling approach, depression is viewed as a particular response to personal circumstances, consequent upon the meanings older individuals attribute to their life-events. The counsellor seeks to elicit these meanings and personal constructs, in order to help clients to interpret their situations (Ricoeur 1981, Allen 1989).

Clients have to be helped to see that their depression is not only a specific response to life-events, but a reflection of their perceptions of, and attitudes towards, themselves. Through gradual unravelling of reality from distorted social construction, clients are confronted with the fact that the conquest of depression lies in themselves. They can then take positive steps to effect improvement (Scrutton 1989).

Health visiting intervention

Apart from collaboration in group work, monitoring of medical regimes and surveillance of clients receiving medical or psychological treatment, health visitors can do much to help reduce the adverse effects of depression. Interventions include preventive, teaching and social support techniques, together with environmental modification where this is possible.

Effort should be made to reinforce non-depressive behaviour, and to provide reassurance, supervision and encouragement to regain well-being, so that older persons are helped to preserve their self-esteem and dignity.

Clients benefit from being taught anxiety-reducing mechanisms, including deep breathing, relaxation, visual imagery and suitable graded exercises (Nash 1988). They often respond to diversional activities, music and drama.

Socio-economic measures to relieve any financial distress, and actions to improve general circumstances, are of course necessary. Social contact should be encouraged, as should the use of such amenities as clubs, day centres, libraries and leisure interest groups. Voluntary visiting can be helpful.

Intervention at community level

In addition to individual and group interventions, health visitors can assist at the community level to increase public awareness about depression and its psychosocial origins. They can discuss how it can be combated and can emphasise the increased risk faced by older people. The assumption is that as the public become more aware, and involved in discussing the emotional and social needs of older people, they are more likely to foster meaningful roles for them.

Working with voluntary agencies interested in mental health not only provides support for older sufferers but allows health visitors to extend their health promotion activities as well.

CARING FOR ELDERLY PEOPLE WITHIN ETHNIC MINORITY GROUPS

Traditionally Britain has had a variety of ethnic minority groups within its population. This process accelerated during and after the Second World War, so that today many different races and cultures are represented within the United Kingdom.

Some of the elderly persons within such groups have been here for many years. Others have arrived recently, having come to join their families or find refuge. The extent to which they have settled down, met with favourable social and economic circumstances, and achieved some level of integration within the host country, will likely be reflected in their health and social needs.

As with all other older individuals, it is important to appreciate that those from differing ethnic minorities are a heterogeneous group. The cultural diversity between different ethnic groups may be as great, or greater, than that shown between them and the indigenous population. This is stressed by Qureshi (1989), and is significant in view of the fact that the NHS was designed to cater for a more homogeneous population. Consequently it has been slow to recognise that a multi-cultural society calls for multi-cultural services (Mares et al 1985, McNaught 1985, Fenton 1987).

Migration patterns

Because migration is rarely random, it is often helpful to examine the historical associations of each group in Britain. Discovering the reasons why they have come, and the circumstances prevailing at, or since, their arrival, may highlight the nature of their actual or potential health and social needs.

For example, one of the largest groups who have maintained a steady influx to Britain over many years are the Irish. Their arrivals are usually young, economically active persons. Many settle in major cities, though there is frequent dispersion throughout the country. Although close contact is maintained with Eire, long-term living in Britain is a strong feature. Thus many Irish older adults have been here for many years, and most health visitors are likely to encounter someone from this group. Similarities in some customs and lifestyles facilitate assimilation.

Religious influences are usually strong and ritually adhered to. Patterns of health and disease frequently resemble those of the indigenous population. Susceptibilities are reputed to be homocystinuria, schizophrenia and tuberculosis. Alcohol-related diseases are a risk for some, which can lead to nutritional anaemia and risk of vitamin deficiencies, especially in men.

Nevertheless, apart from the travelling tinkers who maintain distinctive features, and hence have specific needs, most elderly Irish differ little from indigenous older adults. Their health care therefore follows a similar pattern.

Others who have deliberately chosen migration, usually for work reasons, are ethnic Italian and Spanish persons. Most came to Britain post-war. They have established strong and identifiable communities, and usually have well-developed social networks for supporting their elderly members.

Many older persons within these groups cherish

the hope of returning to their country of origin at retirement, but a number remain here. Although there may be some language difficulties, and certain culture patterns and customs differ from British ones, they are usually familiar with the health and social services. Many are cared for within extended families, although one should not assume this to be so. Employment opportunities, especially for women, and housing pressures, may lead to cultural change.

Other arrivals on a relatively planned basis include Afro-Caribbeans, who came in response to post-war calls for their labour. They work in essential services, especially transport, catering and the health service, many being ancillary workers.

They were joined in the late 1960s to early 1970s by Asians, either from the Indian subcontinent or seeking refuge from East Africa. Thus their social circumstances are very diverse. It is noteworthy, that while the elderly from the New Commonwealth or Pakistan currently form less than 2% of the population 65 years and upwards, a 'bulge' of those now aged 45–59 years predicts a considerably increased proportion by 2000 AD. Hence there is likely to be an increased demand for health, social and other services.

In contrast to deliberate migration patterns, some other groups have arrived here as refugees. Many Jewish persons came at the turn of the century, seeking refuge from persecution in Eastern Europe. They were than joined by others, prior to, and during, the Second World War. Their strong cultural bonds and corporate concern are well demonstrated. For these reasons, and possibly because of reluctance on the part of authorities to provide them with culturally appropriate services, the Jewish Welfare Board was set up. It serves as an example of ethnic initiative to formalise help. It therefore provides for a number of needs encountered among elderly Jews.

Although certain genetic and environmental influences are manifest in the patterns of health and disease (such as a reputed tendency to higher levels of depression and maturity-onset diabetes), their health states resemble national norms.

However, Polish immigrants appear to have fared less well. They, and the former displaced persons from Estonia, Latvia and the Ukraine, have been isolated from their kin for many years, because of post-war political decisions. Second-generation ethnic minorities may have lessened cultural ties with their parents' country of origin. They may, therefore, be less ready to learn and speak their own language. This may entail that older people who have never mastered English may be 'communication deprived'. This can lead to social isolation and depression — experiences which may well have been repeated for successive waves of refugees from Hungary, Cyprus, China, Turkey and Vietnam.

Nevertheless recent momentous political events, notably in eastern Europe, may create change for some of these elderly, often 'forgotten', persons.

Furthermore, freer mobility within the EEC could also have an influence on future demographic trends, as could an increased amount of trade with countries in the Middle East and Japan. Health visitors thus have to be prepared to meet a range of different ethnic groups in their practice, depending on their locality and the social structure of their community.

Compounded vulnerability

However, whatever the circumstances surrounding their arrival in this country, all first-generation ethnic minority groups are likely to have undergone considerable social dislocation and cultural shock. In addition to the risks of ageism, with which all elderly persons may have to contend, ethnic minority elderly are also at risk of encountering subtle or overt prejudice and discrimination. Some of this may be health-services-related. For although the NHS has instituted some initiatives in response to ethnic minority needs (such as funding projects, providing interpreters and appointing a few Ethnic Advisers), racial discrimination *is* experienced (The Guardian 1984, Mares et al 1985, McNaught 1985). Examples include:

- addressing ethnic elderly persons in derogatory terms
- giving inadequate explanations regarding treatments
- undertaking inadequate examinations before offering prescriptions or treatment

- using parameters or behavioural models culturally specific to white British persons (Fenton 1987; Bhat et al (1988).

Most of these strictures may of course represent communication failures, or poor professional practice, which may be experienced by all older adults, but they carry overtones of covert racial discrimination for many ethnic minority elderly persons.

Location problems

There is a tendency for specific minority groups to settle in close proximity with each other. This often means they are located in inner cities, where, like many indigenous residents, they may share the effect of 'urban decay'. Housing is often substandard and frequently overcrowded. Ethnic minority elderly rarely have the residential qualifications required for local authority housing, and in any case this is in extremely short supply. Few authorities make available 4/5 bedroom houses suitable for an extended family. Furthermore transport and other facilities in the locality are often poor, creating further social isolation or deprivation (Glendenning 1979).

Unless they have accumulated capital, or have worked in this country long enough to qualify for contributory Retirement Pension, many ethnic minority elderly may find themselves on low income. Even when they have long work histories and residence qualifications, the posts they have filled rarely carry occupational pensions.

The complicated claims procedure for Income Support, which places onus on the claimant, may prove bewildering, acting as a disincentive to apply. Explanation, guidance and advocacy are therefore frequently required.

Dietary aspects

While Europeans and some other ethnic minority elderly may have little difficulty obtaining their accustomed foods, others may have problems. Many shops or markets now sell staple Afro-Asian foods, but the cost of such products, or mobility difficulties, may entail that some older people cannot obtain them easily. This can mean dietary restriction, superimposed on religious constraints and/or food taboos.

It is important for health visitors to understand dietary customs, as they can considerably affect well-being in different realms.

Muslims for instance may eat only halal meat, which has been ritually slaughtered and blessed. They are forbidden to eat pork or pork products, but their diet is nourishing and few problems are experienced.

However, there may be problems when older Muslims are admitted to hospital, or advised to attend Day Centres, or Luncheon Clubs, where specific provisions are rarely made for them. Meals-on-wheels may similarly be regarded as unacceptable.

Sikhs, mostly Punjabi speaking, may be vegetarian; Hindus almost always are. Some are strict vegans, although males will often eat eggs. They may be at risk of insufficient protein, iron, Vitamins D and B_{12}, unless acceptable substitutes for their preferred foods can be found. For this reason luncheon clubs or meals on wheels services may be refused.

Health visitors can do much to interpret their elderly clients' wishes to dieticians and service providers. Where home helps are provided, practitioners may offer appropriate guidance to enable these workers to prepare and serve suitable food, in line with cultural acceptability.

Dress

Devout Sikh adult males traditionally wear turbans, which, together with the other 'K' signs (uncut hair, a special comb, a symbolic dagger and special underpants), are worn constantly, even when washing or ill. Sikh women traditionally wear shalwar Kameez (trousers and shirt), suitable for day or night use. They may fear to accept services which they consider may compromise their dress, or cut across their personal modesty.

Muslim and Hindu women are equally strict. Muslim women in purdah are usually clothed from head to toe in garments which do not reveal the shape of the body. The items of jewellery worn often have great social or religious significance, so older women may greatly fear their removal. Because these women often remain in the home, and therefore may not be regularly exposed to sunshine, they are at risk of Vitamin D deficiency, unless dietary sources compensate.

Medical and nursing services which involve examinations, or intimate personal care, should, whenever possible, be undertaken by a person of the same sex. Hence older women may need help to arrange examination by a female doctor, preferably one of similar caste (Karseras & Hopkins 1987).

Religious factors

There are also, of course, specific religious observances to note. These are usually highly valued by ethnic minority elderly.

They may fear that their spiritual well-being will be culturally violated when they are too feeble to insist on conformity (Karseras & Hopkins 1987).

Most Christians will follow similar practices to the indigenous population, although some groups have specific beliefs affecting times of worship, diet and conduct (e.g. Seventh Day Adventists who observe Sabbath, are vegetarian and avoid all stimulants).

For Jewish elderly persons their customs are relatively well understood. Kosher food is usually available in hospitals and similar institutions, and there is often a high level of social welfare provision, which meets the cultural beliefs and values.

For those of the Muslim faith, symbolic cleansing and set times for prayer (five times a day) are strictly observed. The left hand is used for washing and the right for eating. This can have important implications when clients sustain paralysing conditions, or when rehabilitation is required.

Fasting is another firm feature. Apart from Ramadan, many older Muslims fast weekly, often on Fridays — holy day. Thus it is inadvisable to visit on such days, except in emergency. Muslims aim to pay at least one visit to Mecca in a lifetime — Haj; there are also charitable obligations. Muslims approve of blood transfusions, but not transplant operations or post-mortems. When dying, a Muslim aims to face Mecca. After death, ritual washing should be undertaken by a Muslim of the same sex, and burial takes place within 24 hours, usually in a reserved area of a cemetery. Mourning lasts 40 days, and white is worn.

Sikhs have no prohibition against blood transfusions, organ transplants or post-mortems. They value prayers, and at death are cremated with their five signs of Sikhism. The ashes are sometimes taken to the sacred Temple in Amritsar. Mourning usually lasts 1 month.

Hindus aim to sip holy water from the Ganges, when dying; they concentrate their thoughts on The Creator. Ritual washing after death is followed by cremation, the ashes being scattered either on the Ganges, or other water, by a priest. Mourning is short, since death is viewed as a stage to achieving unity with God.

All groups have their sacred scriptures, specific festivals and recognised clergy. It is wise to discover the salient features for each group, and to understand the meaning ascribed to attendant customs, in order to show appropriate respect. Further details on Asian cultures can be found in Karseras & Hopkins (1987), and on Black cultures in Bhat et al (1988).

Family networks and elderly support

An impression is often given of extended family networks supporting ethnic minority elderly, especially among Asians and Afro-Caribbeans. While older people undoubtedly do command great respect, and are readily helped, one cannot assume that this is always so, or that it will continue.

Furthermore not all ethnic minority elderly have families in Britain. Among East African Asians 25% are estimated to be without kin in the UK. Current housing and employment policies militate against large families, and some are no longer prepared to try to cope with elderly members in cramped, overcrowded conditions, with limited help. Hence it is likely that heavier demands will be made on health and social services in future. This may require differing cultural provision. The importance for health visitors of obtaining accurate and comprehensive health and sociocultural histories, as part of systematic assessment, cannot be over-emphasised. This allows vulnerable ethnic elderly persons to be promptly identified.

HEALTH NEEDS

Although race was one dimension affecting health which the Black Report identified (DHSS 1980, Townsend & Davidson 1982), there are problems in examining different minority groups on this basis. This is because 'race' is rarely assessed in official statistics. Instead country of origin is used, which means that white persons born abroad, or ethnic minority group persons born in the UK, confound the data. Nevertheless,

> there is sufficient evidence from individual studies and official sources, to confirm that ethnicity is a relevant dimension of health inequality.
>
> (Bhat et al 1988)

Using mortality as a comparative measure, Marmot et al (1984a) produced the first comprehensive study on immigrant mortality. Figure 10.4 shows the comparative findings based on a standard mortality rate (SMR) of 100. Although these data apply to all age groups, the high SMR for all causes, and both sexes, for those from the African Commonwealth, should be noted. For females born either in the Caribbean, or the Indian subcontinent, the SMR is also high. These figures are largely accounted for by a higher level of deaths from circulatory disease, and also cancer, especially in males. Such work is supported by studies from Cruikshank et al (1980), Blakemore (1982), Marmot et al (1984b), McNaught (1987).

It is thus possible to identify specific morbidity risks for the different groups:

- *Africans*: hypertensive and cerebrovascular disease; liver cancer; tuberculosis
- *Asians*: ischaemic heart disease; diabetes; tuberculosis; cancer of liver, buccal cavity, and throat; diabetes
- *Caribbeans*: hypertensive disease; stroke; diabetes; tuberculosis; liver cancer.

Thus it is clear that 'common' disorders, rather than 'exotic' or hereditary ones, are chiefly responsible for mortality in all three groups. This refutes the belief that 'imported' diseases constitute a public health threat. The conditions for which specific ethnic groups are at risk are comprehensively given in Qureshi (1989), and the preventive actions for these various states are outlined in Smith & Jacobson (1988).

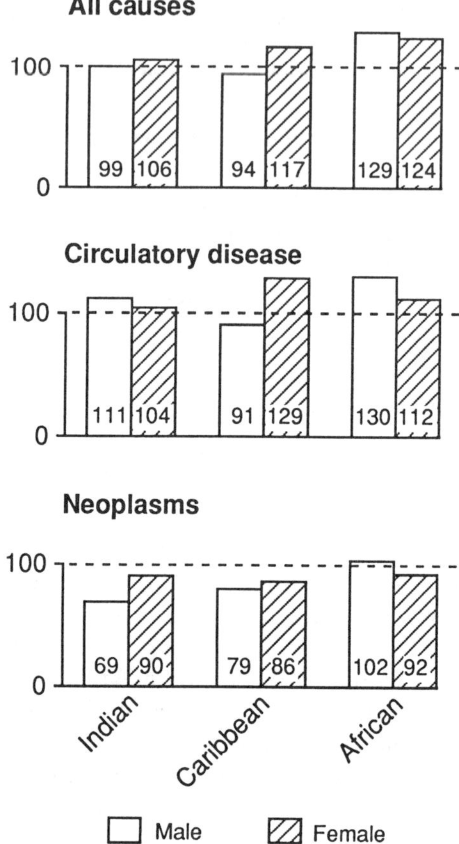

Fig. 10.4 Immigrant mortality in England and Wales standard mortality rates by geographical region of birth, and by sex, for all causes, for circulatory disorders and for neoplasms (for adults aged 20 years and upwards). (Based on material from Townsend & Davidson (1982); Marmot at al (1984a) and Bhat et al (1980).)

Patterns of consultation

There is some evidence to suggest that Afro-Caribbeans and Asians make high use of general practitioner services, with an average 90% consultation each year. Older Asians tend to be under-represented in hospital services. This may be because they resort to Hakims or Vaids, healers practising traditional forms of Eastern medicine. The Ayurvedic or Unani systems of medicine, used by some, are based on the humoral theory of disease, with the need to ensure body balance. Consequently herbal treatment, diet and some psychotherapy will likely be prescribed. It is always necessary to enquire from older ethnic minority persons if alternative therapies are being used, as drug interactions can occur, or certain conditions may be misdiagnosed. Drug compliance becomes an increasing challenge when natural forgetfulness is compounded by poor comprehension of English. Care must be exercised to ensure that basic principles of drug administration and monitoring are clearly grasped, and that side-effects are quickly detected, reported and dealt with.

Mental health

It is difficult to find confirming evidence for the suggestions, in some studies, that Africans and Caribbeans exhibit greater levels of mental illness than other minority groups or the indigenous population (Ineichen 1980). The Hospital Inpatient Mental Health Inquiry does not give data by ethnic origin. There is also the question of whether the medical model is a relevant cultural paradigm for use in mental illness Transcultural psychiatry is a comparatively recent study in Britain (Rack 1982, Helman 1984). Distressed persons from ethnic minority groups may have difficulty communicating about their impaired state with someone from a differing culture, so that although there has been an identified high problem of psychosis attributed to Asians and Afro-Caribbeans, this may be explained on sociocultural grounds (Karseras & Hopkins 1987, Bhat et al 1988, Qureshi 1989).

What seems to be important for health visitors is that they seek to establish good communication with their older ethnic minority clients, and obtain full sociocultural histories (Dobson 1987, 1989). They should also seek to offer support to families when psychiatric treatment has to be provided, since this is often regarded as a stigma.

THE MISTREATMENT OF ELDERLY PEOPLE

Violence towards older people is receiving increasing, if reluctant, attention since its early identification in the late 1960s. Both Baker (1975) and Burston (1975) described incidents, mainly of confused elderly persons being abused by an overwrought carer.

The numbers of recorded cases bear little relationship to the estimated prevalence, especially those of later researchers, probably because of a lack of professional awareness about the problem.

Literature shows inconsistencies in terminology, with 'granny abuse', 'elderly abuse' and 'non-accidental injury' all being used. Hence Johnson (1986) introduced the term 'mistreatment' to cover all the circumstances of abuse or neglect of old people.

Abuse and/or neglect can be *intentional* or *unintentional*, although it is sometimes difficult to classify events quite so clearly. So far, little attention has been given to unintentional abuse or neglect.

Mistreatment can take the form of abuse (physical, psychological, or financial/material), or neglect, which is either passive or active (Breckman & Adelman 1988).

Abuse

Physical abuse

Physical abuse of an elderly person is defined at present as 'any physical harm or injury, resulting from assault, inflicted by someone, on an older individual, usually 65 years or more'. It includes beating, kicking, knocking, restraining, shaking, or shoving an older person, as well as burning, scalding, or wounding them. Sexual abuse also falls into this category, as does the imposition of unreasonable physical demands, such as excessive or prolonged toileting.

Nutritional abuse occurs when older persons are given inappropriate food, which is either infantile or which they cannot chew properly or digest without discomfort. Additionally, older persons may be subjected to physical drug abuse, either with unnecessary purgatives or to induce drowsiness, greater compliance and submission.

Psychological abuse

Psychological abuse means 'any behaviour which causes emotional harm, cognitive distress, or undue stress to an older person' (Quinn & Tomita 1986). It incorporates belittling, denigration, ignoring, insults, prolonged silence, rejection, threats, verbal abuse and yelling. It also encompasses patronisation, ageist behaviour, infantilisation (treating an old person as a child), competence erosion and the creation of learned helplessness (see Ch. 3 pp. 52–53 and Ch. 8, p. 178).

Financial and/or material abuse

This is defined as 'the misappropriation of possessions, property or money; extortion; theft; exploitation and/or confidence trickery, undertaken for the benefit of an abuser and the deprivation of an older person' (Breckman & Adelmann 1988). It thus covers a range of unfavourable actions, including deception, fraud, falsification, forgery and masquerading.

Neglect

This is regarded as 'failing to provide basic necessities or minimal care for an older person'.

The passive form is inadvertent, occurring when food or drink, clothing or medications are forgotten, or misgiven, but the action is without malice or intent to harm. This can occur when an elderly caregiver becomes confused.

Active neglect, however, is the deliberate withholding of necessary care, with intent to punish or harm an older person. It can arise from emotional conflict, excessive hostility, rejection, or the ingrained effects of inter-generational violence.

Epidemiology of mistreatment

Epidemiological studies are still sparse in the UK (O'Brien & Piper 1990). An American study of over 2000 randomly selected older persons identified certain patterns (Pillemer & Finklehorn 1988) but these may not all apply to the UK. Abused older persons had poor levels of health, concomitant disabilities, and rarely lived alone, whereas neglected persons lived alone more often, but had few social supports. Contrary to other findings of a predominance of female victims, these researchers found that elderly men were often abused, mostly by their wives. Cognitive incompetence was more common in neglect.

Incidence and prevalence

The incidence rate of frank abuse or neglect in the Pillemer & Finklehor (1988) survey was 32 per 1000 of the population 65 years and over. This is much higher than earlier studies. It may not apply to the UK.

Prevalence, on the other hand, has been estimated to be around 10%. Potential abuse/neglect has not been calculated, being too problematic. Table 10.5 gives some impression of a composite profile of abusers (perpetrators), while Table 10.6 shows a picture of victims. These profiles are based on cumulative characteristics drawn from several research studies.

Predisposing causes

Much abuse arises from caregiver stress, especially when care is being given to confused, disabled, often incontinent old people, on a round the clock basis, without respite (Hocking 1988).

It is exacerbated when caregivers experience one or more of the following:

- poor health, or excessive fatigue
- emotional insecurity and/or low self-esteem
- lack of social support or respite care
- social deprivation, or unmet dependency needs.

However, other researchers contend that elderly mistreatment is largely an extension of general family violence, and often the result of role-modelling, through subsequent generations. They therefore see more analogy between spouse viol-

Table 10.5 Characteristics of persons involved in the mistreatment of elderly people (perpetrators), shown by type of mistreatment

Demographic, biographic and social factors	Psychological mistreatment	Physical mistreatment	Financial/material mistreatment	Passive neglect	Active neglect
Sex	Either	Often male, but wives attack husbands	Either	Either	Often female; can be either
Age	Any age	Any age; often 65+	Often young	Mostly older	Any age
Marital status	Married/divorced or single	Often a spouse	Either	Either	Either
Socio-economic status	Any group	Any group	Often lower group	Any group; often low	Any group
Physical health status	Often poor; history of drug or alcohol abuse; may be disabled	Often poor; may be disabled or chronically sick; alcohol or drug abuser	Usually good or fair	Often poor; may have chronic illness	Often good
Psychological health status	Adverse stress reactions; emotionally dependent; history of drug/alcohol abuse or mental illness; recent decline in cognitive ability	Poor self-control; labile/violent outbursts; unrealistic expectations; may be dependent	Often dependent; emotionally unstable	Arrested development; depressed; may be mentally ill; apathetic; recently bereaved or suffered loss	Immature; often dependent; emotionally unstable; weak coping skills; history of inter-generational violence
Financial status	Often poor; usually dependent	Often dependent	Often dependent on victim; may be in debt	Often poor	May be dependent on victim
Lives with victim	Usually	Probably	Often does not	Usually; may live alone	Usually so, but may live alone
Dependent on victim for basic needs, love, security, interaction	Often heavily so	Dependency may have increased recently	Often so	Often so	May or may not be
Quality of relationship with victim	Often poor or ambivalent	Often ambivalent; may be hostile	Variable; may be covertly hostile	Usually quite good	Indifferent, poor or hostile
Stress levels	Frequently stressed; often maladaptive in stress situations	Variable; often reacts strongly to stress situations	May have lost job; recent redundancy; some crisis situation e.g. prison or lost status	Easily stressed; worn down by prolonged caring	May react sharply to stress; Often is not stressed

Based on material from Hardie (1986), Wolfe (1986), Breckman & Adelman (1988), Hocking (1988), Eastman (1988) and Stanhope & Lancaster (1988).

Table 10.6 Characteristics of elderly victims of mistreatment, shown by types of mistreatment

Demographic and social factors	Psychological and verbal abuse/ mistreatment	Physical mistreatment	Financial and material mistreatment	Passive neglect	Active neglect
Sex	Mainly female	Male or female; if over 75, usually female	Mostly female	Male or female	Either, but more often female
Marital status	Married or single	Often widowed	Single or widowed	Either	Either
Socio-economic status	All classes	Tends to be lower groups	Often higher group	All groups	All groups
Physical health status	Fair or poor; may or may not be disabled	Poor; often incontinent; often disabled	Fair; may or may not be disabled	Poor; often disabled	Poor; often disabled
Psychological health status	Poor emotional health; cognitively oriented; affect low	Poor emotional health; may have cognitive impairment	Often loss of cognitive competence; poor memory	Some loss of cognitive competence	Low mental health; often disoriented
Financial status	Often dependent	Often independent, but can be dependent	Either; usually independent	Either	Often independent
Social support systems	Often lacking or unstable	May be stable	Often loss of support has occurred recently	Often lacking	Often lacking
Living arrangements	Often lives with abuser	Often stable/lives with abuser	May not live with abuser; often recently relocated	Lives with abuser	Lives with abuser
Dependency on abuser for basic needs, love, security, social interaction	Heavily so	Often so	Has become more so recently	Heavily so, but may not be aware of this	Usually heavily so

Based on material from Podnieks (1985), Hardie (1986), Wolfe et al (1986), Breckman & Adelman (1988), Eastman (1988), Pillemer & Finklehor (1988) and Stanhope & Lancaster (1988).

ence and elder abuse than between the latter and child abuse (Stearns 1986).

The case studies of Mrs M and Mr J illustrate some of the intricate factors which influence mistreatment.

CASE STUDIES

Mrs M, widowed, aged 83, was cantankerous, confused, and aggressive. She had partial hearing loss, difficulty in walking, and was frequently incontinent. She had lived for 3 years with her daughter and son-in-law and their three children, in a three-bedroom house, having severed earlier social ties.

Her daughter, Mrs D, stopped work to care for her mother. In spite of state Benefits, income was lost. Over 3 years, Mrs D curtailed her social activities, becoming socially isolated and increasingly stressed. Her husband sought social support outside the home and her children became resentful of her divided attentions.

One day, after a particularly unco-operative episode, Mrs D pushed her mother to the floor, breaking her left arm.

Mr J, aged 85, with mild Alzheimer's disease, lived close to his niece, who had a busy career, often travelling abroad. Following his discharge from hospital, several 'no access' follow-up visits were recorded. Two months later he was found to be increasingly confused, underweight, dehydrated and unkempt. His niece had made arrangements for his care during a time of her absence, but had not been informed that the plans had broken down. The elderly man had been left to fend for himself, with dire result.

Detection of mistreatment

Detection is often problematic because victims are frequently unwilling to admit mistreatment. This may be because of pride, shame, fear, bewilderment or confusion. They may fear to seek help because of heavy dependence on their abuser, and may blame themselves for the situation.

Other barriers to detection lie in the ageist attitudes of staff and lack of professional awareness of risk situations. Professional workers may have preconceived notions about likely perpetrators, and therefore may not notice clues and cues in situations. They may attribute reasons only to caregiver stress, without appreciating that the mistreatment is sometimes a continuation of family violence. On occasions the victim may participate, instigate or acquiesce.

Alerting signs which may guide health visitors are given in Table 10.7 and Figure 10.5.

The health visiting role

Primary prevention

Working with a family on a long-term basis, and strengthening their coping skills in general, enabling them to face multiple stresses, may be the most effective way to contribute to the prevention of elderly mistreatment. Primary prevention therefore comprises encouraging the provision and utilisation of a range of amenities which help persons learn acceptable ways of handling frustrations.

It includes promoting healthy development at all ages and stages of life; assisting older people to plan effectively for retirement, improve their stamina and fitness, and retain their independence; raising their self-esteem and enhancing their contribution to family and community life.

Primary prevention also encompasses the education of individuals, families and communities re-

Table 10.7 Possible signs of mistreatment of elderly persons, shown by type of mistreatment

Psychological or verbal abuse	Anxiety or aggression displayed by elderly person or ?abuser; ambivalence	Elderly person is unusually passive; has low self-esteem, or self-reproach	Elderly person seems excessively tired; confused; has insomnia; is tearful; resigned; afraid of ?abuser	Unexplained weight loss or gain; appetite changes; restlessness or withdrawal
Physical mistreatment	Unexplained injuries; bruising, often over shoulders, buttocks, thighs or forearms; genital infection or damage	Weals; wounds; chafing; burns; scalds; under-scalp haemorrhages; delay in seeking help	Contractures resulting from restraint or prolonged immobility; fear of ?abuser	Signs of over-medication: slurred speech, confusion, drowsiness, passivity, excessive acquiescence, reduced responsiveness
Financial or material abuse	Sudden unexplained withdrawal of money from accounts; unaccountable disappearance of goods and chattels	Sudden/unusual inability to meet bills	Changed lifestyle; excessive reticence regarding expenditure	Unusual interest shown by others in elderly person's possessions/assets; restricted access to elderly person; private conversation prevented
Neglect, passive or active	Unexplained weight loss or dehydration; signs of malnutrition; unkemptness; soiled clothing and linen; untidy environment; lack of evidence of foodstuffs or cooking	Untreated sores; excoriation; infection or injury; absence of prescribed aids: spectacles, hearing aids, dentures	Signs that medication has been withheld; unsafe environment ignored; inadequate heating or lighting; elderly person withdrawn or passive	Refusal to deal with hazards or unhygienic surroundings on part of ?abuser; restricted access to old person; old person left for long periods without care; caregiver hostile or aggressive

Based on material from Podnieks (1985), Hardie (1986), Breckman & Adelman (1988), Pillemer & Finklehor (1988), Stanhope & Lancaster (1988).

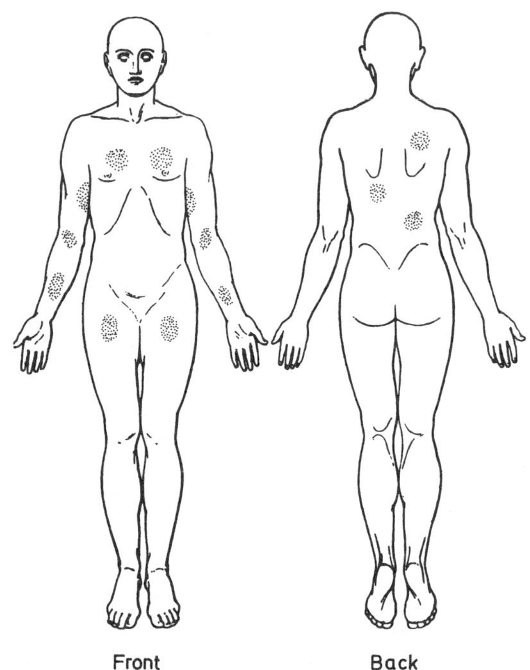

Fig. 10.5 Some areas of bruising suggestive of possible mistreatment of elderly persons.

garding the needs of older people and effective ways of caring for them.

By generating positive attitudes towards older people, and promoting healthy living at all ages, health visitors can assist families to approach their difficulties in a collaborative and problem-solving manner. Through working in schools, clinics, and employing organisations, practitioners can encourage stimulation, empowerment, interdependence and appropriate outlets for the release of anger and associated emotions. Anticipatory guidance techniques, and the mobilisation of relief services in fraught situations, are also of value.

Secondary prevention

Secondary prevention is required when abuse or neglect is incipient. Health visitors can then initiate measures to help reduce potential mistreatment. For action to be effective, practitioners need to explore their own feelings about the issue, and resolve any negative attitudes towards potential perpetrators. This is not an easy task. However, it is the only way that acceptance of a perpetrator is possible; and is an essential prelude to effective communication and work with both parties. Such communication rests upon trust in the relationship and is helped if practitioners convey warmth, understanding, empathy, compassion and care. It requires time, patience and the investment of considerable energy, so worker-support systems are essential.

Both parties need to talk out their feelings in a 'safe' climate, explore possible causes and seek, through mutual respect and problem-solving, to resolve these. Workers will probably need to mobilise a range of support services, such as home help, nursing services, or day centres, to provide respite and relieve tension. Voluntary visiting and befriending may sometimes prove helpful. Surveillance, the use of telephone 'hot lines' when tensions rise, and the effective treatment of any disabling or chronic condition, are also crucial.

Multi-disciplinary case conferences may be required at this stage, and key workers may be appointed. Such workers can assist carers to offer improved care to older people, encouraging co-operation rather than provoking resistance. Promoting continence, mobility and independence in the older person, as far as possible, can also help.

Paramount is ensuring that the caregiver's needs are recognised and met in an acceptable manner.

Tertiary prevention

This is needed when frank abuse has occurred and secondary prevention has failed. It will involve help for both victim and perpetrator. Protection of the victim is the primary goal, following reporting of the situation to the general practitioner and health visiting manager. Protection is usually best achieved by removal from the home situation, either to hospital or a place of refuge. This may be a LASS residential establishment or voluntary provision. Ameliorative treatment should be given as indicated.

Legal action against the perpetrator may be taken. Practitioners should ensure all records are accurate; current; comprehensive, but concise; legible; signed and dated. They should be made available as appropriate. Health visitors may be required to attend any subsequent court proceedings, and they should seek legal advice, in concert with their nursing manager.

Thereafter therapeutic interventions will be required by both parties, to help them rebuild their lives. This will include dealing with the psychosocial accompaniment of the mistreatment, such as anger, guilt, shame and/or blame. The aim is to facilitate independent healthy lives and the maintenance of caring relationships, without further mistreatment situations.

SUMMARY

In this chapter the needs of specific groups of elderly people and their carers have been explored. The high prevalence of impairment, disability and, sometimes, handicap has been shown, with reference to recent research. The impact of pain, restriction, immobility and loss of self-respect on elderly people and their significant others has been discussed. The purpose has been to highlight the action needed from health visitors.

The importance of transcultural issues in influencing the health visiting role has been examined, and the needs of specific ethnic minority elderly persons considered.

Finally the problem of elder mistreatment has been looked at, with particular reference to health visiting interventions at primary, secondary and tertiary levels. With shrinking family size and increasing numbers of older people, this is an aspect that may increase in the future, unless we can take steps now to provide our elderly population with adequate physical and psychosocial care, and the economic means to enable them to exercise choice in later maturity.

REFERENCES

Allen M N 1989 The meaning of visual impairment to visually impaired adults. Journal of Advanced Nursing 14: 640–646

Arie T 1988 Questions in the psychiatry of old age. In: Evered D, Whelan J (eds) Research and the ageing population. Ciba Foundation Symposium No 134. Wiley, Chichester

Baker A A 1975 Granny battering. British Medical Journal 3: 592

Bhat A, Carr-Hill R, Ohri S 1988 Britain's Black population: a new perspective, 2nd edn. Gower, Aldershot

Blackburn J 1988 Chronic health problems of the elderly. In: Chilman C S, Nunally E W, Cox F M (eds) Chronic illness and disability. Families in trouble series, vol 2. Sage, Newbury Park, California

Blakemore K 1982 Health and illness among the elderly of ethnic minority groups in Birmingham. Health Trends 14 (3) (August): 69–72

Blumenthal M D 1980 Depressive illness in old age: getting behind the mush. Geriatrics (April): 34–43

Branch L G 1985 Health practices and incident disability among the elderly. American Journal of Public Health 75 (12) (Dec): 1436–1439

Breckman R S, Adelman R D 1988 Strategies for helping victims of elder mistreatment. Sage, New York

Brown G W, Harris T O 1978 Social origins of depression. Tavistock, London

Burston G R 1975 Granny battering. British Medical Journal 3: 592

Bury M 1982 Chronic illness as biographic disruption. Sociology of Health and Illness 4 (2): 167–181

Charlesworth A, Wilkin D, Durie A 1983 Carers and services: a comparison of men and women caring for dependent elderly people. Equal Opportunities Commission, Manchester

Charmaz K 1983 Loss of self. Sociology of Health and Illness 5 (2): 168–194

Cruikshank J K, Beavers D G, Verdelle L O, Haynes R, Corbett J C R, Selby S 1980 Heart attack, stroke, diabetes and hypertension in West Indians, Asians and Whites in Birmingham, England. British Medical Journal 281: 1108

Darnbrough A, Kinrade D 1988 Directory for disabled people: a handbook of information and opportunities for disabled and handicapped persons. Faulkner-Woodhead, Cambridge, in association with The Royal Association for Disability and Rehabilitation

Davies S, Stewart A 1987 Nutritional medicine. Pan, London

DHSS (Department of Health and Social Security) 1980 Inequalities in health. Report of a Committee, Chairman: Sir Douglas Black. HMSO, London

Disability Alliance Briefings 1989 Comments on The Disability Prevalence Survey. Disability Alliance (ERA), London

Dobson S 1987 Transcultural nursing: the role of the health visitor in multi-cultural situations. Unpublished Ph D Thesis, University of Edinburgh, Edinburgh

Dobson S 1989 Conceptualizing for transcultural health visiting: the concept of transcultural reciprocity. Journal of Advanced Nursing 14: 97–102

DSS (Department of Social Security) 1989 Caring for people: community care in the next decade and beyond. Government White Paper, November. HMSO, London

Eastman 1988 The elderly at risk of abuse. Primary Health Care 6 (9) (Oct): 4

Fenton S 1987 Ageing minorities: Black people as they grow old in Britain. Commission for Racial Equality, London

Glendenning F (ed) 1979 The elders in ethnic minorities. A Beth Johnson Foundation publication, in association with the Department of Adult Education, University of Keele, and the Commission for Racial Equality, London

Gray M, McKenzie H 1980 Take care of your elderly relative. Allen and Unwin, London

The Guardian newspaper 1984 Report on racial discrimination in the National Health Service. 4th January
Hall J H, Zwemer D 1979 Prospective medicine. Methodist Hospital of Indiana, Indianapolis
Hanley I, Baikie E 1984 Understanding and treating depression in the elderly. In: Hanley I, Hodge I (eds) Psychological approaches to the care of the elderly. Croom Helm, London
Hardie J 1986 Violence and the elderly. Journal of District Nursing (April): 4–6
Harris A 1971 Handicapped and impaired. OPCS, HMSO, London
Health Promotion 1986 The Ottawa Charter. Report of the First International Conference on Health Promotion, Ottawa, Canada. Health Promotion 1 (4): iii–v. Oxford University Press, Oxford
Helman C 1984 Culture, health and illness. John Wright, Bristol
Herbst K, Humphrey C 1980 Hearing impairment and mental state in the elderly living at home. British Medical Journal 281: 903–905
HMSO 1968 Report of the Committee on Local Authority and Allied Personal Social Services (Seebohm Report). HMSO, London
Hocking E 1988 The elderly at risk. Primary Health Care (4th Oct): 4
Ineichen B 1980 Mental illness among new Commonwealth migrants to Britain. In: Boyce A (ed) Mobility and migration. Taylor & Francis, London
Ingham J, Miller P 1982 Consulting with mild symptoms in general practice. Social Psychiatry 17: 77–88
Jenkins C D 1985 Life's crises. World Health (August/September): 10–12
Johnson T 1986 Critical issues in the definition of elder mistreatment. In: Pillemer K A, Wolfe R (eds) Elder abuse: conflict in the family. Auburn House, Dover, Massachusetts
Karseras P, Hopkins E 1987 British Asians: health in the community. H M & M Publications, Topics in community health series. Wiley, Chichester
Kline N 1976 Incidence, prevalence and recognition of depressive illness. Diseases of the Nervous System 37: 10
Klingbeil K 1986 Interpersonal violence: a comprehensive model, in a hospital setting: from policy to program. Public Health Report of the Surgeon-General: DHHS No HRS-D-MC-86-1 Health Resources and Services Administration. US Public Health Service, US Dept of Health and Human Services, Washington DC
Knight S, Gann R 1988 Self help guide: a directory of self help groups in the UK. Chapman and Hall, London
LeMay A C, Redfern S J 1987 The nature and frequency of nurse–patient touch, and its relationship to the well-being of elderly patients. In: Sorvettula M (ed) Collaborative research and its implementation in nursing: Proceedings of the Working Group of European Nurse Researchers Conference, Helsinki 1986. Finnish Federation of Nurses and Nursing Research Institute, Helsinki
Lewis C B 1985 Ageing: the health care challenge: an inter-disciplinary approach to assessment and rehabilitation. Davis, Philadelphia
Littlewood R K, Lipsedge M 1982 Aliens and alienists. Penguin, Harmondsworth
MacLean U 1989 Dependent territories: the frail elderly and community care. Nuffield Provincial Hospital Trust, London
MacLeod Clark J 1985 The development of research in interpersonal skills in nursing. In: Kagan C M (ed) Interpersonal skills in nursing: research and application. Croom Helm, London
McNaught 1985 Race and health care in the United Kingdom. Occasional Paper No 2. Health Education Council, London
Mares P, Henley A, Baxter C 1985 Health care in multi-racial Britain. Health Education Council/National Extension College, Cambridge
Marmot M G, Adelstein A, Bulusu L 1984a Immigrant mortality in England and Wales. Studies in Medical and Population Subjects (47): HMSO, London
Marmot M G, Adelstein A, Bulusu L 1984b Lessons from the study of immigrant mortality. The Lancet (30th June): 1455–1457
Minassian D C, Mehra V, Jones B R 1984 Dehydrational crises from severe diarrhoea or heat stroke, and the risk of cataract. The Lancet 8380 (1): 751–753
Murphy E 1982 The social origins of depression, in old age. British Journal of Psychiatry 141: 135–142
Murphy E 1983 The prognosis of depression in old age. British Journal of Psychiatry 142: 111–119
Nash W 1988 At ease with stress: the approach of wholeness. Darton, Longman Todd
Nichols K 1984 Psychological care in physical illness. Croom Helm, London
O'Brien J G, Piper M E 1990 (in press) Elder abuse. In: Pathy M S J (ed) Principles and practice of geriatric medicine. Wiley, Chichester
OPCS 1988a Surveys of disability in Great Britain. Report No 1: The prevalence of disability amongst adults. HMSO, London
OPCS 1988b Surveys of disability in Great Britain. Report No 2: The financial circumstances of disabled adults living in private households. HMSO, London
OPCS 1989 Surveys of disability in Great Britain. Report No 4: Disabled adults: services, transport and employment. HMSO, London
Orem D 1980 Nursing: concepts for practice, 2nd edn. McGraw Hill, New York
Ottawa Charter for Health Promotion 1986 Health Promotion 1 (4): iii–v. Oxford University Press, Oxford
Petty R, Sensky T 1987 Depression: treating the whole person. Unwin Hyman, London
Pillemer K A, Finklehor D 1988 The prevalence of elder abuse: a random sample survey. The Gerontological Society of America 28 (1): 51–57
Podnieks E 1985 Elder abuse: it's time we did something about it. The Canadian Nurse 81 (Part II): 36–39
Post F 1981 Affective illnesses. In: Arie T (ed) Health care of the elderly. Croom Helm, London
Quinn M, Tomita S (eds) 1986 Elder abuse and neglect: causes, diagnosis and intervention strategies. Springer, New York
Qureshi B 1989 Transcultural medicine. Kluwer Academic Publishers, Dordrecht
Rack P 1982 Culture and mental disorder. Tavistock, London
Redfern S 1989 Key issues in nursing elderly people. In: Warnes A M (ed) Human ageing and later life:

multi-disciplinary perspectives. Edward Arnold, London

Ricoeur P 1981 Hermeneutics and the human sciences. Translated and edited by Thompson J. Cambridge University Press, New York

The Royal College of Physicians 1986 Physical disability in 1986 and beyond. Journal of Royal College of Physicians of London 20 (3) (July): 160–194

Saunders P 1989 The A–Z of disability: directory of information, services, organizations, equipment and manufacturers. Crowood Press, Ramsbury, Marlborough, Wiltshire

Scrutton S 1989 Counselling older people: a creative response to ageing. Age Concern Handbooks, Edward Arnold, London

Smith A, Jacobson B (eds) 1988 The nation's health — a strategy for the 1990s. Report from an independent Multi-disciplinary Committee, Chairman: Sir Alwyn Smith. King Edward's Hospital Fund for London, London

Stanhope M, Lancaster J 1988 Community health nursing: process and practice for promoting health, 2nd edn. Mosby, St Louis

Stearns P J 1986 Old age family conflict: the perspective of the past. In: Pillemer K, Wolfe R (eds) Elder abuse: conflict in the family. Auburn House, Dover, Massachusetts

Townsend P, Davidson N 1982 Inequalities in health (The Black Report). Penguin Books, Harmondsworth

Twining C 1988 Helping older people: a psychological approach. Wiley, Chichester

Wade D T, Langton-Hewer R, Skilbeck C E, David R M 1985 Stroke: a critical approach to diagnosis, management and treatment. Chapman and Hall, Medical, London

Weale 1989 Eyes and age. In: Warnes A M (ed) Human ageing and later life: multi-disciplinary perspectives. Age Concern Institute of Gerontology and Edward Arnold, London

WHO (World Health Organization) 1978 Alma Ata declaration on primary health care. WHO, Geneva

WHO (World Health Organization) 1980 The international classification of impairments, disabilities and handicaps. WHO, Geneva

WHO (World Health Organization) 1981a Preventing disability in the elderly: report of a WHO Working Group (Euro Reports and studies No 65). Regional Office for Europe, WHO, Copenhagen

WHO (World Health Organization) 1989 Health of the elderly. Report of a WHO Expert Committee. Technical Report Series 779. WHO, Geneva

Wolfe R S 1986 Major findings from three medical projects on elderly abuse. In: Pillemer K, Wolfe R S (eds) Conflict in the family. Auburn House, Dover, Massachusetts

Zigman S 1981 Photochemical mechanisms in cataract formation. In: Duncan G (ed) Mechanisms of cataract formation in the human lens. Academic Press, London

FURTHER RECOMMENDED READING

Fuller J H S, Toon P D 1988 Medical practice in a multi-racial society. Heinemann Medical, London

Tomlin S 1989 Abuse of elderly people: an unnecessary and preventable problem. A public information Report from The British Geriatrics Society

CHAPTER CONTENTS

11

What of the future?

The reality of an ageing population is with us. This fact can no longer be ignored, whether we adopt the stance of a professional worker likely facing an increased workload; consider it from the viewpoint of a family, aware of longevity in relatives or family friends; or regard it from a personal angle, with a degree of self-interest, realising that we too may one day be old. The implications of a rising proportion of older people in the population affect us not only as individuals, but also as citizens. For, whereas many of the decisions which affect how we live our lives in our later years, are our own, it is society which often affords us the chance to do so with dignity and independence.

Throughout this book, we have endeavoured to present positive attitudes towards the care of older people, believing that these adults constitute a great human resource to be wisely utilised. However, their full utilisation depends on their maintaining functional independence, high-level wellness and quality of life, which includes ultimately a dignified and peaceful death. These qualities, which allow for participation in family and community affairs, are unlikely to be achieved by and for older persons through high technology. Instead these older clients are more likely to depend on a repertoire of self-care competencies, and on the complementing care of well-informed families, friends and neighbours. They will also require the perceptive, but unobtrusive, assessment of practitioners who are aware of the complex nature of ageing and the specific needs generated. Additionally they will require programmes of co-ordinated, progressive and continuing care, often of an innovatory nature, provided by multidisciplinary teams.

In 1980 WHO indicated the direction for future research and social policies for older people, emphasising the services and systems needed by the elderly world-wide:

1. services subserving basic vital needs, such as housing and money
2. life-enhancing services, e.g. clubs, education, health promotion, transport and leisure
3. compensating services when there is difficulty or impairment
4. care services when function is lost.

A decade later the need for such services remains substantially the same.

Within such programmes, we believe the health visiting service can play a major part, provided there is a corporate professional decision to do so. This implies a willingness to re-appraise methods and techniques used. In this connection we welcome the National Standing Conference report (1989), with its proposals for curriculum change for future health visitors.

Four other drastic and far-reaching programmes are likely to affect the way in which such a contribution can be offered and utilised. These are:

1. the implementation of Project 2000 and the reform of pre-registration nursing education
2. the reform of the National Health Service
3. the reorganisation/reform of community care
4. the Strategy for Nursing, for the UK, set within the overall WHO Strategy, Health for all by the year 2000.

THE REFORM OF PRE-REGISTRATION NURSE EDUCATION

Project 2000 offers student nurses a new preparation for practice, leading to a qualification at Diploma level, recognised within higher education. Courses based upon a health model, with a strong emphasis on health promotion, aim to prepare first-level practitioners to work in a range of care settings. This requires students to gain ex-

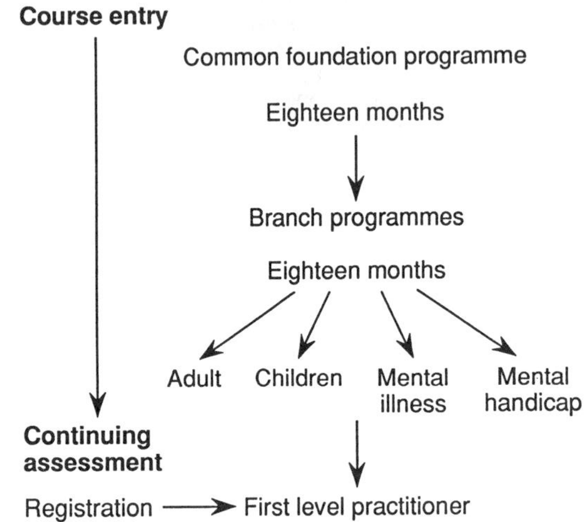

Fig. 11.1 General course design for Nurse Education, under Project 2000.

perience both inside and outside institutions, the latter necessitating different forms of exposure to work in the community (Orr 1990). Courses are designed for progression from a common foundation of 18 months duration to branch programmes of similar length which allow for concentration in an area of special interest. Thus at registration the first-level practitioner will be qualified to work in either adult, children, mental illness or mental handicap fields (see Fig. 11.1).

During preparation students are expected to achieve certain learning outcomes which incorporate specific skills, knowledge and attitudes, which will enable them to give competent nursing care. They are also expected to develop their ability to understand the sociocultural, political and emotional influences which affect individuals, families and communities.

In the context of this book, they are required to identify the social and health implications of ageing for the individual, his/her friends, family and community. Thus at registration, such first-level practitioners are expected to meet the nursing needs of older adults at any point along the health–illness continuum. Individualised care to patients, at all stages of dependency and in a variety of care settings, is also expected (ENB Circular 1989).

Implications for future health visitor preparation

The changes mentioned above hold considerable implications for future nurse and health visitor preparation. In consequence, care of the older client should be improved. Future health visitor practitioners will be drawn from a pool of nurses with a broader-based knowledge. Because these practitioners will qualify at Diploma level, it is reasonable to assume that the second-level practitioners will be educated to Degree level, thus paving the way for the much-needed Masters and Doctoral programmes. Thus at the second level (Specialist), and in Advanced practice, research will become a marked activity.

The Credit Accumulation Transfer Scheme (CATS), presently being developed within higher education, will allow existing practitioners, who pursue approved post-registration studies, to accumulate points towards a degree. This is likely to give an impetus to the need for continuing education.

The project 2000 document recognises that second-level practitioners will be either Clinical Specialists, or Specialists in Health Promotion. The latter therefore provides a new brief for future health visitors. Because prospective health visitor students will be drawn from four branch programmes, future health visiting course design should probably foster a modular approach, to cater for the variety of learning needs and experiences. In turn this will necessitate a common core content, which will incorporate a professional dimension that will enable all students to appreciate and identify with the professional practitioner role as health promotion specialist.

This need to address the issues of post-registration preparation forms the basis of investigations currently being undertaken by the UKCC Post-Registration Education and Practice Project (PREPP). The three main planks of the project, encapsulated by the UKCC standards framework, are depicted in Fig. 11.2. The project report will be eagerly awaited by existing and future health visitors.

The significance of these radical educational re-

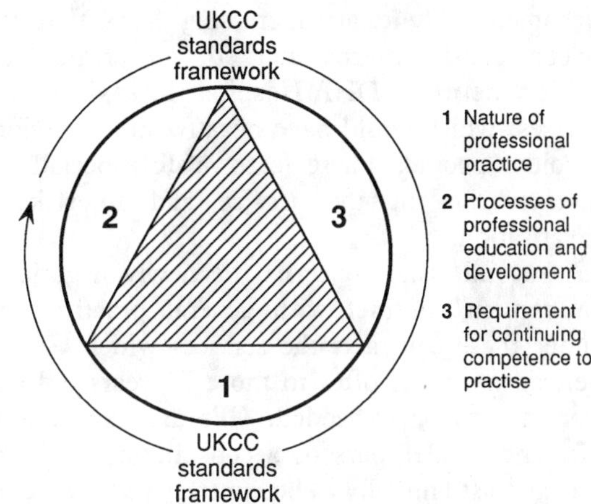

Fig. 11.2 The United Kingdom Central Council for Nurses, Midwives and Health Visitors' Standards Framework Model, based on information from The Post-Registration Education and Practice Project (PREPP), August 1989.

forms is likely to be far reaching. They imply that in future there will be further improvements in the research content on which care for older clients is based, and an even more critical approach to practice and evaluation. The knock-on effect should be seen in more comprehensive selection procedures for entrants to nursing and in the eventual impact on general education. Other issues affecting practice include the implications of first-level practitioners working in the community, which will doubtless require health visitors to act as team leaders heading up skill-mixed teams. In addition pre-registration students will require health visitors to plan, co-ordinate and/or provide structured learning opportunities, as well as the assessment and evaluation of their student progress. All the above will call for enhanced skills, especially in marketing the health promotion specialist role.

THE NATIONAL HEALTH SERVICE REFORMS

A number of earlier references have already been made to proposed NHS reforms and to health visitor concerns about their potential effects on care for older clients (DHSS 1989). The bill to introduce the new legislation is currently before

Parliament. There are increasing fears that the concept of 'the internal market', will create competition between DHA/Hospital Trusts and GP services, which could have negative repercussions for older people. These fears relate especially to fragmentation of the service and to risk of privatisation.

A second issue concerns the newly negotiated government contract with general practitioners. Under these contracts the services which GPs or their agents must offer to those 75 years old and over, are to be expanded. GPs are expected to offer these older persons a consultation or home visit at least annually. The contract requires a social assessment, a mobility and mental assessment, an assessment of the senses and continence, a functional assessment, a review of medication, and a consideration of the availability of home carers or relatives (Tremellen 1990). This is a commendable development but it raises the question as to who will undertake the tasks. Many directly employed practice nurses are already required by GPs to undertake home visiting 'if asked to do so'. However, in many instances they lack community preparation to undertake this duty. Hence their professional accountability could be compromised.

By contrast, health visitors are well able to offer this service to older people. However, for them direct employment by GPs would constitute a threat to their practitioner autonomy. Professional organisations are advocating the negotiation of joint FPC/DHA contracts as an acceptable alternative to such direct employment. There is no guarantee that such negotiations will be successful, and some health visitors fear that their future work with the older elderly will be under some threat.

A counter-view, however, is that some GPs will recognise the advantages of utilising the services of DHA-employed health visitors, because of their specialist skills. Nevertheless, even where other agents do undertake contractual tasks for the GP, it should be recognised that this relates to an assessment within the medical model only. Hence this does not preclude health visitors from offering their health promotion services to the 'older elderly'. Furthermore, the 'younger elderly' will still continue to provide great scope for health promotion and health education activity, as one important aspect of the health visiting role.

THE REORGANISATION OF COMMUNITY CARE

The government proposals for the reorganising of community care have as their main emphasis the provision of home care whenever possible (DSS 1989). With our wish to see a high quality of care for older people, we do not take issue with such an aim. Rather our concerns for the future lie in the following.

1. That while there are no proposed standards for monitoring the care provided in clients' own homes, quality cannot be assured. One possible solution might be the devising of joint, professionally determined and agreed criteria, which are client centred.
2. That there is insufficient detail regarding the funding of the proposed services and in particular no ring-fencing of the budget, except in relation to mentally ill clients. This highlights the need for political awareness and continual monitoring of resources.
3. That while the input from the community nursing services is regarded as vital, there is no indication as to how this is to be safeguarded. Collaborative practice would seem to be indicated, and a possible role for health visitors as key workers, or case managers, in certain instances.
4. That there is no mention in the proposals regarding how the rights of service users in the future are to be guaranteed. There would seem to be a case for advocacy or representation.

Thus the potential for future developments between health visitors and social services staff, especially in relation to older clients, would seem to be considerable. However, it requires concerted action to determine how far the health visiting profession can make this challenge become an opportunity.

THE STRATEGY FOR NURSING, AND THE WHO STRATEGY: HEALTH FOR ALL BY 2000

The Strategy for Nursing (DHSS Nursing Division 1986) set out a plan for the overall nursing profession in the UK, within the context of the international strategy for Health for All by 2000 (WHO 1978, 1985). Targets set for the early 1990s focus on manpower, management, education, practice and leadership. In this last category the authors of the UK report had clearly taken note of the comments made by Dr Mahler, Director General of WHO, when he said in relation to the programme 'Health for All', 'NURSES SHOULD LEAD THE WAY' (Mahler 1985).

We have already signified that we believe the nursing profession in general, and health visiting in particular, can play a leading part in health promotion, at all ages, and particularly for older people. However, stating what should be done and what can be done *does not ensure that things will be done*. Individual and collective action has to be taken to translate stated targets into reality. Issues such as recruitment and retention of staff have to be faced. The principles of health promotion have to be applied to ourselves as well as to our client/patients. The early health visitors were imbued with pioneer spirit. They initiated and developed schemes in conjunction with lay personnel; there is an urgent need for a resurgence of this approach. In this, Managers have a vital role in facilitating health visitors, so that they can play their part, especially in relation to older people. There are distinct areas for development, especially within the 'family visitor' function, in work within groups and in community development, which staff should be assisted to undertake.

Others, too, have to help health visitors achieve their aims in relation to the ongoing care of older people. In particular, community medical staff, within the 'new public health movement', can do much to encourage and help.

Most of all the future of health visiting care for older adults depends upon the ability of this present generation of practitioners to demonstrate conclusively that they can substantiate their professional claims to offer a unique service to elderly people.

REFERENCES

DHSS (Department of Health and Social Security) Nursing Division 1986 A strategy for nursing. HMSO, London

DHSS 1989 Working for patients. HMSO, London

DSS 1989 Caring for people: community care into the next decade and beyond. HMSO, London

ENB (English National Board for Nursing, Midwifery and Health Visiting) 1989 Circular: Project 2000: a new preparation for practice. Guidelines and criteria for course development and the formation of collaborative links between approved training institutions within the NHS and centres of Higher Education. ENB, London

Mahler H 1985 Nurses should lead the way. WHO Features 97: 1–3

National Standing Conference of Representatives of Health Visitor Education and Training Centres 1989 Health visitor education and training: the way forward. Report of a Study Conference Weekend, May 1989. NSCHETC, Sheffield

Orr J 1990 Project 2000 and the specialist practitioner. Nursing Standard 4 (7) (17th Jan): 35–37

Tremellen J 1990 Assessing the elderly in the community. Health Visitor 63 (2) (Feb): 49–51

WHO (World Health Organization) 1978 Alma Ata Declaration. Report of the International Conference on Primary Health Care. WHO, Geneva

WHO (World Health Organization) 1980 Services and systems of care for the elderly. (document 1CP/ADR 015) Helsincki

WHO (World Health Organization) 1985 Targets for health for all. WHO Regional Office for Europe, Copenhagen

Appendix 1

Guide to community assessment, with special reference to the elderly

Increasingly health visitors and other community nursing staff are required to utilise community profiles. Consequently community assessment is a necessary prelude. Initial assessment is required when providing baseline data, or when moving to new areas; regular updating of material is required in 'familiar' communities. Much material may be provided through new computerised information systems, but sometimes practitioners may be required to provide their own data. Student health visitors are expected to produce neighbourhood studies as part of their background assessment material.

Familiarisation with the epidemiological perspective and community dynamics, can prove invaluable to health visitors, helping them to take a population perspective and enabling them to slot work with families and individuals into context.

The following guide is therefore provided, to assist readers to think about those aspects of community life which impinge on members and which can profoundly affect the quality of living.

The framework is not claimed to be exhaustive; it can, of course, be adapted to individual need. Acknowledgement is freely made to many other publications which have helped guide thinking.

ASSESSMENT

Give the name of the community, especially the root derivative and the meanings assigned to this; boundaries as defined both geographically and administratively; size, shape, demarcating characteristics.

Community characteristics

Topographic features. Describe nature of terrain; presence of hills/valleys and similar natural features — their implications for community health and safety.

Geographic features. Give brief description of main geographic features; main climate, rainfall, mean temperature and seasonal variations. Note the import of these features for community health and well-being.

Historic features. Make brief reference to major historical features, especially those that have direct bearing on current care for older people in the particular community, and the relevance of these historical features for general community health today.

Demographic features. Note population size and structure. Consider trends in population over past 20 years; note major changes, especially those affecting older people. Identify the proportion of older adults within the total population, and relate this information to social class and ethnic distribution, where possible. Compare and contrast with forward projections. Identify the likely implications of these population trends for the health and social services in general, and the health visiting service in particular.

Identify the main mortality and morbidity statistics, noting general trends within the total population and the age-specific death rates. Ascertain and consider the major causes of death and the main morbidity patterns, with particular reference to elderly people. Specify which programmes, if any, have been commenced to deal with these various major causes of death and disease among the general population and especially amongst older adults. Outline specific evaluation of such programmes, to determine effectiveness/impact. Identify major deficits in programme-planning in this sector: determine priorities for action.

Community health services

Ascertain and analyse the major health services in terms of stated criteria. Are bed ratios appropriate for the population (especially older adults), in hospital and residential establishments? Identify short-fall in provisions and give priority rating. Identify the manpower establishments in terms of stated criteria, indicating funded and filled posts in hospital and domiciliary services. Relate to standardised staff–population ratios, where available. Ascertain deficits and consider implications of same, especially affecting the care of elderly adults.

Determine the accessibility and availability of services, especially obtaining the views of older persons on this issue.

Note how the Community Health Council and other similar local 'watchdog organisations', view the adequacy/inadequacy of services. Specify any areas of unmet need.

Collect data relevant to the pattern of hospital admissions and discharges, especially relating to older people. Examine the use of accident and emergency departments, identifying where possible any local problems which cause clients, especially, elderly clients, to use these services in preference to general medical and community nursing services. Consider the efficiency/effectiveness of any follow-up systems, following hospital admission or use of outpatient or accident and emergency services. What improvements, if any, need to be made?

Community nursing services

Review the data pertaining to the number of visits paid by (a) District Nurses (b) Health Visitors to different sections of the population. Draw the inferences from these patterns of service, as set against the age-specific population groups. Identify the percentage of persons served and not served, particularly noting the short-fall in service for older persons. Consider what needs to be done to remedy any marked deficits in care.

Where possible relate the service given to the various settings, viz: home visits; consultations in clinics, surgeries, and health centres. What inferences can be drawn? Note the proportion of service accorded to day centres, residential establishments, sheltered housing and other places where care may be given. Obtain the 'feel' of the distribution of activities; identify where inadequacies appear. Note the formal recorded health education activities designed especially for elderly people, and the approximate proportion of the elderly so contacted. Determine what improvements require to be made.

Evaluate the health visiting service given to this community over the past 5 years, related to major goals, and particularly identify the service accorded older adults. Compare/contrast with the major goals of the health visiting service, *for this community*, for (a) the next year, (b) the next 5 years, with particular reference to the goals set for care of older clients. Determine how far the goals set accord with the wishes of clients and any client/carers; what degree of involvement in planning and implementing such care is forthcoming from this community? Could these levels of involvement be improved? How?

Environmental health services

Note standards of environmental health care with specific reference to water supplies, sewage and refuse disposal, pollution, nuisance abatement, housing, public lighting, street cleaning, supervision of shops/markets/restaurants, food hygiene and supervision. Note particularly the attention paid to the needs of older persons within the environment, especially related to the incidence of infectious diseases, food poisoning and accidents.

Consider the adequacy of environmental health services in relation to community needs; staff–population ratios and the extent to which staff are involved in multi-disciplinary activities with health visitors and community health staff, e.g. in health education/promotion activities.

Ascertain machinery for determining joint goals; how far can improvements be effected?

Social services

Briefly describe the services available, identifying adequacy/inadequacy in relation to community needs. Note staff–population ratios in relation to recommended establishments and identify any short-fall. What steps are being taken to remedy such short-fall? Identify the lines of communication between health and social services personnel and the existence of any arrangements for improving these, e.g. regular liaison groups.

How will current proposals for reforming community care services impinge upon existing liaison arrangements? How will they affect existing services?

Briefly describe the specific services for the elderly available within this community, e.g. clubs; leisure facilities; services for the impaired, disabled and/or handicapped; provision of day centres in relation to need; proportion of services allocated to elderly persons by the home help service; meals on wheels services; laundry services; transport services; any specific home care assistant scheme?

Discover the details of short-term admission facilities for elderly persons, within the social services sector; numbers of places in residential accommodation, in relation to need; the existence of special programmes designed to facilitate rehabilitation in the case of disability. Discover any specific social problems affecting the community, which call for particular action, especially affecting the older population.

Voluntary services

Is there a directory of voluntary services available in the community? Identify particularly those societies with interest in the care of older people. Note how to contact these. Are services well-staffed? Are there arrangements for older persons who wish to engage in voluntary service? Are there specific gaps in the service? Is there a co-ordinating body, and, if so, do health visitors liaise? How far will proposals to increase the contribution of voluntary organisations in community care modify existing arrangements?

Private services

What private provision exists in the community; especially relating to the care of older people? What contact do health services personnel have with these various services?

Educational services

Briefly describe the services available, in relation

to population need. Are educational establishments easily accessible to older clients? Are there any special programmes available for the older population, or concessions for participation in general programmes? Discover what proportion of older persons avail themselves of educational provisions. Can any improvements be effected? How?

Details of local government

State the composition of the local council and note the electoral machinery and patterns. Note the sources of local authority finance and the disbursement of funds against stated community needs. What proportion of available monies is used for services affecting older clients? What changes are envisaged in view of proposed legislative reforms?

Does the civic authority pursue any specific policy affecting older people?

Identify the key figures in public life and community affairs. Does the community show a keen interest in electing and lobbying its leaders? What degree of interest and support is shown by these key persons, especially in relation to the care of older persons?

Communication measures

State the local newspapers and any local radio stations or other media. How far do health visitors use these forms of communication to put across health promotion measures; are they afforded adequate scope to do so? To what extent do the media appear to influence policies affecting the care of older people?

Housing and associated amenities

Briefly examine the general housing layout, noting the overall design in terms of accessibility, structure, personal convenience and aesthetic appeal. Does housing overall enhance the quality of community living? Describe the major types of dwelling, noting the proportion of home owners to public and private tenants. Identify the pattern of living for the older population. Is this appropriate?

What is the percentage of sub-standard housing? What proportion of older persons live in such sub-standard housing? Outline the proposed programmes for dealing with local housing problems, noting the adequacy/inadequacy of such. Examine trends in waiting lists. Are there specific provisions for elderly persons within this community's housing programmes? Do these provisions meet the needs of the older population? Can persons in larger accommodation obtain exchange to smaller accommodation relatively easily? What sheltered accommodation is provided? Is this an adequate proportion and is the housing located within reasonable proximity to other accommodation? Is it near to other amenities, including transport services, shops and churches?

What avenues of communication exist between housing department personnel, wardens, and health service staffs? Are these channels well used? Can communication be improved, and, if so, how?

Note the general distribution of shops, markets, post offices, public libraries and places of worship. Is there adequate neighbourhood provision for elderly persons unable to travel to town centres? Is public transport available, accessible and suitable for older persons? Are there concessionary fares for older persons?

Are leisure facilities available to older persons and can they easily avail themselves of these? Do they do so? Is the range of recreational clubs and peer-group interests appropriate for older persons? Can elderly housebound persons be transported easily and regularly to these leisure facilities? What action, if any, is being taken to improve any inadequacies in common amenities, for community members, especially the aged?

Protective services

Briefly describe the availability of fire, ambulance and police services. Note lines of communication. Consider the distribution of services in relation to community needs. Are there specific schemes for protecting older persons?

Employment facilities

Briefly review the major types of employment available in the community. Is there a broad diversification of employment? What is the percentage of unemployed persons? How does the trend compare with 5 years ago? How with the national average? What action, if any is being taken to effect any improvement?

Is there any specific provision for the employment of older persons in this community? If so, briefly describe the schemes, noting the lines of communication and systems of referral of elderly persons who may wish to work. If there are no schemes, can any be mooted? Is there support for such new development?

Community dynamics

Identify the levels of interest shown by community members in community affairs. Can 'Key individuals' be identified? How far can the community be described as a caring community? Why is this so? Identify particularly the degree of community interest and support for programmes and policies affecting the care of older people.

SUMMARY OF HEALTH AND SOCIAL NEEDS WITHIN THE COMMUNITY

Summarise the main unmet health needs of the community arising from:

a. community composition and structure
b. community resources
c. community dynamics.

Identify the major unmet health needs of the older population. Set out the priorities for meeting:

- general community health needs/problems
- the specific health needs/problems of the elderly in this community.

List which of these problems are amenable to health visiting intervention. Outline the action proposed to deal with these health visiting concerns.

State with which of the other problems health visitors may be able to assist. Which of these main health problems should be referred to other health or social agencies? Outline how this can be done. State the evaluation criteria being used to ascertain whether (a) health visiting action or (b) other action proves effective.

Appendix 2

Guide to family assessment, with special reference to elderly people

It should of course be borne in mind that all records are confidential. They must be able to be seen by the client without causing any offence, and the collection of data should never be undertaken in an obtrusive manner. The purpose of ascertainment of family health and well-being should be explained and family wishes respected. The activity should be participative, and family members made aware that their views and involvement are paramount. Goals set should represent family choice and should be realistic and relevant. All the administrative aspects of record keeping should be borne in mind.

ASSESSMENT

Family characteristics

Composition of family; name; address; date of birth; sex; occupation; relationship to household head; ethnic group; socio-economic group.

Health status of family members

Ascertain the current health status of each family member, identifying any deviation from the norm regarding growth, development and health. Consider indices of physical measurement if available, e.g. height, weight, body mass, and relate these to standards such as centiles, height and weight charts/ponderal indices. Does any action need to be taken? Are any family members concerned about specific health needs? Are the health needs of older persons understood and considered by other family members?

List significant past accidents or illnesses affecting members; state current ones and consider any implications for health visiting. Ascertain family history regarding any allergies, use of prostheses, or appliances, including spectacles and hearing aids. State patterns of specific therapy regarding medications taken by family members.

Obtain current immunisation status of members, and their habits in relation to eating, drinking, smoking and any other addictions. Consider nutritional status, outlining levels of family nutritional knowledge, group eating patterns, facilities for the preparation and storage of food, cooking facilities and significant shopping behaviour.

Ascertain family patterns of consultation with health services personnel and level of use of services. Note any implications. Observe and consider relationship with personnel and areas where improvement might be effected.

Family housing

Ascertain the type of home and its size in relation to family needs, particularly those of older members. Note if home is rented/owner occupied, and if there are any specific related difficulties with either type.

Ascertain standards of domestic hygiene and home management; note if facilities such as heating, ventilation, lighting, toilet arrangements, hot water supply, bathroom and laundry provisions are adequate for family needs. Can older family members utilise these facilities appropriately?

Check if there are specific accident hazards, such as unlighted passageways, halls, steps; unprotected windows; unguarded fires, stoves, and similar appliances; unsafe steps/stairs or walkways; loose floor coverings; inappropriately sited shelves, cupboards, hooks and so on.

Ascertain what aids, gadgets and other adaptations have been utilised to assist family with care of older persons in home. Identify any short-fall in provision, and action necessary to meet need.

Consider housing location in relation to civic amenities, shops, markets, post office, banks, places of worship, public libraries, telephones, public transport and leisure facilities. How convenient is access to educational establishments, ambulance services, health centres, hospitals, social services, police and fire services, and voluntary organisation centres? Relate accessibility to these services to the use made, and note any particular difficulties.

Family transport

Ascertain forms of family transport, including whether family owns a car or other vehicle. If public transport is used, identify frequency and adequacy of services and their suitability/accessibility for older family members. Determine any specific transport needs and outline action to remedy same if possible.

Family income

Where possible, ascertain levels in relation to family needs, especially for older persons. Consider adequacy/inadequacy in relation to family budgeting, specific expenditure such as disability-related costs, and whether benefits and entitlements are being received. Note relative socio-economic status against family peer group. Is there any evidence of financial deprivation? What action, if any is needed to remedy same?

Family resources

Consider family physical, psychological, social, spiritual and economic resources. How far can family as a unit meet present demands in each of these realms?

Identify usual family coping mechanisms. How far can family group be regarded as effective? Consider particularly in relation to stages of family development and the developmental tasks family members have to achieve. How well does family manage to supply the needs of different members, especially older persons?

Family dynamics

Identify levels of family care for each other, with particular reference to older members. Can a 'main carer' be identified? Is this the same individual as the family health care manager? Is there adequate support available for persons filling these roles? Identify any action required to improve the situation.

Consider levels of family stability and interaction and the pattern of family decision making. Are these democratic or authoritarian patterns? Are family members flexible/able to interchange roles if and when required.

Observe and consider family attitudes towards elderly member(s). Are there aspects of family care and understanding which give rise to concern? How can family be assisted to achieve greater growth and enhanced well-being?

Family relationship with the community

Consider how family members interact with others within the community. Is family well integrated? Are members active in civic affairs? Are they involved with any specific groups, clubs, or voluntary services? Outline the particular involvement family have with activities designed for older people.

Family perception of present health and social needs

How does family perceive their present health and social needs? What priorities in care can be set in the light of family goals? Specify particularly those priorities which directly impinge on older members. How far can family meet these needs? Are they willing to do so? Of remaining needs, which are amenable to health visitor intervention? Which needs require referral? Has family consent to referral been obtained?

How perceptive are family members to possible future needs? Is anticipatory guidance welcome?

SUMMARY OF FAMILY HEALTH CARE PLAN

Summarise the main goals of family health care; if possible, state same in behavioural terms. Specify the actions agreed with family, and the allocation of responsibility agreed between family members and practitioner. State the criteria set for determining action-outcomes. Are family members clear about these and willing to participate in evaluation? In particular are older family members aware of goals, action and evaluation criteria and do they approve/have they exercised free choice? It should be remembered that the health care plan belongs to the family and not to the practitioner, who acts as a facilitator.

In subsequent visits when action has been evaluated, new goals in care will be set with family, particularly concerning older members, and family care will be re-organised as indicated and desired.

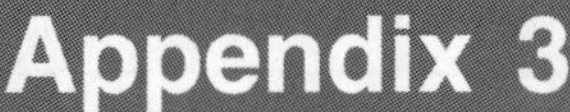

Appendix 3

Models and frameworks used in nursing and health visiting practice

MODELS RELATED TO THE CONCEPT OF HEALTH AS ADAPTATION

Crisis intervention model

Caplan (1964, 1974) proposed a model, based on adaptation theory, which he felt had particular application to community health personnel, in that it was intended to be used as a preventive measure, but chiefly at primary prevention level. He perceived this model as a crisis-intervention device. The model assumes the following.

a. Individuals are holistic beings who throughout life react to environmental stress in a total-person fashion. Since through the life-span persons encounter constant internal or external stressors, they are constantly engaged in a struggle to achieve homeostasis and meet their energy needs. Such adaptation is brought about by a series of inborn and learned coping strategies.

b. At certain times in individuals' lives they encounter events which constitute overwhelming stress. Such experiences constitute 'crisis'. The labelling of an event as a 'crisis' is, however, highly personal; since it is the *significance* of the experience for the individual and the *impact* it makes upon them, that causes them to regard an event so. Thus what constitutes 'crisis' for one person, may appear relatively trivial to another person. However, there are certain events which appear to be regarded as crisis by many people; these include death of a loved person, pet or object; loss of health or functional ability; loss of home and valued personal possessions.

c. Crises constitute 'turning points' in people's lives. They can cause such adaptation and change that it is possible for individuals to emerge from them stronger and enriched. This is considered a healthy outcome and hence becomes the overall goal of interventionist-care.

d. Certain events, such as developmental transitions, can also come to be regarded as crises, e.g. retirement. It is possible to anticipate such events, and sometimes to predict the probability of others. Where practitioners can invoke probability, they have a clear role in primary prevention. They can assist the individual to take 'avoidance action', as in advocating prophylaxis to reduce the chance of encountering the crisis of infectious disease, or to become a non-smoker to prevent smoking-related disease or disability. When the event cannot be avoided, it is possible through the technique of *anticipatory guidance*, so to prepare persons that they are able to cope with the experience in a healthy manner.

e. Where an event has occurred and the use of primary preventive techniques has proved unsuccessful, secondary or tertiary level prevention can be practised, depending on the stage of the reaction. Such intervention depends upon practitioners being able to recognise specific stress-reactions, and the characteristic pattern of reaction, to crisis is thought to be shown as: shock; disbelief and numbness; defensive retreat; sad acknowledgement of reality; adaptation and change; integration and enrichment. The aim of the intervening practitioner is to enable the person to move through these stages in a healthy fashion and complete the last one satisfactorily.

f. Thus during the acute phase of shock the practitioner aims to nourish, protect, sustain and comfort.

During the time of defensive retreat the practitioner aims to promote healthy grieving and 'worry-work', within a supportive relationship. As the individual moves into an acknowledgement of reality the practitioner assists the person to problem-solve and gradually withdraws intensive support as the person implements his/her decisions, adapts and changes. Finally through supportive discussion, the practitioner helps them to discover meaning in their experience and integrate this realisation into their life.

The model is thought to have value for older people as they are susceptible to potential and actual crises, some of which can be predicted. For this reason it has been used in this book in connection with intervention during bereavement (see Ch. 7).

The relationship between the model and the health visiting process may thus be seen as shown in Table A3.1.

Table A3.1

Crisis intervention model	Health visiting process
Rests on adaptation theory	*Assessment* Collects data pertinent to stress events and identifies client perception of their significance.
Takes account of Crisis theory Probability theory	Identifies client's normal coping patterns and any variation in present state. Determines phase of reaction and associated needs and problems, sets out these priority order and decides direction of care required, in order to achieve positive adaptation.
Perceives interventionist as assuming roles as supporter; protector; helper; motivator; counsellor	*Planning* Assists client to identify goals. Selects actions to support and care for client whilst he is in state of disequilibrium. Plans with client for eventual self-help and autonomy, following healthy grieving, for loss of any kind.
Perceives intervention as following a distinct pattern, intensive at first then tapering off as balance is regained	*Implementing* Executes care plan to help client cope with crisis and regain balance.
	Evaluating Monitors progress; judges outcomes against goals and relevant criteria. *Reorganising* Re-plans and implements as needed.

The Roy adaptation model

The Roy adaptation model is primarily a systems model with interactionist elements. It is based on adaptation theory, derived from Helson (1964). It is applied to nursing (Roy 1970, Riehl & Roy 1980). The model assumes the following.

a. People are bio-psychosocial beings, in constant interaction with matching environments. They respond to internal and external stimuli by a process of adaptation and change. The innate and acquired mechanisms of response constitute a unique pattern for each individual, which Roy suggests constitutes an '*adaptive zone*'. Stimuli falling within this 'adaptive zone' will be responded to positively; those which, by reason of amount or strength, fall outside this 'adaptive zone' cannot be responded to positively and therefore the 'steady state' will be lost. Individuals will then likely require help to assist them to achieve homeostasis, whenever possible.

b. Roy classifies the types of stimuli individuals encounter as *focal*, *contextual* and *residual*.

Focal stimuli are immediate and confronting events/experiences, and include any which cause physiologic or psychosocial disturbance.

Contextual stimuli are regarded as background events which occur alongside the novel focal stimuli and can affect these.

Residual stimuli are those which relate to the beliefs, attitudes and traits held and the emotions culled from earlier experiences, which may affect the way an individual responds to current stimuli.

For example, an elderly man may fall whilst visiting the toilet during the night. He is unable to rise or contact help, and lies there feeling pain in his right leg and hip (focal stimuli). Whilst on the floor he is affected by the lowered environmental temperature (contextual stimuli). He may, or may not, be aware that the latter is partly related to his socio-economic state (also contextual stimuli) as well as to his attitudes towards economy and habits of thrift, which cause him to turn off his heating at night, even during very severe weather conditions (residual stimuli).

c. Roy sees the individual as reacting in four ways to these three different forms of stimuli. These ways or modes she classifies as:

1. *Physiologic mode* — encompassing changes in temperature; oxygen exchange; electrolyte balance; or sensorimotor response.
2. *Self-concept mode* — whereby adjustments are made in the way an individual sees and conducts himself, as he interprets the way others perceive him.
3. *Role function* — alterations in the way an individual fulfils specific roles, as a result of changes in the role behaviour of others with whom he is in a role-relationship.
4. *Interdependence mode* — behavioural adjustments in light of changing circumstances, in order to maintain relative balance in interpersonal relationships.

Roy sees intervention by the practitioner as therefore occurring whenever a need or deficit exists in client or client-resources, in any one of these four modes. Such intervention is two-pronged and demands the exercise of professional judgement. It is directed towards manipulating the stimuli, to prevent stress encounters, or to minimise their effect. Stimuli may be singly manipulated, or in combination. The other action is directed towards strengthening and extending the client's 'zone of adaptation'. For example, returning to our earlier example of the elderly man who sustains a fall: health visiting intervention would aim to determine the probability of falling; prevent the risk by advising a commode near the bed at night; would point out the need to maintain an even temperature during the day and night and would discuss with and educate client on the need to temper thrift during periods of excess cold, in favour of survival. This manipulation of stimuli would be accompanied by efforts to extend the client's adaptive level, by helping him to work out an emergency plan to cope with such an eventuality, so that help could be promptly summoned.

Although, as with other conceptual models, there are distinct differences between the framework used and the health visiting process, the link between them might appear as shown in Table A3.2.

Table A3.2

Roy adaptation model	Health visiting process Data collected on personal and social level
Theory of adaptation	*Assessment* Identify risk of encountering stimuli. Classify stimuli and decide on forms of client reaction and adaptation.
Postulates of client bio-psychosocial response to stress	*Planning* Identify client goals. Select behaviour which will achieve goals; then clarify actions which meet goals, modify stimuli and increase client coping ability.
Goals to care	*Intervention/Implementing* Execute plan and alter stimuli which fall within client adaptive zone. Extend client adaptive zone to cope with stimuli. *Evaluating* Scrutinise client and practitioner action in terms of outcome against desired goals and process used. *Re-organising* Review plan and re-organise in light of evaluation

Stress-adaptation model

This model was described by its authors, Saxton & Hyland (1979) as based on adaptation theory. The model assumes the following.

a. Throughout life an individual must constantly face stressors, to which he must adaptively respond as a total person. Such stresses may be environmental — namely, physical, chemical, microbiological or social — or may be personal physical, developmental, or emotional stressors. Whilst the normal adaptive responses to stress can cause an individual to grow and develop, extra stress, such as that arising from accident, illness, infection or loss, can overwhelm and impair balance.

b. Whilst adaptations are usually appropriate, there are times when individuals act inappropriately, and these maladaptations are not only ineffective, but can themselves impose further stress so compounding the original disturbance. An example of this might be when an elderly widow reacts to the death of her husband by refusing to eat or make any social contact.

c. This chain reaction of primary stress-reaction →secondary stress-reaction can be repeated, so that the person is increasingly preoccupied with endeavours to cope with cumulative stress.

Saxton & Hyland (1979) describe five levels of adaptive behaviour:

(i) normal responses to stress, including reflex action
(ii) more conscious adaptation; individual aware of attempts to change and cope
(iii) individual reacts and displays adaptive signs and symptoms
(iv) secondary-level stress adaptive reactions appear
(v) life-threatening stress reaction takes place.

d. Practitioners are therefore seen as intervening:

(i) to reduce the extent and intensity of the stress encountered
(ii) to limit the individual's attempt to restrict compensatory responses
(iii) to deal with the symptoms of response
(iv) to interrupt and re-direct secondary stress reactions
(v) to supplement individual responses to maintain life-function.

Thus in the example of the elderly woman, recently bereaved of her husband, a health visitor practitioner might try, where possible, to prepare her beforehand for the inevitability of such a loss, would encourage anticipatory grieving and limit the individual's efforts to deny the likelihood of such an event. When the death actually occurred, the practitioner would deal with the ensuing symptoms of shock, through comforting and sustaining the individual and limiting the client's attempt to ignore hunger needs, by arranging for light appetising food and drink to be unobtrusively served to her frequently during the shock-phase. Furthermore she would subtly circumvent her client's attempts to withdraw totally from social contact, by allowing some time for solitude and respecting the client's need to be alone, yet paying short visits to her, to support and supervise her, and encouraging suitable others to do so. Additionally the practitioner would marshall resources to see that shopping, cooking, and personal care activities which sustain life, could be suitably continued on the client's behalf, until the widow could re-assert adequate personal control. The practitioner would then gradually withdraw help as the client's coping mechanism improved.

The links between the model and the processes of care are shown in Table A3.3.

Table A3.3

Stress-adaptation model	Health visiting process
Based on adaptation theory, taking account of physiological and psychological theories.	*Assessment* Collects personal, family and community data to enable identification of causal stress-agents and client reaction patterns.
Postulates innate and acquired adaptive responses	Recognises adaptive needs and sets these out in priority order.
Emphasises the dynamic relationship between organism and environment and personal coping behaviour.	*Planning* Determines care goals with client as far as possible. Selects actions designed to strengthen adaptive responses and prevent or modify maladaptive ones.
Sets out indicators related to 5 levels of stress-reaction.	*Implementing* Acts to modify stressors and execute plan. Actively seeks to improve client coping ability through involving client in responsibility for care. *Evaluating* Estimates progress with client, assessing outcome against desired goals and judging process against valid criteria for efficiency and effectiveness. *Re-organising* Re-arranges intervention in accordance with evaluation and continues to scrutinise and re-plan as needed.

Orem's self-care model

This is a systems model, designed specifically for nursing and based on Orem's conceptualisation of man as an independent and self-governing individual (Orem 1971). It is based on the values of self-help and service to others. The model assumes the following.

a. All persons function in bio-psychosocial-spiritual dimensions, and initiate and perform activities on their own behalf, in order to sustain life and health in each of these realms.

b. Self-care is learned behaviour, developed through curiosity, instruction and spaced repetition. The successful performance of self-care activities rests on an individual's level of cognitive awareness, their degree of maturity, and the extent of their knowledge and skill concerning what constitutes suitable activities to sustain life and health.

c. To engage in effective self-care the individual must be able to initiate and maintain actions which will sustain life processes, regulate hazards and promote normal growth and development.

Additionally Orem sees self-care as divided into two categories:

- universal self-care needs
- health-deviation self-care needs.

Universal self-care needs require concern about the common elements we all need to sustain life, such as air, food, fluid, activity, rest, solitude and social interaction. They also relate to the promotion of normal age-phase behaviour through conformity. On the other hand health-deviation needs only require attention when changes have occurred as a result of injury, illness, disability, deprivation or loss and/or through the changes brought about by any medical diagnosis and treatment.

Intervention is, therefore, seen as identifying an individual's self-care needs, through the exercise of professional judgement. Determining any deficit in an individual's capacity to meet such needs, it also seeks to design action to help persons bridge this self-care deficit, either through teaching the person new coping mechanisms and self-care techniques, where this is possible, or in teaching and supporting lay-carers, who may meet the self-care deficit for the person. Where these two courses of action are inappropriate, the practitioner may actively supply the self-care deficit by doing for the person what he cannot do for himself, or arranging for some other agency to do this and then monitoring its fulfilment. Other intervention includes structuring the environment in such a way as to support the fulfilment of identified self-care needs and so guiding, supporting and helping the individual as to lead them to assume that level of self-care which is appropriate for them.

The link between the model and the health visiting process is possibly as shown in Table A3.4.

Table A3.4

Orem's self-care model	**Health visiting process**
Self-maintenance and self-care are basic values, needed for effective functioning in human society.	*Assessment* The practitioner identifies the extent to which the client *does* practice self-care activities normally, and the ways in which present circumstances cause *deficit* in his self-care ability. Furthermore practitioner identifies what potential for self-care the client possesses; how far any deficit could be met by other lay-carers; what knowledge and skill a person requires in order to meet the client's self-care needs and, if they are unable to do this at present, what action the practitioner needs to take to enable them to learn to do so.
The individual who is normal will wish to engage in self-care, and in all circumstances will strive to do this.	*Planning* Specifies care measures, resources and co-ordinating activities. With client and other carers determines different responsibilities for action, allocating these, in line with the goals of care. Monitors each stage.
Perceives care goals as related to autonomy through self-care activities. Regards practitioners as identifying self-care deficits and remedying these.	*Implementing* Initiating, controlling and delivering care according to the detailed plan.
	Evaluating Determining the results of action taken, against the desired goals of personal independence in self-care. *Re-organising* Scrutinises evaluation data, decides how to redesign the care given and then adjusts same.

Goal-attainment model

The goal attainment model can be said to be a systems model with interactional elements. It is concerned with evaluation, and its conceptual advantages are seen to lie in its action-setting. For the elderly its significance is that it focuses on short-term services to a community-based group, rather than to the institutionalised or severely mentally impaired aged. It is based on personal and social values, including the belief that people should have the opportunity to assess their own capacities, needs and interests, and should make the decisions that affect their well-being.

Assumptions underlying the model are as follows.

a. Most people, including the elderly, are able to determine what they need, can make decisions about how best to achieve these needs, and want to make such decisions for themselves. Furthermore they need to make such decisions if they are to remain functional in contemporary society.

b. Persons who have the decision-making power taken away from them stagnate, become apathetic and eventually lose touch with reality.

c. Professional intervention is of value since it is seen as facilitating the individual to achieve his/her goals, and not perceived as imposing goals on individuals.

d. Such professional intervention is likely to be most effective if concentrated on helping clients achieve specific and limited goals of their own choosing, within brief bounded periods of service.

e. It is possible to determine the success or failure of such intervention, because outcomes can be related to pre-determined objectives.

Thus such a model emphasises the strengths of an elderly client as well as taking account of his/her limitations. Furthermore, by causing the worker to be tuned in to the client's definitions of his/her problems, through the use of a framework which stresses the client's ability to cope with these, and to work towards solutions within a limited time-period, engenders a more positive view of the client-system (Cormican 1977). Where an older person has a positive self-image and perceives himself/herself to be positively viewed by others, and seen to be self-directing, he or she is likely to use their potential to achieve satisfactory outcomes. In societies where ageism is a constant risk, such positive elements are highly constructive.

Although the model is not synonymous with the health visiting process it may be operationalised through the latter, as Luker (1982), was able to show. The links between them are shown in Table A3.5.

Table A3.5

Goal-attainment model	Health visiting process
Recognises personal and social values, including those of the organisation of which the practitioner forms part.	Recognises underlying values. *Assessment* Collects relevant data in effort to identify client goals, values and problems. Analyses steps needed to be fulfilled in order to achieve goals. Helps client prioritise goals.
Recognises desire for independence present in individuals and asserts their ability to make and follow through on decisions, despite age.	*Planning* Structures tasks, so that the primary responsibility for reaching goals rests with the client and not the worker, thus promoting independence.
Respects the right of the older individual to cope with life-activities, test out action and make other plans, should initial actions fail to meet desired objectives.	*Implementing* Describes and explains the action taken and by whom
Supports evaluation as a highly complex activity, which seeks to determine observed change, and relationship to actions taken and/or other causes.	*Evaluating* Measures the degree of change which has taken place, relating these to the action taken. Determines both process and outcome.

The most marked differences between the model and the operational tool which seeks to utilise it, lie in the fact that the model assumes evaluation research against set goals for a predefined population, whereas the health visiting process describes care given to one individual, for the express purpose of helping that one person; hence the measurement of the effectiveness of that care becomes a secondary activity, albeit a very important one. However, the use of the model has been said to increase client motivation (Kastenbaum 1973).

CLARK'S MODEL FOR HEALTH VISITING

This model was derived from health visitors' '*private images*' as presented in the documents of health visiting organisations, and as they were reflected in the practice of a group of health visitors who tape-recorded their home visits and clinic consultations with families for 1 year as part of a research study (Clark 1985). It was further tested by the author over a 2-year period of practice, but is considered to need further refinement and testing, in work with other client groups.

Unlike other nursing models, which mainly assume that

- the focus of care is an individual person
- nursing is concerned with people's problems
- nursing goals almost always are intended to achieve change
- nursing begins at the point of a discrete illness episode and ends at the point of discharge following that episode,

health visiting models focus on

- the group as an object of care, as well as an individual
- needs rather than problems, since health visiting practitioners do not assume the existence of problems, although these may sometimes be present
- seeking to achieve stability, rather than always creating change, although change in behaviour may be required. This is because, unlike nursing, health visiting is undertaken with healthy persons, and the object of intervention is to assist them to remain so and to improve their well-being
- interaction that is a serial activity, taking place over time, often several years, and in such a way that each intervention or interaction builds on, and is determined by, the previous one.

Hence any model for health visiting must: focus on the family or group as a unit, aim for stability rather than change, and provide continuity over time. Like nursing it must define and relate concepts which constitute nursing and those which constitute the paradigm of health visiting within nursing, including health, prevention, needs and coping (Fawcett 1984, Clark 1985).

In Clark's model the unifying framework which links together these aspects is *general systems theory* (von Bertalanffy 1968), which has been used as a means of understanding the dynamics of both nursing and of families. The person, family or community who/which is the object of concern, is perceived as a system — that is, a whole, which functions as such by virtue of the interdependence of its parts. In particular it functions as an open system, affecting and being affected by its environment, within which it must maintain a state of balance or equilibrium if it is to survive.

Within this framework the elements of the model can be defined as follows.

- *Health* is a dynamic equilibrium, a state of balance between the person and his or her environment, in which the balance is held at the level which allows the person to function physiologically, psychologically and socially, at his or her optimum level.
- *Needs* are 'those tangible and intangible items, which the person must have in satisfactory amounts in order to attain and maintain . . . the physical and psychological balance we call health' (Johnson & Davis 1975).
- *Problems* — 'if a person's needs are over- or under-fulfilled, the balance is disturbed; this disturbance is referred to as a patient problem' (Johnson & Davis 1975).
- *Coping* is the activity by means of which the person strives to maintain equilibrium (Antonovsky 1979).
- *Prevention*. The model uses the concepts of primary, secondary and tertiary prevention as developed by Caplan (1961) and by Neuman (1982). By primary prevention is meant the processes involved in reducing the risk that people in the community will fall ill. Secondary prevention within the model refers to the activities in reducing the duration of established cases of . . . disorder, thus reducing their prevalence in the community. Tertiary prevention means the prevention of defect and crippling, which involves rehabiliting services which aim at returning sick/injured persons as soon as possible to a maximum degree of effectiveness.
- The goal of health visiting — *to promote health* — is to maintain and, over time, improve the level of the dynamic equilibrium called health, by heading off harmful stressors and enhancing the client's resistance resources and coping abilities. It also aims to facilitate the entry of beneficial inputs, in the process of prevention at all three stages.

The diagrams, Figures A3.1–5 present the health visitor and client as two open systems interacting with each other through an activity called health visiting. This follows Peplau's definition of nursing as 'a significant therapeutic interpersonal process' (Peplau 1952) and was used by King (1981). It should be noted that the interaction is represented as a two-way process which, following systems theory, affects both systems.

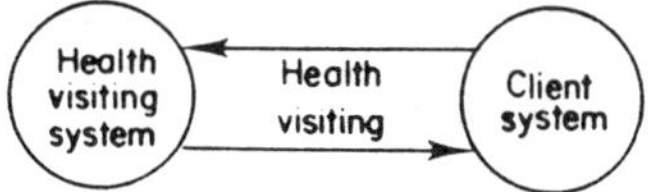

Fig. A3.1

The health visiting system may represent the health visiting service or an individual health visitor. The client system may represent an individual client, a family or any group, or a community. Each system may contain several subsystems. When the system is a group as opposed to an individual, the only difference in the model is the different set of subsystems which make up the system. The two systems are set within a shared environment, within which they constantly interact (Fig. A3.2).

Following Neuman (1982), each of the two systems is represented as a *'core'* surrounded by *'rings'*, which protect the core against harmful

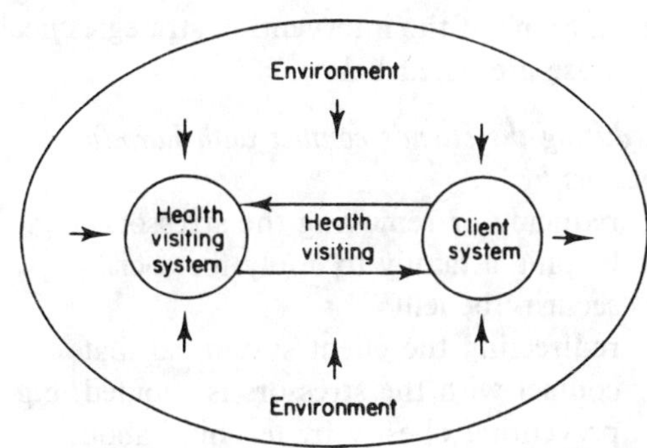

Fig. A3.2

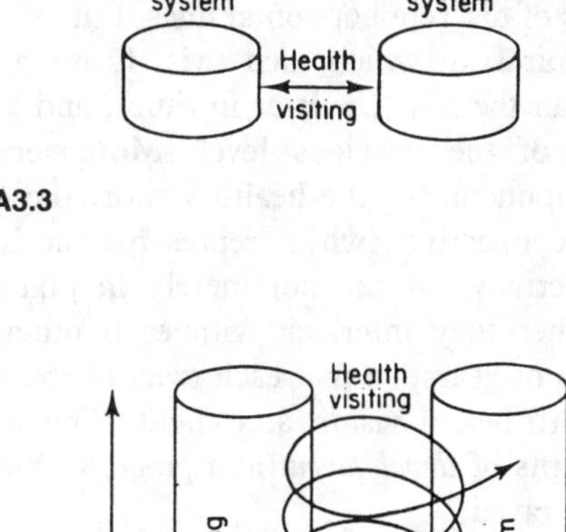

Fig. A3.3

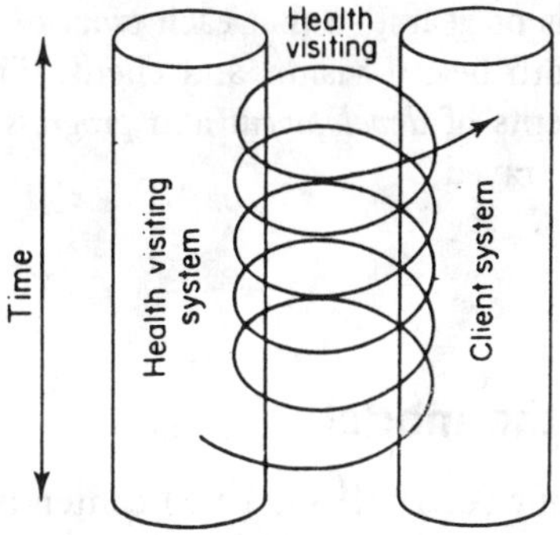

Health visiting
Time
Health visiting system
Client system

Fig. A3.4

stressors, while admitting the beneficial inputs necessary to meet needs. When needs are properly met the system is able to maintain equilibrium. Over time it improves the level at which it is held. This is achieved by influencing the stressors which threaten the system's integrity and by building up the client's (or group's or community's) resistance resources. It is reinforced through the processes of primary, secondary and tertiary prevention (Fig. A3.5).

Figure A3.3, which is the same as Figure A3.1 but viewed from a different perspective (having been turned through 90°, from a vertical to a horizontal plane), is intended to show the relationship between Figures A3.1 and A3.4.

Figures A3.1–3 show health visiting at a moment in time. Figure A3.4 is intended to show a cumulation over time, to highlight the point that health visiting is a 'serial activity'. The significance of Figure A3.4 is that it presents the

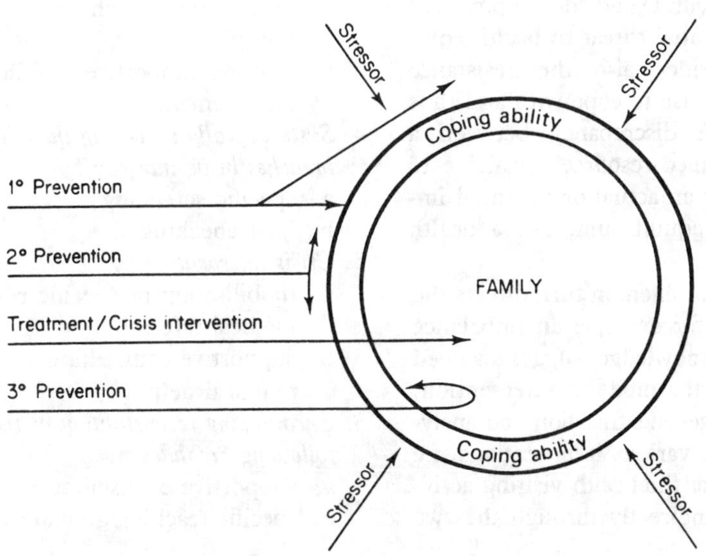

Fig. A3.5

interaction between health visitor and client, not as a series of discrete horizontal lines, but as a continuous spiral, in which each twist forms a level higher than the last (i.e. later in time), and a continuation of the previous level. Moreover, the three components — the health visitor, the client and the 'connective' (which represents the health visiting activity) — are not merely in juxtaposition. Rather they interlock with each other like cogwheels or gears, so that each twist of the spiral moves both health visitor and client. This allows the concepts of *development* and *progress over time* to be portrayed.

Using the model

The author (Clark 1985, 1986) contends that the value of any model should be measured not by the way it looks on paper, but by its usefulness in practice. The purpose of this model is to provide a framework for health visiting practice. It suggests what kind of information the health visitor should collect, in order to make an assessment of the client's needs and to plan and carry out appropriate interventions. This model directs the health visitor to look at the client's needs in terms of the stressors (physiological, psychological and social; environmental, behavioural and developmental) which constitute a potential threat to health equilibrium, and to consider also the resistance resources the client can use to cope with and thus prevent breakdown. A discrepancy between a stressor and the resistance resources available to cope with it constitutes an actual or potential imbalance in the health equilibrium, i.e. a health problem (Clark 1985).

The definition of the problem in turn directs the choice of intervention; for example an imbalance which is due to lack of knowledge, suggests a need for specific teaching as the mode of intervention. The model also encourages identification and analysis of the constraints on various interventions, i.e the stressors which affect the health visiting activity, both directly and indirectly through the two systems. Some of the intervention strategies health visitors use are listed below.

1. *Reducing the client's contact with harmful stressors by*
   a. reducing or removing the stressors: e.g. helping a family to apply for social security benefit
   b. redirecting the client system so that contact with the stressors is avoided: e.g. preventing obesity by teaching about family nutrition
2. *Improving the client's generalised resistance resources by*
   a. anticipatory guidance
   b. health teaching
   c. developing confidence and self-esteem
   d. enhancing general coping behaviour
3. *Improving the client's response to specific stressors by*
   a. anticipatory guidance: e.g. preparation for retirement
   b. specific measures: e.g. influenza vaccination
   c. specific teaching: e.g. on maintaining fitness via exercise and deep breathing
   d. mobilisation of appropriate services: e.g. referral for home help services, or respite care in certain circumstances
   e. enhancing specific mechanisms: e.g. putting into touch with a specific support group
   f. offering support, e.g. following bereavement
4. *Systematically surveying the client system for breaches in its integrity by*
   a. specific screening
   b. 'just checking'
5. *Crisis intervention by*
   a. mobilisation of specific resources, e.g. medical referral
   b. supportive counselling
   c. practical help
6. *Encouraging reconstitution of the system, following breakdown, by*
   a. supportive counselling
   b. specific teaching/guidance.

An example

The Brown family consisted of Mrs Anne Brown (78), her niece Margaret Brown (57), and a friend Cora Butler, aged 72.

The first contact with the family came when Miss Margaret Brown asked for help with her aunt, who suffered from Alzheimer's disease (2nd February 1984). Initial family assessment was recorded on 4th February 1984, and completed three weeks later, after scrutiny of data obtained subsequent to enquiries. Detailed results of assessment are *not* shown here.

Using the model to consider the household group as a unit (the client system), it was deduced that the major stressors with which it had to cope were the deteriorating cognitive state of Mrs Anne Brown, the relative frailty of Miss Cora Butler, who acted as 'carer' while Miss Margaret Brown was at work, and Miss Brown's need to maintain her job for the next 3 years, pending retirement. The unit's financial resources were rather low, but just outside the level of social security benefits.

Reduction of contact with harmful stressors was brought about by arranging Day Centre placement 3 times weekly for Mrs Brown, and by teaching simple management techniques to both Miss Butler and Miss Margaret Brown.

Client's generalised resistance resources were improved by increasing reality-orientation, raising self-esteem, establishing routine and via diversional therapy.

Improving the unit's response to specific stressors was brought about by referral to a support group for carers of the elderly and mentally frail, and by supportive visiting, including help from a voluntary visitor from The Alzheimer's Disease Society.

Systematic surveying of the client system for breaches in its integrity was maintained by regular health visiting surveillance (checking). Crisis intervention was given on three occasions, when family resources were strained, through arranging short-term respite — recuperative holidays for Miss Butler and Miss Margaret Brown, and admission for Mrs Brown to residential accommodation for a few weeks; by medical referral of Miss Butler, for an acute respiratory episode; and by liaison with occupational health services at Miss Brown's place of work, to arrange for some leave of absence. Reconstitution of the system following breakdown was achieved by providing supportive counselling while decisions were reached about the full-time admission of Mrs Brown to a nursing home, for the last 3 weeks of her life, and by bereavement support for both Miss Brown and Miss Butler, following Mrs Brown's death on 7th September 1989.

It is presently continued by the ongoing but unobtrusive surveillance of Miss Butler and Miss Brown.

The couple remain a relatively healthy unit at present, but there is a potential risk of disturbance since Miss Brown continues to care for Miss Butler, who has now developed maturity-onset diabetes.

REFERENCES

Antonovsky A 1979 Stress, health and coping. Jossey Bass, New York

Von Bertalanffy L 1968 General systems theory. Brazillier, New York

Caplan G 1961 An approach to community mental health. Tavistock, London

Caplan G 1964 Principles of preventive psychiatry. Basic Books, New York

Caplan G 1974 Support systems and community mental health. Mental Health Behavioural Publications, New York

Clark J 1981 What do health visitors do? A review of the research 1970–1980. Royal College of Nursing, London

Clark J 1985 The process of health visiting. Unpublished PhD thesis, Polytechnic of The South Bank, London

Clark J 1986 A model for health visiting. In: Kershaw B, Salvage J (eds) Models for nursing. Wiley, Chichester

Cormican E J 1977 Task-centred model for work with the aged. Social Casework (October): 490–494

Fawcett J 1984 Analysis and evaluation of conceptual models of nursing. F A Davis, Philadelphia

Helson H 1964 Adaptation level theory. Harper and Row, New York

Johnson M, Davis M 1975 Problem solving in nursing practice. Wm Brown & Co, Dubuque

Kastenbaum 1973 The foreshortened life perspective. In: Brantl V M, Raymond-Brown (ed) Readings in gerontology. Mosby, St Louis

King I 1981 A theory for nursing. Wiley, New York

Luker K 1982 Evaluating health visiting practice. Royal College of Nursing, London

Neuman B 1982 The Neuman systems model: application to nursing education and practice. Appleton-Century-Crofts, Norwalk, Connecticut

Orem D 1971 Nursing: concepts of practice. McGraw Hill, New York

Orlando I 1961 The dynamic nurse–patient relationship. Putnam, New York

Peplau H 1952 Interpersonal relations in nursing. Putnam, New York

Riehl J P, Roy C 1980 Conceptual models for nursing practice, 2nd edn. Appleton-Century-Crofts, New York

Roy C 1970 Adaptation: a conceptual framework for nursing. Nursing Outlook 18 (3): 42

Saxton D F, Hyland P A 1979 Planning and implementing nursing intervention: stress and adaptation applied to patient care, 2nd edn. Mosby, St Louis

Appendix 4

Community Adult Record: the Health Visiting Assessment Form devised by the HVA Special Interest Group for the Elderly

This appendix represents the *Health Visiting Assessment Form* devised by the members of the HVA Special Interest Group for the Elderly, and validated by Ms Sue Phillips in her research, including the research project undertaken for Southwark and North Lewisham Health Authority and discussed in Chapter 6.

Guidance notes for those utilising this assessment form are given below but are not exhaustive. If problems are encountered in use, practitioners are urged to contact the Special Interest Group.

Notes on Community Adult Record

Type of Accommodation should include whether owner-occupied, council-owned, housing association, etc., as well as recording whether it is a house, bungalow, flat or other type of dwelling.
Community Services — to include contact with district nurses, home care workers, meals on wheels service, Community Psychiatric Nurses, voluntary organisations, day hospitals, and so on.
Next-of-kin/other is intended mainly for practitioner information. Details of significant people in client's life, e.g. neighbour if appropriate, or main carer.

The remainder of the form is largely self-explanatory, but a check list is given at the end to offer further guidance.

COMMUNITY ADULT RECORD

NAME ______________________ D.O.B. ____________

ADDRESS ______________________ PHONE ____________

____

____

RELEVANT CULTURAL FACTORS ______________________

TYPE OF ACCOMMODATION ______________________

OTHERS IN HOUSEHOLD:

Name	**Relationship**

Person to contact in case of emergency:

Name ______________________

Address ______________________

____

Phone ______________________

Any other Carer:

____

____

____

____

Community Services Involved:	**Name**	**Phone**
General Practitioner		
District Nurses		
Health visitor		
Home Care		
Meals on Wheels		
Social Worker		
Voluntary Organisations		
Others		

Dates of Assessment

1) .... 2) .... 3) ....

ASPECTS OF POSITIVE HEALTH

Level of Independence

☐☐☐

Fully independent 1
Has help with shopping/housework 2
Has help with personal care 3
Needs help with shopping/housework 4
Needs help with personal care 5

Mobility

☐☐☐

Fully mobile 1
Some difficulty, but can get out 2
Fully mobile within home 3
Some difficulty within home 4
Bed/chair bound 5

Exercise

☐☐☐

Regular deliberate exercise 1
Normal daily activities 3
No exercise 5

Hobbies/Interests

☐☐☐

Specify: Stimulating 1
Some 3
None 5

Diet

☐☐☐

Varied diet 1
General dietary advice required 3
Specialised diet. advice required 5

Fluid Intake

☐☐☐

Adequate (6–8 cups daily) 1
Barely adequate 3
Evidence of dehydration 5

Smoking

☐☐☐

Never 1
Less than daily 3
1–15 daily 4
More than 15 daily 5

Alcohol

☐☐☐

Never 1
Within recommended limit 2
Over recommended limit 3
(HEC guide = 10 units/week women
20 units/week men)

Weight Maintenance

☐☐☐

Normal range 1
Up to 1 stone overweight 3
2 stones or more over/under wt 5

Bowels

☐☐☐

Regular without laxatives 1
Occasional constipation/diarrhoea 3
Takes medication to control 4
Uncontrolled and severe problem 5

Continence

☐☐☐

Fully continent 1
Continent with aids 2
Stress incontinence 3
Urinary incontinence 4
Doubly incontinent 5

LIVING ENVIRONMENT

Accommodation

☐☐☐

Suitable for needs 1
Slightly unsuitable for needs 3
Grossly unsuitable for needs 5
Specify problem:

Home Safety

☐☐☐

No apparent hazards 1
Slight hazard/risk 3
Serious hazard/risk 5
Specify hazard:

Income

☐☐☐

Adequate for needs 1
Barely adequate for needs 3
Not managing 5

Heating

☐☐☐

Adequate 1
Barely adequate 3
Inadequate 5

Awareness of Benefits

☐☐☐

Not eligible 1
Claiming relevant benefits 2
Aware but not claiming 4
Not aware of all relevant benefits 5

Tick benefits received

Retirement pension	Housing benefit
Income support	Attendance allow.
	Other

FAMILY RELATIONSHIPS AND SOCIAL CONTACTS

Family Relationships

☐☐☐

Happy 1
Slight stress 3
Severe stress 5

Bereavement/Significant Loss Event

☐☐☐

None 1
Adjusting appropriately 2
Could benefit from extra support 4
Barely coping 5

Specify event and date:

Responsibilities as Carer

☐☐☐

None 1
Some, coping well 2
Slight strain 3
Severe strain 5

Social Contacts

☐☐☐

Often enough as perceived by client 1
Complains of some loneliness 3
Complains of severe loneliness 5

Life Satisfaction

☐☐☐

Enjoying this period of life 1
Resigned to life stage 3
Rejecting of life stage 5

ASPECTS OF DEVELOPMENTAL AGEING

Hearing

☐☐☐

No difficulty 1
No difficulty with aids 2
Some difficulty, has no aid 3
Some difficulty with aid 4
Completely deaf 5

Vision

☐☐☐

Good 1
Good with glasses 2
Poor vision with glasses 3
Partially sighted 4
Blind 5

Teeth

☐☐☐

Teeth/dentures — comfortable 1
No teeth/dentures — comfortable 2
Has problems eating or talking 3
Teeth causing pain/discomfort 5

Feet

☐☐☐

Comfortable, no problems 1
Receiving treatment 2
Minor problems, needs treatment 3
Major problems, needs urgent treatment 5

Speech

☐☐☐

Normal 1
Slight impairment 3
Severe impairment 5

Breathing

☐☐☐

Normal 1
Occasional difficulty 3
Severe difficulty 5

Sleep Pattern

☐☐☐

Normal 1
Disturbed occasionally 2
Disturbed regularly 3
Sleeps with medication 4
Disturbed even with medication 5

Memory and Orientation

☐☐☐

No impairment 1
Slight memory impairment 3
Impairment interfering with ability to cope 4
Severely confused with serious risk 5

SIGNIFICANT LIFE EVENTS/HOPES FOR THE FUTURE

ASPECTS OF ILL HEALTH/DISABILITY

MEDICAL CONDITIONS with dates	RELATED DISABILITY	TREATMENT
1	....	....
2	....	....
3	....	....
4	....	....
5	....	....
6	....	....
7	....	....
8	....	....

Understands Condition/Treatment

☐☐☐

Yes 1
No 5

Complies with Treatment

☐☐☐

Yes 1
No 5
Specify reason if No:

RELEVANT HOSPITAL ADMISSIONS/CASUALTY ATTENDANCES
1.
2.
3.
4.

UNREPORTED/UNDIAGNOSED SYMPTOMS (Using Symptom Sheet if Necessary)
1.
2.
3.
4.
5.
6.

DATE + CONTACT POINT*	HEALTH FOCUS	1) NEEDS IDENTIFIED BY ASSESSOR AND/OR CLIENT	ACTION TAKEN & FUTURE PLAN	HAS ACTION MET NEED

* CONTACT POINT: H — HOME VISIT; B — BASE OF HV; C — CLINIC; E — ELSEWHERE.

CHECKLIST OF SYMPTOMS THAT MAY BE OF USE IN THE OVERALL ASSESSMENT

Mental health
Orientated in time and place
Short term memory loss
Long term memory loss
Lack of motivation
Anxiety
Depression
Change in normal behaviour pattern

Nervous system
Headaches
Dizziness/Faints
Visual disturbances
Hearing disturbances

Circulatory system
Pallor
Ankle swelling
Pain in chest on exertion
Tiredness/lethargy/weakness
Cramp/tingling in limbs
Varicose veins
Leg ulcers

Respiratory system
Breathlessness day/night
Productive cough
Wheezing
Nasal congestion

Digestive system
Indigestion/heartburn
Abdominal pain/discomfort
Vomiting/nausea
Recent weight change
Change in bowel habit
Painful or bleeding piles

Genitourinary system
Pain/difficulty passing urine
Frequency/urgency
Bleeding/discharge
Irritation
Prolapse

Skin
Irritation
Boils/lumps
Any lesion slow to heal

Musculo-skeletal system
Backache
Pain/swelling in any joint
Limitation of movement

Reproduced by permission of the HVA Special Interest Group for the Elderly.

Appendix 5

The multi-dimensional scale for the Health Locus of Control construct

The original Health Locus of Control (HLC) Scale was developed by Wallston et al (1976), as a uni-dimensional measure of people's beliefs that their health is, or is not, determined by their behaviour.

Individuals with high scores on the 11-item HLC scale are 'health-externals'; they are presumed to have generalised expectancies that the factors which determine their health are such things as luck, fate, chance, or powerful others — factors over which they have little control. On the other end of the dimension are the 'health internals', who believe that the locus of control for health is internal and that one stays or becomes healthy, or sick, as a result of his or her behaviour.

This original HLC scale was designed to yield a single score similar to Rotter's Internal–External scale (Rotter 1966). The higher the score on this HLC scale, the more external the belief in locus of control. However, evidence supporting the multi-dimensionality of the generalised locus of control scale suggested the need to explore the dimensionality issue (MacDonald 1973).

Further questioning of the conceptualisation of locus of control as a uni-dimensional construct came from Levenson (1975). She developed three 8-item Likert-type scales (Internal, Powerful Others, and Chance I:P:C:) to measure generalised locus of control beliefs, and demonstrated initial evidence of their discriminant validity. This pointed to the need to explore this approach in predicting health behaviours.

The reconceptualisation of the health locus of control along multi-dimensional lines was undertaken by Wallston et al (1978). A total item pool was constructed, with 25 IHLC items, 30 PHLC and 26 CHLC items.

Tested through a research study described in Wallston et al (1978), 6 new items were identified for each of the three new scales. Forms A & B, which each incorporate a version of these 18 items are shown on pages 307 and 308. The results of testing for reliability are given in the quoted literature and subsequent research studies.

Acknowledgement is made to Professor Wallston, Vanderbilt University, Nashville, Tennessee 37240; further information can be obtained from the authors from this address.

Items 1, 6, 8, 12, 13, 17 identify Internality in relation to the health locus of control (a high score indicates internality).

Items 3, 5, 7, 10, 14, 18 relate to Powerful Others Health Locus of Control (a high score represents the belief that the health locus of control is vested in the action of powerful others).

Items 2, 4, 9, 11, 15, 16 relate to Chance Health Locus of Control (a high score indicates the belief that the health locus of control is the result largely of chance).

The authors discuss the development of these new scales, considering that health researchers have at their disposal a set of instruments with far greater potential usefulness than the original unidimensional HLC scale. It might be utilised by the assessment of more than one dimension of health locus of control, with the probability of increasing understanding and prediction of health behaviours. Examples quoted include an investigation where the dependent variable is delay in seeking care following observation of a possible cancerous mass. With other factors controlled, persons scoring high on the Chance HLC should theoretically delay longer than those scoring high on Powerful Others HLC, or Internality HLC.

A second example covers the situation of a person experiencing unpleasant side-effects following taking medication prescribed by a physician. A person with high scores on the Powerful Others HLC section of the Scale might be expected to continue taking the medication, especially if he/she also has high trust in physicians. Conversely a person with a high score on the Chance HLC might be expected to abandon the medication entirely. A person with strong beliefs in internal health locus of control might carry out a self-study by going off the medication for a day or two, noting the difference, then resuming the medication to see if the side-effects disappear. Other examples are included in the quoted literature.

How far the measurement of health locus of control will provide more precise and conceptually relevant predictions than previously possible remains an empirical question, which depends for its answer on further research.

REFERENCES

Levenson H 1975 Multidimensional locus of control in prison inmates. J Appl Soc Psychol 5: 342–347

MacDonald A P 1973 Internal–external locus of control. In: Robinson J P, Shaver P (eds) Measures of social psychological attitudes. Institute for Social Research, University of Michigan, Ann Arbor

Rotter J B 1966 Generalized expectancies for internal versus external control of reinforcement. Psychol. Monogr. 80: 609

Wallston K A, Wallston B S, Kaplan G D, Maides S A 1976 Development and validation of the Health Locus of Control (HLC) scale. J. Consult. Clin. Psychol. 44: 580–585

Wallston K A, Wallston B S, DeVellis R 1978 Development of the Multidimensional Health Locus of Control (MHLC) Scales. Health Education Monographs 6 (2) (Spring): 160–170

MULTI-DIMENSIONAL HEALTH LOCUS OF CONTROL — FORM A

MHLC Form A
This is a questionnaire designed to determine the way in which different people view certain important health-related issues. Each item is a belief statement with which you may agree or disagree. Beside each statement is a scale which ranges from strongly disagree (1) to strongly agree (6). For each item we would like you to circle the number that represents the extent to which you disagree or agree with the statement. The more strongly you agree with a statement, then the higher will be the number you circle. The more strongly you disagree with a statement, then the lower will be the number you circle. Please make sure that you answer every item and that you circle *only one* number per item. This is a measure of your personal beliefs; obviously, there are no right or wrong answers.

Please answer these items carefully, but do not spend too much time on any one item. As much as you can, try to respond to each item independently. When making your choice, do not be influenced by your previous choices. It is important that you respond according to your actual beliefs and not according to how you feel you should believe or how you think we want you to believe.

	Strongly Disagree	Moderately Disagree	Slightly Disagree	Slightly Agree	Moderately Agree	Strongly Agree
1. If I get sick, it is my own behaviour which determines how soon I get well again.	1	2	3	4	5	6
2. No matter what I do, if I am going to get sick, I will get sick.	1	2	3	4	5	6
3. Having regular contact with my physician is the best way for me to avoid illness.	1	2	3	4	5	6
4. Most things that affect my health happen to me by accident.	1	2	3	4	5	6
5. Whenever I don't feel well, I should consult a medically trained professional.	1	2	3	4	5	6
6. I am in control of my health.	1	2	3	4	5	6
7. My family has a lot to do with my becoming sick or staying healthy.	1	2	3	4	5	6
8. When I get sick, I am to blame.	1	2	3	4	5	6
9. Luck plays a big part in determining how soon I will recover from an illness.	1	2	3	4	5	6
10. Health professionals control my health.	1	2	3	4	5	6
11. My good health is largely a matter of good fortune.	1	2	3	4	5	6
12. The main thing which affects my health is what I myself do.	1	2	3	4	5	6
13. If I take care of myself, I can avoid illness.	1	2	3	4	5	6
14. When I recover from an illness, it's usually because other people (for example, doctors, nurses, family, friends) have been taking good care of me.	1	2	3	4	5	6
15. No matter what I do, I'm likely to get sick.	1	2	3	4	5	6
16. If it's meant to be, I will stay healthy.	1	2	3	4	5	6
17. If I take the right actions, I can stay healthy.	1	2	3	4	5	6
18. Regarding my health, I can only do what my doctor tells me to do.	1	2	3	4	5	6

MULTI-DIMENSIONAL HEALTH LOCUS OF CONTROL — FORM B

MHLC Form B

This is a questionnaire designed to determine the way in which different people view certain important health-related issues. Each item is a belief statement with which you may agree or disagree. Beside each statement is a scale which ranges from strongly disagree (1) to strongly agree (6). For each item we would like you to circle the number that represents the extent to which you disagree or agree with the statement. The more strongly you agree with a statement, then the higher will be the number you circle. The more strongly you disagree with a statement, then the lower will be the number you circle. Please make sure that you answer every item and that you circle *only one* number per item. This is a measure of your personal beliefs; obviously, there are no right or wrong answers.

Please answer these items carefully, but do not spend too much time on any one item. As much as you can, try to respond to each item independently. When making your choice, do not be influenced by your previous choices. It is important that you respond according to your actual beliefs and not according to how you feel you should believe or how you think we want you to believe.

	Strongly Disagree	Moderately Disagree	Slightly Disagree	Slightly Agree	Moderately Agree	Strongly Agree
1. If I become sick, I have the power to make myself well again.	1	2	3	4	5	6
2. Often I feel that no matter what I do, if I am going to get sick, I will get sick.	1	2	3	4	5	6
3. If I see an excellent doctor regularly, I am less likely to have health problems.	1	2	3	4	5	6
4. It seems that my health is greatly influenced by accidental happenings.	1	2	3	4	5	6
5. I can only maintain my health by consulting health professionals.	1	2	3	4	5	6
6. I am directly responsible for my health.	1	2	3	4	5	6
7. Other people play a big part in whether I stay healthy or become sick.	1	2	3	4	5	6
8. Whatever goes wrong with my health is my own fault.	1	2	3	4	5	6
9. When I am sick, I just have to let nature run its course.	1	2	3	4	5	6
10. Health professionals keep me healthy.	1	2	3	4	5	6
11. When I stay healthy, I'm just plain lucky.	1	2	3	4	5	6
12. My physical well-being depends on how well I take care of myself.	1	2	3	4	5	6
13. When I feel ill, I know it is because I have not been taking care of myself properly.	1	2	3	4	5	6
14. The type of care I receive from other people is what is responsible for how well I recover from an illness.	1	2	3	4	5	6
15. Even when I take care of myself, it's easy to get sick.	1	2	3	4	5	6
16. When I become ill, it's a matter of fate.	1	2	3	4	5	6
17. I can pretty much stay healthy by taking good care of myself.	1	2	3	4	5	6
18. Following doctor's orders to the letter is the best way for me to stay healthy.	1	2	3	4	5	6

Appendix 6

Sample examination questions

The following are samples of some examination questions, which have been set for student health visitors, pertaining to the care of older people. They serve to indicate the scope and range of the health visiting course content, in relation to elderly people; but, of course, such questions by no means form a comprehensive list. Not all may be answered from this book.

SECTION 1: THE DEVELOPMENT OF THE INDIVIDUAL

Part A: Psychosocial development

1. Outline the major psychological and social developments in later life. How does an understanding of the psychology of ageing affect the work of health visitors?

2. Retirement . . . crisis point or stepping-stone? Discuss this statement, illustrating your answer with reference to the role of health visitors in relation to retirement.

3. Briefly describe the major learning theories. What modifications, if any, are likely to occur in later life? What effect might a knowledge of learning theories and theories of ageing, have on the work of health visitors?

4. Bereavement may be a common experience for the old. Briefly describe the impact of bereavement in later life, showing how health visitors might assist older persons to cope with loss, grief and mourning.

5. Outline the main psychosocial theories of ageing. How might you, as an health visitor, utilise a knowledge of these various theories, to help you in your work with elderly persons.

6. Analyse some of the myths and stereotypes related to sexuality in later life. How might these be (a) prevented, (b) overcome? Discuss the main facets of the health visiting role, in relation to sexual development in persons in later maturity.

7. Discuss how health visitors might assist elderly people to achieve successfully the developmental tasks of ageing.

8. Briefly describe the cognitive changes that occur in normal ageing. What factors would you take into account when assessing the cognitive state of an elderly client. Outline the goals of care.

9. Explain how you would approach the task of teaching staff in a Day Centre for older people, about cognitive and emotional functions in old age. How would you assist the staff to promote cognitive and emotional well-being in their elderly members?

Part B: Physical and physiological aspects of growth and development

1. Describe the main physical changes which normally present in old age. How would you use this knowledge to assess the care an older person might require from a health visitor?

2. Compare and contrast the normal physical changes that occur in sensory fields in older persons, with those pathological processes which may occur. Why is it important for an health visitor to try to differentiate these? Give examples to justify your answer.

3. Outline the main principles of locomotor development in human life. What changes may occur in old age? How can health visitors help to prevent/reduce adverse locomotor changes in later maturity?

4. Describe the nutritional needs of the over-60s. What principles would guide you when checking the diet of an elderly couple whose sole income is derived from Income Support?

5. Explain the changes which normally occur in the digestive tract as a result of ageing. How would you use this knowledge when giving guidance on the nutritional management of a 75-year-old man, who has recently come to live with his daughter?

6. Biological rhythms are an integral part of human life. Discuss how such rhythms may influence the ability of older people to adapt. How would you use this knowledge to assist you when assessing, planning and implementing care for a male octogenarian, who has been referred to you for follow-up care following a period in hospital?

7. Discuss the psychological aspects of disability, in the light of the prevalence rates of disabling conditions among older people.

8. 'Most people prefer to die in familiar surroundings.' Discuss this statement and the role of the health visitor in understanding and meeting the needs of older persons who are dying, and of their families.

SECTION 2: THE INDIVIDUAL IN THE GROUP

1. In the past when an Eskimo mother became old her family expected her to wander off into the snow. In contemporary society when an English mother becomes old, her family expect her to enter a Home. Discuss this statement, with reference to the role of the family in the care of older people.

2. Compare and contrast the structure and functions of the ageing family, with those of (a) the young adult family, (b) the middle-aged family. How might these differences in structure and function affect your work as a health visitor with an ageing family?

3. Analyse some of the changing cultural norms which may affect older people. How does a knowledge of culture and change, affect health visiting professional activity?

4. What difficulties, if any, are likely to be encountered by elderly members in ethnic minority families? How can health visitors help?

5. Define and differentiate moral and spiritual development. How might cultural differences affect such development? Discuss how an health visitor might foster spiritual development in an older client.

6. What characteristics would you look for, when assessing the social competence of elderly people? How can health visitors help to promote and maintain social competence in the later years?

7. Discuss the sociological aspects of housing the elderly. What part can health visitors play in relation to housing and health?

8. What is significant to health visitors in the relationship between epidemiology and sociology? Illustrate your answer with reference to the care of elderly people.

SECTION 3: THE DEVELOPMENT OF SOCIAL POLICY

1. Define and discuss the concept of 'social need', with particular reference to the development of social policy, for either the older disabled person, or the old person dependent on social security benefits.

2. 'Care in the community, must increasingly mean care by the community' (DHSS 'Growing older' 1981). Discuss this statement in the light of current and proposed policies for older persons.

3. 'Poverty is the giant from which our older citizens would feign escape.' Discuss this statement with reference to social policy developments in income maintenance since 1980.

4. Discuss the role of (a) the home help service and (b) the chiropody service, in the care of older people. How can health visitors facilitate the work of members of these services and improve their liaison with them?

5. Discuss the notion that poverty or inequality are less likely to concern older persons than are ageism and dependence.

6. How far do gender-stereotypes affect the development of social policies for lay-carers of elderly people? Is this issue of any consequence for health visitors? Why?

7. Discuss the concept of voluntary service in relation to older people (a) as volunteers; (b) as recipients of voluntary service. What part can health visitors play in such services?

SECTION 4: SOCIAL ASPECTS OF HEALTH AND DISEASE

Part A: Epidemiology, social aspects of health and disease and health service administration

1. What do you understand by the term 'food poisoning'? Differentiate between the main types. What guidance would you give to the staff of a Day Centre, for elderly people, concerning the prevention of food poisoning?

2. Describe the various sources of health information. Discuss the sources you might utilise more often, including specific publications. How would you render such information effective in your health visiting practice?

3. Of what use to an health visitor is a knowledge of epidemiology? Explain how you would apply an understanding of this discipline, to enable you to work effectively with older people in your locality?

4. Differentiate between the incidence rate and the prevalence rate in community assessment of diseases. Discuss the relative merits of each of these two rates, in (a) evaluating preventive efforts and exploring the natural history of disease among older people, and (b) planning services to meet needs encountered in populations of older persons.

5. Compare and contrast the relationship between the health visiting process and the epidemiological process. Show how you could use this awareness of the inter-relationship to help you assess the health needs of older persons in a community.

6. Discuss the role of the health visitor in the Primary Health Care Team. How would you organise health visiting services in the care of the 75-year-old group and upwards, within a general medical practice setting?

7. Discuss the respective roles of health visitors and community psychiatric nurses in the care of the older mentally frail.

8. You are moving to a new locality to work as an health visitor, and find you are working in a practice which has a population of 9000. You discover there are 1350 persons aged 65 years and over, registered with the practice. There are 2 health visitors, 3 district nurses and 4 general practitioners in the team. What information would you seek and how would you organise your health visiting and health promoting work within this team, with particular reference to the care of the older practice population?

Part B: Current medical problems

1. Mr H, aged 64 years, is disabled by chronic bronchitis and emphysema. His wife, aged 70 years, suffers from generalised osteo-arthritis and congestive cardiac failure. Neighbours and friends seem unwilling or unable to help. Can a health visitor do anything? How?

2. Discuss the investigation and management of dementing illness among older people. What can the health visitor contribute to care of dementia sufferers and their carers?

3. What are the likely problems faced by elderly diabetics? How may they be overcome? Illustrate your answer with reference to the role of health visitors in the management of diabetes among older persons.

4. Discuss the management role of the health visitor in cases of self-neglect (Diogenes syndrome).

5. 'Depression is different from unhappiness'. Discuss this statement, outlining its relevance to the health visiting care of an older person, diagnosed as depressed, 6 months after retiring.

6. Discuss the role of the health visitor where it is suspected that an elderly grandfather, within a household, has been abused.

7. What are the common psychiatric problems encountered in persons in later life? Discuss the role and function of the health visitor in the prevention and control of such disorders? How would you support and help a family coping with one such problem?

8. State the causes of transient confusion in older persons. How can this state be differentiated from dementia? Discuss the treatment of transient confusion, stressing the part health visitors can play in the prevention and management of such a condition.

9. Discuss the respective roles of health visitor, district nurse and social worker, in the care of an elderly couple, where the wife is suffering from Parkinson's disease and the 80-year-old husband has maturity-onset diabetes, and a history of three myocardial infarctions in the past 5 years. How can the couple be enabled to function as independently as possible, without feeling either over-protected or unsupported?

SECTION 5: PRINCIPLES AND PRACTICE OF HEALTH VISITING, INCLUDING HEALTH EDUCATION

Part A: Principles and practice of health visiting

1. Describe an age–sex register and discuss its uses and limitations. What are the implications of such a register in terms of: (a) identification of vulnerable groups, including older persons; (b) health promotion activity among the well elderly practice population?

2. 'Records are a vital part of health visiting practice'. Discuss this statement with particular reference to responsibility, authority and accountability, in health visiting.

3. State the objectives of health visiting care for older clients. How far do you consider the present preparation of practitioners fits them for effective care with this section of the population?

4. A 64-year-old woman who has had a right mastectomy for malignant breast disease, seeks your help about her subsequent care. How would you handle this situation and plan care with her?

5. Discuss the view that health visitors use 'lack of time' as an excuse for avoiding work with older adults, when in fact it is 'because they have no appropriate frame of reference' for caring for older people (Luker 1981).

6. Discuss the notion that care of older persons has a lower priority amongst members of the caring professions than work with most other age groups.

Part B: Health education

1. Discuss imaginative and effective ways of presenting budgeting knowledge and nutritional guidance to a group of older persons whose incomes are limited.

2. Discuss the purpose and content of a short course for wardens of sheltered accommodation for older persons, on 'Our senior citizens and how to care for them'. How far do you consider health visitors should be involved in such courses?

3. You are asked to participate in a support group for lay-carers of elderly people. What important principles would you consider, regarding group work? What emphases would you encourage and how would you see the group developing?

4. Accidents are a major cause of mortality and morbidity in later life. What knowledge would you utilise to enable you to plan a relevant programme of accident prevention for the older population in your locality? How would you design and execute such a programme?

5. You are working as an health visitor in an inner city area. A student nurse is seconded to you for her community experience. Show how you would plan a programme for her that would enable her to grasp the purpose and scope of the health visiting role, in the context of community health and social care for older people. What steps would you take to confirm that learning had taken place?

Appendix 7

List of useful addresses for those caring for older people

ENGLAND

ABBEYFIELD SOCIETY, 186/192 Darkes Lane, Potters Bar, Herts. EN6 1AB (Tel 0707 448445). Provision of purpose-built accommodation, and adaptation of suitable houses, to offer housing (usually bed-sitting rooms) to older people. Resident housekeepers and voluntary helpers mostly available in these homes.

ACCESS COMMITTEE FOR ENGLAND, 35 Great Smith Street, London SW1P 3BJ (Tel 071 222 7980). National focal point on access to the built environment.

ACROSS TRUST, Crown House, London Road, Morden, Surrey SM4 5EW (Tel 081 540 3897). Operates a transport scheme for chronically sick, disabled or elderly persons, going on holiday or pilgrimage. Uses Jumbulances — trained helpers.

ACTION FOR BENEFITS, c/o NUCPS, 124–130 Southwark Street, London SE1 0TU (Tel 071 928 9671). National campaign fighting against social security cuts.

ACTION FOR DYSPHASIC ADULTS, Northcote House, 37a Royal Street, London SE1 7LL (Tel 071 261 9572). Information and advice for all dysphasics; acts to facilitate the rehabilitation of adults with speech impairments following strokes or associated conditions. Publishes literature.

ADVOCACY, NATIONAL CITIZEN, 2 St Paul's Road, London N1 2QR (Tel 071 359 8289). National resource and advisory centre for people involved in citizen advocacy — independent, voluntary representation for persons not able to defend and exercise their rights. Publishes a useful handbook, 'A Powerful Partnership'.

AGE CONCERN (ENGLAND), Astral House 1268 London Road, London SW16 4ER (Tel 081 679 8000). See also telephone directory for local branches. A centre of policy, research, information and social advocacy on all subjects regarding the welfare of elderly people. Local Age Concern Groups throughout the UK help with provision of day centres, luncheon clubs, meals-on-wheels and other services. Produces many publications.

AGE ENDEAVOUR FELLOWSHIP, 'Willowthorpe', High Street, Stanstead Abbotts, Nr Ware, Herts. SG12 8AS (Tel 0920 870158). Small but growing charity encouraging activity and employment for retired and elderly people.

AGEING, THE CENTRE FOR POLICY ON, 25–31 Ironmonger Row, London EC1V 3QP (Tel 071 253 1787). Encourages better service for older people, through informed debate and encouraging good practice. Has a reference library and information service publications.

ALZHEIMER'S DISEASE SOCIETY, Bank Buildings, Fulham Broadway, London SW6 1EP (Tel 071 381 3177). Offers advice/information and support to families with a sufferer from this disease. Supports local groups; encourages and finances research into the condition. Useful publications.

ARTHRITIS CARE, 6 Grosvenor Crescent, London SW1X 7ER (Tel 071 235 0902). Provides a wide range of services for persons suffering from arthritis/rheumatism. Offers advice, financial and practical help. Runs specially adapted holiday hotels for members. Publishes 'Arthritis News'.

ARTHRITIS AND RHEUMATISM COUNCIL FOR RESEARCH, 41 Eagle Street, London, WC1R 4AR (Tel 071 405 8572). Finances research into causes and cure of rheumatic diseases; publishes handbooks for sufferers; runs prostheses club for persons who have had replacement joints fitted.

ALCOHOLICS ANONYMOUS, PO Box 1, Stonebow House, Stonebow, York YO1 2NJ (Tel 0904 644026). National organisation helping those who wish to control alcohol addiction.

BACK PAIN ASSOCIATION (NATIONAL), 31–33 Park Road, Teddington, Middx TW11 0AB (Tel 081 977 5474). Offers an information service on all forms of back pain.

BLIND, ASSOCIATION FOR THE GENERAL WELFARE OF THE, 37–55 Ashburton Grove, Holloway, London N7 7DW (Tel 071 609 0206). Offers a welfare service and advice for all blind persons, particularly elderly.

BLIND, GUIDE DOGS FOR, Alexandra House, 9 Park Street, Windsor, Berks. SL4 1JR (Tel 0753 855711). Some elderly people may benefit from the use of a guide dog, especially if they were blinded earlier in life.

BLIND, NATIONAL LIBRARY FOR, Cromwell Road, Bredbury, Stockport, Cheshire SK6 2SG (Tel 061 491 0217). Offers a comprehensive library service for the blind and partially sighted. Is the main source of reading material in Braille; also offers books in Moon Type and has its own series of large-print books. Gives advice on services for the blind; publications, aids and access to some welfare funds.

BLIND, ROYAL NATIONAL INSTITUTE FOR, 224–228 Great Portland Street, London W1N 6AA. Offers an advisory service: guidance on welfare provisions, rehabilitation, residential homes. Offers Publications; runs Talking Book Library; sells aids and equipment.

BLIND, TELEPHONES FOR THE, 'Mynthhurst', Leigh, Reigate, Surrey RH2 8RJ (Tel 0293 862546). Grants towards telephone installations and/or rental for registered blind persons.

BLIND, WIRELESS FOR THE, 224 Great Portland Street, London W1N 6AA (Tel 071 388 1266). Provides radio sets for blind persons free of charge.

BRITISH ASSOCIATION FOR THE HARD OF HEARING, 7–11 Armstrong Road, London W3 7JL. Publishes the magazine 'HARK' quarterly, offers advice, runs clubs, encourages self-help groups.

BRITISH ASSOCIATION FOR SERVICE TO THE ELDERLY (BASE), 119 Hassell Street, Newcastle-under-Lyme, Staffs. ST5 1AX (Tel 0782 661033). Advocates the multi-disciplinary approach to caring for elderly people. Membership is open to anyone who has an interest in service to elderly persons. Runs courses and conferences.

BRITISH DIABETIC ASSOCIATION, 10 Queen Anne Street, London W1 (Tel 071 323 1531). Offers advice on diet, aids, holidays. Publishes a monthly journal 'Balance'.

BRITISH GERIATRICS SOCIETY, 1 St Andrew's Place, London NW1 4LB (Tel 071 935 4004). The only medical organisation in the UK specifically concerned with the medical problems of elderly persons. Promotes developments in geriatric medicine; encourages research, independence in elderly people; campaigns for improved facilities for older sick persons.

BRITISH RED CROSS SOCIETY, National Headquarters, 9 Grosvenor Crescent, London SW1X 7E (Tel 071 235 5454). (See local directory for nearest branch.) An advisory, instructional and welfare service, running clubs for disabled and elderly people; holidays; escort services; access to some funds and gives advice on aids, equipment and resources.

BRITISH LEGION, THE ROYAL, 48 Pall Mall, London (Tel 071 930 8131). Offers information, social and supportive contact; has some welfare funds for ex-service personnel. Limited accommodation for older persons formerly engaged either in HM Forces, or in work of national importance.

CANCER AFTERCARE AND REHABILITATION SOCIETY, 21 Zetland Road, Redland, Bristol BS6 7AH (Tel 0272 427419/232302). Self-help group for cancer patients, their families and friends, offering support/help/advice.

CANCER HELP CENTRE, Grove House, Cornwallis Grove, Clifton, Bristol BS8 4PG (Tel 0272 743216). An holistic programme, based on healing diet, counselling, relaxation and meditation.

CANCER RELIEF/MACMILLAN FUND, Anchor House, 15/19 Britten Street, London SW3 3TZ (Tel 071 351 7811). Offers support, advice and help to cancer sufferers and their families. Purpose-built short-stay homes, home-based support services/financial aid. Applications via hospital, community health, or social services.

CANCER UNITED PATIENTS, BRITISH ASSOCIATION OF, (BACUP), 121/123 Charterhouse St, London EC1M 6AA (071 608 1661). Offers help and advice on care/treatment.

CARERS NATIONAL ASSOCIATION, 29 Chilworth Mews, London W2 3RG (Tel 071 724 7776). Helps carers who have, or have had, the care of elderly or disabled dependants. Gives advisory service by letter; campaigns for increased support and benefits. Formed through a merger of Association of Carers and The National Council for Carers and their Elderly Dependants.

CHEST HEART AND STROKE ASSOCIATION, Tavistock House North, Tavistock Square, London WC1H 9JE. Major information centre on chest and cardiac conditions. Encourages local stroke clubs; publishes a range of helpful literature. Organises a postal Emphysema club for sufferers.

CHRISTIAN CORRESPONDENCE GROUPS, 8 Dukes Close, North Weald, Epping, Essex CM16 6DA. Postal group correspondence for older and disabled persons; produces a magazine 3 times per year.

CITIZENS' ADVICE BUREAUX, NATIONAL ASSOCIATION OF, Myddleton House, 115–123 Pentonville Road, London N1 9LZ (Tel 071 833 2181). Co-ordinates the work of the local Bureaux throughout the country, which offer free, impartial and confidential advice, to anyone on any subject. NACAB trains volunteer workers and produces a wide range of leaflets etc.

COLOSTOMY ASSOCIATION, BRITISH, 38–39 Eccleston Square, London SW1V 1PB (Tel 071 828 5175). Provides a free advisory service, applicable to older persons, on colostomy, its care and rehabilitation.

COMMUNICATION FOR THE DISABLED FOUNDATION, Foundation House, Church Street West, Woking, Surrey GU21 1DJ (Tel 04862 27848). Offers disabled persons alternatives to conventional methods of writing or communicating.

COMMUNITY HEALTH COUNCILS, ASSOCIATION OF, IN ENGLAND AND WALES, 30 Drayton Park, London N5 1PB. Provides a forum for discussion and exchange of concerns on health matters. Has produced a leaflet 'Patients' Rights' in Punjabi, Hindi, Bengali, Gujerati, and Vietnamese. Will investigate matters of concern referred to them.

CONSUMERS' ASSOCIATION, 2 Marylebone Road, London WC2N 6DS. Research, information and campaigning body on behalf of consumers.

CONTACT, 15 Henrietta Street, Covent Garden, London WC2E 8QH (Tel 071 240 0630). Service providing companionship and outings for elderly housebound persons, living alone.

CORRESPONDENCE, CARE AND SUPPORT GROUP, 14 Windsor Terrace, East Herrington, Sunderland WR3 3SF. Puts ill and housebound persons, including elderly, in touch with each other, by letter, for support/self-help.

COUNSEL AND CARE FOR THE ELDERLY, Twyman House, 16 Bonny Street, London NW1 9LR (Tel 071 485 1566). Provides a free advisory service to elderly people on any matter of concern, and a counselling service to help with particular problems. Information on nursing and residential care homes. Financial help towards the cost of nursing at home.

CROSSROADS CARE ATTENDANT SCHEMES, LTD, ASSOCIATION OF, 10 Regent Place, Rugby, Warwickshire CV21 2PN (Tel 0788 73653). Paid attendants care for elderly or disabled people in their homes, thus avoiding admission to hospital and easing the strain on relatives. Local schemes available in different parts of the country.

CRUSE—BEREAVEMENT CARE, Cruse House, 126 Sheen Road, Richmond, Surrey TW3 1UR (Tel 081 940 4818/9407). Offers a service of counselling, advice and opportunities for social contact, for all widows and widowers, whether alone or with children, to relieve suffering after bereavement and encourage rehabilitation.

DEAF ASSOCIATION, THE BRITISH, 38 Victoria Place, Carlisle, Cumbria CA1 1HU (Tel 0228 48844). Concerned with the welfare and education of deaf persons of all ages. Provides holidays and residential homes for elderly deaf persons.

DEAF/BLIND HELPERS LEAGUE, NATIONAL, 18 Rainbow Court, Paston Ridings, Peterborough PE4 6UP (Tel 0773 73511). Organises social functions; provides links; material help towards holidays, equipment, and during sickness; has self-contained flats, a guest home and a holiday flat. Publishes 'The Rainbow', quarterly.

DEPARTMENT OF HEALTH, Richmond House, 79 Whitehall, London SW1A 2NS (Tel 071 210 3000) and Alexander Fleming House, Elephant and Castle, London SE1 6BY (Tel 071 407 5522).

DEPRESSIVES ASSOCIATED, PO Box 5, Castletown, Portland, Dorset DT5 1BQ. Offers help and support to persons of all ages, suffering from depression. Builds up local support groups, promotes an understanding of the condition, and the removal of stigma associated with it.

DIAL UK, 117 High Street, Clay Cross, Chesterfield S45 9DZ (0246 250055). Telephone information service for the disabled. Has 75 local groups for disabled persons.

DISABILITY ALLIANCE, 25 Denmark Street, London WC2H 8NJ (Tel 071 240 0806). A federation of organisations for disabled people who have joined together to press for a comprehensive income scheme for disabled people. Publishes an annual 'Disability Rights Handbook'; other helpful publications.

DISABLED LIVING FOUNDATION, 380–384 Harrow Road, London W9 2HU (Tel 071 289 6111). Is a premier information service on all aspects of living with a disability (physical, mental, sensory, or problems of old age). Has a permanent exhibition of aids and equipment; publishes information bulletins and undertakes research.

ELDERLY AND GENTLEFOLKS, FRIENDS OF, 42 Ebury Street, London, SW1W OLZ (Tel 071 730 8263). Provides permanent residential accommodation for elderly people and gives grants to help others to remain in their own homes. Manages 11 homes in the south of England.

EPILEPSY, BRITISH ASSOCIATION FOR, Anstey House, 40 Hanover Square, Leeds LS3 1BE (Tel 0532 439393). Runs an advice service, providing help for people with epilepsy and their families, and supports research. Publishes a journal 'Epilepsy Now'.

EXTEND (EXERCISES FOR THE ELDERLY AND DISABLED), 1a North Street, Sheringham, Norfolk NR26 8LJ (Tel 0263 822479). Has an exercise plan available, but send SAE.

FORUM ON THE RIGHTS OF ELDERLY PEOPLE IN EDUCATION (FREE), 60 Pitcairn Road, Mitcham, Surrey CR4 3LL (Tel 081 640 5431). Acts as a clearing house for information on all aspects of education for the elderly. Publishes regular bulletins; encourages local groups and offers assistance and advice in the development of new programmes for older people.

FRIENDS BY POST, 6 Bollins Court, Macclesfield Road, Wilmslow, Cheshire SK9 2AP (Tel 0625 527044). Encourages penfriends for older people, especially housebound.

HEALTH EDUCATION AUTHORITY, Hamilton House, Mabledon Place, London WC1 (Tel 071 631 0930). A special health authority responsible for health promotion within England. Produces a range of health education materials.

HEALTH INFORMATION SERVICE, Lister Hospital, Corey's Mill Lane, Stevenage, Herts SG 14AB. (Tel 0438 314333). Offers a comprehensive health information service on all topics and on self-help groups. (NHS approved).

HEALTH VISITORS' ASSOCIATION, 50 Southwark Street, London SE1 1UN (Tel 071 378 7255). (Has a Special Interest Group for Health Visitors working with elderly people.)

HELP THE AGED, 16–18 St James' Walk, London ECIR OBE (Tel 071 253 0253). Works to improve the quality of life of elderly people in the UK and overseas. Provides day centres, day hospitals, minibuses, rehabilitation units, and some sheltered housing. Campaigns for fair provision for the elderly.

INVALIDS AT HOME TRUST, 17 Lapstone Gardens, Kenton, Harrow, Mdx HA3 0EB (Tel 081 907 1706). Helps some older persons remain at home, or leave hospital for home. Supplements the work of specialist charities.

MIND: NATIONAL ASSOCIATION FOR MENTAL HEALTH, 22 Harley Street, London W1N 2ED (Tel 071 637 0741). Promotes mental health and helps the mentally disordered, including older persons. Supports research into mental illness and helps the work of some 2000 mental health associations.

MARIE CURIE MEMORIAL FOUNDATION, 28 Belgrave Square, London SW1 1QG (Tel 071 235 8325). Promotes the welfare of cancer patients and their families. Runs 11 UK Nursing Homes and a nation-wide domiciliary nursing service. Provides urgent welfare needs, advice and general information. Educates professionals and public on cancer.

NATIONAL ASSOCIATION OF WIDOWS, 54–7 Allison Street, Digbeth, Birmingham, West Midlands B5 5TH (021 643 8348). Offers comfort, support and help to all widows, many of whom are elderly. Advises on welfare benefits and publishes a handbook.

OPEN UNIVERSITY, Walton Hall, Milton Keynes MK7 6AA (Tel 0908 74066). Offers home study courses for persons of all ages, but includes a number of older persons among its students.

OSTEOPOROSIS SOCIETY, NATIONAL, Barton Meade House, Radstock, Nr Bristol. Deals with all aspects of osteoporosis.

PARKINSON'S DISEASE SOCIETY, 36 Portland Place, London WC2H 0HR (Tel 071 255 2432). Helps patients and their families with problems arising in the home from this disease. Collects and disseminates information, publishes helpful literature, encourages the formation of local groups, and funds research.

PARTIALLY SIGHTED SOCIETY, Queens Road, Doncaster DN1 2NX (Tel 0302 368998). Particularly concerned with making the most of vision and self-help ways to better vision. Trains people to encourage those prescribed visual aids to use them correctly.

PENSIONERS LINK, 17 Balfe Street, London N1 SEB (071 278 5501). Mainly operates in greater London. Delivers services to, and campaigns for/with, pensioners. 10 local centres.

POPULAR MEDICAL INDEX, Meade Publishing Co., 77 Norton Road, Letchworth, Herts. SG6 1AD. A quarterly index of medical and health topics, mainly from the popular press, the 4th quarter being a cumulative index. Useful for health visitors wishing to see what clients are probably reading, or how/which health subjects are being aired by the popular media

PRE-RETIREMENT ASSOCIATION, 19 Undine Street, London SW17 8PP (Tel 081 767 3225). Provides guidance on retirement: planning, concerns, finance, housing, leisure activities. Runs pre-retirement courses. 36 affiliated associations.

QUIT, The National Society of Non-Smokers, Latimer House, 40/48 Hanson St, London W1P 7DE (071 636 9103).

REACH (Retired Executives Action Clearing House). Victoria House, Southampton Row, London WC1B 4DH (Tel 071 404 0940).

ROYAL COLLEGE OF NURSING, 20 Cavendish Square, London WIM 0AB (Tel 01 409 3333). Has an active Association for the Care of the Elderly (ACE), and an extensive library.

ROYAL SOCIETY FOR THE PREVENTION OF ACCIDENTS, Cannon House, The Priory, Queensway, Birmingham, West Midlands B4 6BS (Tel 021 200 24461). Stimulates interest in accident prevention through local and national organisations, and through training courses. Has a range of publications.

RUKBA, 6 Avonmore Road, London W14 8RL (Tel 01 602 6274). Makes grants or annuities to some professional persons who are in need, infirm or old.

SAGA Embrook House, Sandgate, Folkestone, Kent, CT20 3AY. Arranges holidays on a commercial basis for older persons. Runs clubs and offers a pen-friend service to members of these clubs.

SAMARITANS INCORPORATED, 17 Uxbridge Road, Slough, Berks. SL1 1SN (Tel 0753 32713). Befriends the suicidal and despairing, through many branches throughout UK (consult local directory for telephone numbers). Service is offered on a 24-hour basis, and is confidential.

SEXUAL AND PERSONAL RELATIONSHIPS OF PEOPLE WITH A DISABILITY (SPOD), 286 Camden Road, London N7 0BJ (Tel 071 607 8851). Provides information and advice on problems in sex and personal relationships which disability can cause. General leaflets and reading lists available, and individual advice given on request. Publications list available on request.

TALKING BOOKS FOR THE HANDICAPPED (The National Listening Library), 12 Lant Street, London SE1 1BR (071 407 9417). A library postal service for handicapped people (including dyslexics); tape cassettes on special reproducers, can be operated manually or by remote control. 2000 books on a wide variety of topics. Financial help towards cost of subscription.

TINNITUS, BRITISH ASSOCIATION, c/o Royal National Institute for the Deaf, 105 Gower Street, London WC1 (Tel 071 387 8033). Gives advice, information, and support for sufferers from tinnitus. Encourages formation of local groups and supports research.

THIRD AGE TRUST/UNIVERSITY OF THE THIRD AGE, 6 Parkside Gardens, London SW9 5EY (Tel 071 737 2541). Promotes self-help educational activities among retired people of all ages. Supports new and existing self-help groups. Publishes a journal 'The Third Age' three times yearly, and a pack U3A-DIY to help new groups get started.

WOMEN'S ROYAL VOLUNTARY SERVICE, 17 Old Park Lane, London W1Y 4AJ (Tel 071 499 6040). See also local directories for branches. Offers welfare and emergency work, through a nation-wide network of branches. Works with elderly people, handicapped, families in need etc. Runs day clubs, meals on wheels, home visits, non-medical work in hospitals, work with prisoners etc.

WORKERS' EDUCATIONAL ASSOCIATION (WEA), 9 Upper Berkeley Street, London W1 (Tel 071 402 5608/9). Provides a range of courses for persons of all age groups, often relevant to the

local community and its life. Caters specifically for older people where there is local demand.
There are of course, many other national and local organisations concerned with the care of the elderly. Further details and addresses may be obtained from:

- The Charities Digest (to be found in most reference libraries), and
- Knight S T, Gann R 1988 Self-help guide: a directory of self-help groups in the UK. Chapman and Hall, London

Social Services Departments are usually able to supply details of local branches of organisations.

NORTHERN IRELAND

AGE CONCERN, NORTHERN IRELAND, 6 Lower Crescent, Belfast BT7 1NR (Tel 0232 245729).
ALZHEIMER'S DISEASE SOCIETY, Balyclare, County Antrim (Tel 096 03 22490).

ARTHRITIS CARE, 3 New Forge Lane, Belfast BT9 5NW (Tel 0232 669882).

BLIND, ROYAL NATIONAL INSTITUTE FOR THE, (Tel 0232 663543).

CARERS, NATIONAL ASSOCIATION, Northern Ireland Branch, 2 Annadale Avenue, Belfast BT7 3JR.

CHEST, HEART & STROKE ASSOCIATION, NI, 21 Dublin Road, Belfast BT2 7FJ (0232 320184).

CROSSROADS CARE ATTENDANT SCHEMES, Newtonards (0247 815978).

DIAL, Belfast (Tel 0226 325506).

EXTRACARE FOR ELDERLY PEOPLE, 11a Wellington Park, Belfast BT9 6DJ (Tel 0232 683273).

SCOTLAND

AGE CONCERN, SCOTLAND, 54a Fountainbridge, Edinburgh EH3 9PT (Tel 031 228 5656).

BRITISH LEGION, SCOTLAND, THE ROYAL, Newhaigh House, Logie Green Road, Edinburgh EH7 4HR (Tel 031 557 2782).

CHEST, HEART AND STROKE ASSOCIATION, Glasgow, 103 Clarkston Rd, Glasgow G44 3BL (Tel 041 633 1666).

CROSSROADS (SCOTLAND), CARE ATTENDANT SCHEMES, 24 St George St, Glasgow G2 1EG (Tel 041 226 3793).

CITIZENS' RIGHTS ADVICE SERVICE, 76 Frithside, Fraserburgh (Tel 0346 25307).

DEPARTMENT OF SOCIAL SECURITY, Central Office for Scotland, Argyle House, 3 Lady Lawson Street, Edinburgh EH3 9SH (Tel 031 229 9191).

DISABILITY INFORMATION SERVICE, Stirling, FREEPOST Stirling FK8 2BR (Tel 0786 70300).

RED CROSS SOCIETY, SCOTTISH BRANCH, 204 Bath Street, Glasgow G2 4HL (Tel 041 332 9591).

VOLUNTARY ORGANIZATION, SCOTTISH COUNCIL FOR, 18/19 Claremont Crescent, Edinburgh EH12 5EL (Tel 031 337 2261).

WALES

DIAL (Tel 0685 79797).

DISABLED PERSONS INFORMATION CENTRE, 382–384 Newport Road, Cardiff (Tel 0222 488184).

DSS REGIONAL OFFICE, Block 3, Government Buildings, Gabalfa, Cardiff CF4 4YJ.

WALES COUNCIL FOR THE BLIND, Oak House, 12 The Bulwark, Brecon, Powys LD3 7AD (Tel 0874 4576).

WALES COUNCIL FOR THE DEAF (Tel 0222 887575).

WALES COUNCIL FOR THE DISABLED (Tel 0222 887325).

WALES MIND (National Association for Mental Health), 23 St Mary St Cardiff CF1 2AA (Tel 0222 395123).

Index